The Radiological Diagnosis of
Lung and Mediastinal Tumours

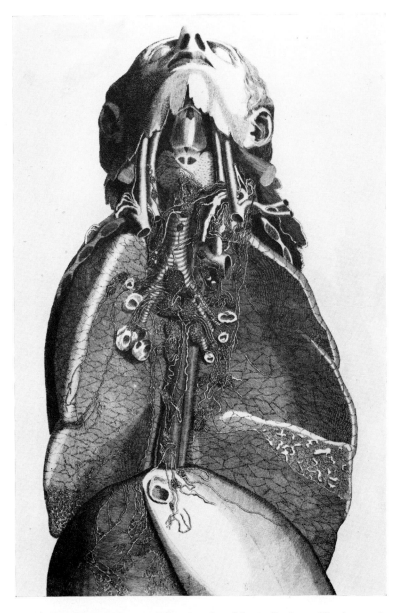

Frontispiece. The lymphatics and lymph nodes of the mediastinum. Woodcut made following the injection of sub-pleural and lung lymphatics with metallic mercury. Plate XXI from Vasorum Lymphaticorum Corporis Humani Historia et Ichno- graphia *(Mascagni, 1787). (All the woodcuts in this book are life size and comprise illustrations of the lymphatics of the whole body)*

The
Radiological Diagnosis
of
Lung and Mediastinal
Tumours

F. W. WRIGHT
M.A., B.M., B.Ch., M.R.C.P., F.F.R.

Consultant Radiologist, United Oxford Hospitals;
Clinical Lecturer in Radiology, University of Oxford

BUTTERWORTHS

ENGLAND: BUTTERWORTH & CO. (PUBLISHERS) LTD.
LONDON: 88 Kingsway, WC2B 6AB

AUSTRALIA: BUTTERWORTHS PTY. LTD.
SYDNEY: 586 Pacific Highway, 2067
MELBOURNE: 343 Little Collins Street, 3000
BRISBANE: 240 Queen Street, 4000

CANADA: BUTTERWORTH & CO. (CANADA) LTD.
TORONTO: 14 Curity Avenue, 374

NEW ZEALAND: BUTTERWORTHS OF NEW ZEALAND LTD.
WELLINGTON: 26–28 Waring Taylor Street, 1

SOUTH AFRICA: BUTTERWORTH & CO. (SOUTH AFRICA) (PTY) LTD.
DURBAN: 152–154 Gale Street

Suggested U.D.C. Number 616–073·75: 616·24–006
Suggested Additional Number 616–073·75: 616·27–006

ISBN 0 407 38385 9

Made and printed in Great Britain by
William Clowes & Sons, Limited, London, Beccles and Colchester

Contents

Preface

The object of this book is to review the various radiological appearances produced by lung and mediastinal tumours, especially those seen on plain radiographs, to illustrate the value of the different forms of tomography both in the further investigation of the tumours and in their differential diagnosis, and to discuss the value of bronchography in the diagnosis of malignant lesions. Chapters are also included describing the lymphatic spread of lung tumours, giving an account of the other radiological procedures (including radio-isotope techniques) which may be employed in the detection or assessment of lung and mediastinal tumours, and discussing the value of radiological surveys for the detection of lung tumours.

At the present time, despite all that has been written about lung and mediastinal tumours, the author has been unable to find any really comprehensive review of their radiological manifestations. The still increasing frequency of bronchial carcinomas, together with their often late diagnosis, has stimulated the present study.

The Churchill Hospital, where the author largely works, is part of the United Oxford Hospitals and is the hospital in the Group in which the Department of Thoracic Surgery, the Chest Clinic and the Radiotherapy Department are situated. Because the United Oxford Hospitals provide the local hospital service for the area and also have many patients referred from a much larger area for treatment or diagnosis, the author has seen about 4,000 patients with such tumours over a period of twelve years.

Most of the illustrations used are from radiographs of patients attending the United Oxford Hospitals, but where a particular abnormality has not been seen or a particular investigation has not been carried out in these hospitals, illustrations have been included which were lent by colleagues in other centres. Their help is gratefully acknowledged.

The author has attempted not only to provide a historical review of the subject and to discuss the radiographic findings in detail, but also to give some figures of the relative incidence of peripheral and central lung tumours, and has analysed the frequency of the various signs in 400 of the cases.

It must be pointed out that in reading radiographs the frequency of individual signs is less important than an awareness of all the many signs which may be present and the ways in which they may vary with the stage of the disease process.

Acknowledgements

I acknowledge grateful thanks to the many colleagues, registrars and former registrars who have helped me in the preparation of this book by referring patients for investigation, helping with the investigations or kindly allowing me to reproduce radiographs. In particular I would like to thank the Chest Physicians and the Thoracic Surgeons of the United Oxford Hospitals, Drs. F. Ridehalgh, J. M. Black, W. S. Hamilton and D. Lane, and Messrs. C. Grimshaw and A. J. Gunning, for their help.

I am also indebted to the following for allowing me to reproduce illustrations as indicated.

The Curators of the Bodleian Library, Oxford—*Frontispiece.*
The Royal College of Physicians and Pitman Medical and Scientific Publishing Co. Ltd.—*Figure 1.2.*
The Editor of *The Sunday Telegraph*—*Figure 1.3.*
The Editor of *Journal of the American Medical Association*—*Figure 2.1.*
Professor L. G. Rigler (U.C.L.A., Los Angeles)—*Figures 2.1* and *3.4* and Tables 2.1 and 2.2.
The Editor of *American Journal of Roentgenology*—Table 2.1 and *Figure 3.102.*
The Editor of *Journal of Thoracic Surgery*—Table 2.2.
Pergamon Press Ltd.—*Figures 3.6, 3.7* and *3.55.*
The Editor of *Clinical Radiology*—*Figures 3.18, 4.1, 4.2, 4.3, 6.9, 7.8a* and *b, 7.11a, 7.13, 7.14, 7.15c and d, 7.17, 7.18c and d, 7.21, 7.22, 7.24, 7.25, 7.29, 7.30, 7.31, 7.34, 7.41, 7.44, 7.45b, 7.50, 7.51, 8.13* and *8.14,* also Tables 7.1, 7.2 and 7.3.
The C. V. Mosby Company, St. Louis, Mo.—*Figure 3.54.*
The McGraw-Hill Book Co., New York—*Figure 3.57.*
The Editor of *Fortschritte auf dem Gebiete der Röntgenstrahlen*—*Figure 3.83.*
Dr. R. B. Illing (Hospital of St. Cross, Rugby)—*Figure 3.117a.*
Dr. W. R. Eyler (Henry Ford Hospital, Detroit, Michigan)—*Figures 3.118, 3.125* and *10.1.*
The Editor of *Radiography* and the Society of Radiographers—*Figures 4.4, 4.5* and *4.10.*
Philips Medical Systems Ltd.—*Figures 4.6, 4.7, 4.9* and *6.4.*
Professor S. Takahashi and Springer-Verlag, Berlin—*Figure 4.8.*
Kodak Pathé and Cercle d'Études et de Recherches Radiologiques, Paris (Professor G. Pallardy and Dr. J. Remy)—*Figure 8.3.*
Dr. M. J. Raphael (Royal Postgraduate Medical School of London) and the Editor of *British Journal of Hospital Medicine*—*Figure 10.3.*
Dr. R. G. Grainger (Royal Hospital, Sheffield)—*Figure 10.8.*
Dr. N. W. T. Grieve (St. Peter's Hospital, Chertsey)—*Figure 10.10.*
Dr. O. Pohlenz (Allgemeines Krankenhaus St. Georg, Hamburg)—*Figures 10.21* and *10.22.*
E. & S. Livingstone—*Figure 10.29* and Table A.8.
The Editor of *British Medical Journal*—Table A.1 and *Figure A.9a.*
The Editor of *Presse médicale* and Vigor Frères, Paris—*Figure A.4.*
The Editor of *Paris médicine*—*Figure A.5.*
H. K. Lewis & Co. Ltd.—*Figures A.6, A.7* and *A.8.*
The Controller of Her Majesty's Stationery Office—*Figure A.9b* (Crown copyright).

ACKNOWLEDGEMENTS

The Department of Medical Illustration, United Oxford Hospitals (Mr. D. Floyd, Miss M. McLarty and Miss S. Barker), Mr. R. L. Emanuel of the Nuffield Orthopaedic Centre, Dr. T. Parry of the Gibson Laboratory, Radcliffe Infirmary, and Dr. K. Maddock gave valuable help with some of the illustrations, the remainder being produced at home.

Finally, I must thank the radiographers of the Churchill Hospital for their assistance with many of the investigations, Mrs. A. Wilkinson and Miss P. J. Healy for typing the manuscript, the publishers for their patience, and my wife and family for their forbearance during the many months of preparation.

1

Introduction

Diagnostic radiology is the most common method of detecting lesions in the chest, particularly when a tumour is suspected. Both miniature radiographs employing photofluorography and full-sized radiographs may be taken for the detection of tumours. The standard of radiography and its interpretation have undoubtedly been gradually improving, but I feel that greater attention to certain points could improve the diagnostic accuracy.

Diagnostic radiology holds a place not only in the demonstration of the suspicious lung shadow but also in its further investigation, and I shall attempt to indicate how far radiology can further the diagnosis and assessment of the disease. It is now fairly widely accepted that not all bronchial tumours can be seen through a bronchoscope, and I shall show that the combination of radiological investigations with bronchoscopy is of considerable value in deciding which patients may be benefited by surgical resection.

IMPORTANCE OF EARLY DIAGNOSIS

The suggestion that diagnostic radiology frequently diagnoses lung tumours only three to six months before the patient's death is unfortunately true in many cases. In some the tumours are rapidly progressive and are unresectable from the onset of symptoms, whilst in others the lesion may have been invisible or unrecognized due to poor radiological technique or poor interpretation (*Figure 1.1*). In some cases, retrospective reviews of the radiographs show that the tumours were obviously present months before they were recognized, and this in particular prompts the search for a better understanding of the radiological abnormalities which may be present, so that such lesions can be detected earlier at a resectable stage.

A particularly well-known victim of lung cancer was the late King George VI who unfortunately, despite a lung resection, lived for only four and a half months after the diagnosis of bronchial neoplasm was made. He had previously had a sympathectomy for ischaemia of the lower limbs (details of the King's illnesses are given in his obituary in the *British Medical Journal*, 1952, and in Appendix 10). According to some newspaper reports, the disease may already have been advanced at the time of his operation (*see* Graham Hodgson, 1972).

The detection of lung tumours at a resectable stage is often difficult, because many bronchial neoplasms tend to involve the hilar and mediastinal nodes at the time of diagnosis. If only plain chest radiographs are taken, these should always be of good quality, underpenetrated and portable examinations usually being inadequate. A radiograph is not a work of art, but a recording of normal and pathological anatomy. Moderate over-exposure is usually better than under-exposure, since with a bright illuminator both lung and mediastinal details can be readily seen. Under-exposure fails to record information which cannot be retrieved by any viewing method.

Earlier diagnosis is unfortunately of increasing importance as the number of cases continues to rise. In 1941 there were 8,597 deaths due to lung cancer, and in 1970 about 30,000. The disease represents approximately one-third of all cancers in males, and in 1968, 11,000 of these men were under the

1

age of 65. In women the incidence is lower but is also rising, although it has not yet reached the figures for cancer of the breast and uterus. (For further details *see Figure 1.2* and Appendix 2.) Similar trends have been found in other countries, including the United States of America.

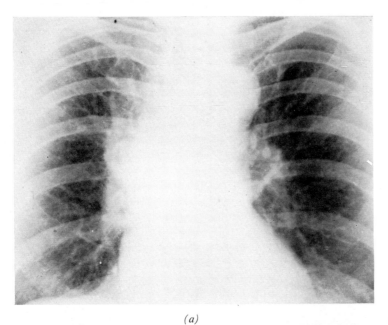

(a)

Figure 1.1. (a) Conventional kV chest radiograph reported as normal. (b) High kV chest radiograph one week later with barium outlining the oesophagus. (c) Inclined frontal tomogram showing massive enlargement of right hilar and subcarinal nodes and narrowing of right lower lobe bronchus

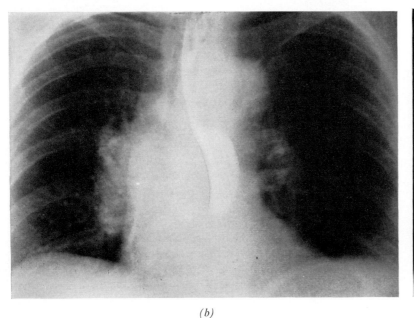

(b)

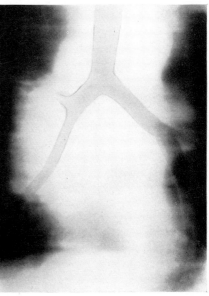

(c)

CAUSES OF LUNG CANCER

The causation of the disease in most cases has been ascribed to smoking habits (Doll and Hill, 1952; Doll, 1953, 1954, 1956, 1964; Royal College of Physicians, 1962, 1971). A similar conclusion was reached by the United States Surgeon General's Advisory Committee (Terry, 1964), although others have incriminated carcinogens in diesel fumes, particularly benzpyrene (Myddleton, 1964). Industrial factors predisposing to lung cancer include the inhalation of nickel, chromates (Baetjer, 1950; Bidstrup, 1964), tar (Hueper, 1957) and asbestos (Bridge and Henry, 1928; Gloyne, 1936; Doll, 1955; Cordova, Tesluk and Knudtson, 1962) and the mining of radioactive minerals, particularly in the cobalt mines of Saxony and the uranium mines of Bohemia (Beyreuther, 1924; Rostoski, Saupe and Schmorl, 1926; Schmorl, 1928). Further details of hazards in these industries and in others where there may be some risk, including coal gas production, haematite mining, isopropyl alcohol manufacture, iron and steel foundries and sandblasting, are given by Raven (1960) and by Boyd et al. (1970). Stocks (1947) found that the death rate from cancer of the lung and larynx was much greater in large towns than in rural areas.

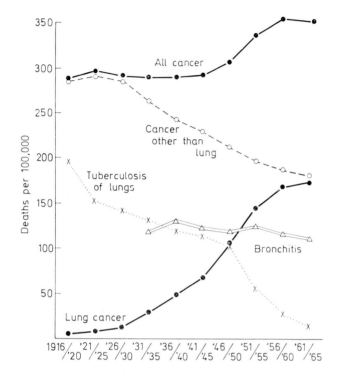

Figure 1.2. Death rates from lung cancer, other forms of cancer, pulmonary tuberculosis and bronchitis in men aged 45–64 years from 1916 to 1965.

Some families show a raised incidence of the disease, and I have personally investigated four brothers who all developed lung cancer under the age of 45. Among non-smokers (approximately one in five patients with lung cancer according to Doll, 1953) and in females the incidence of adenocarcinoma appears to be higher.

Sir George Godber, Chief Medical Officer, Department of Health and Social Security, has estimated that the total number of deaths caused by cigarette smoking in Britain must now be nearly 100,000 per year; this figure also includes deaths due to chronic bronchitis and ischaemic heart disease. As Ball (1970) states, 'there are no countries with an effective programme for the control of smoking, yet in England for every death from tuberculosis there are twenty deaths from cigarette smoking'. Half the lung cancer deaths occur in moderate smokers smoking fifteen cigarettes per day or less. It has been estimated that if nothing is done to reduce smoking, 250,000 of the children now at school will die from the disease. There is now a ban on the advertising of cigarettes on commercial television and a warning on cigarette packets that 'smoking can damage your health', but Government expenditure on advertising the dangers of smoking amounts to only £100,000 per year in contrast to the £50 million spent on advertising each year by the tobacco industry. Government revenue from tobacco duty (*Figure 1.3*) totals £1,000 million annually from 23 million smokers, and it has been suggested that no government can afford to allow such revenue to disappear.

The Royal College of Physicians in 1971 set up a company, ASH (Action on Smoking and Health Ltd.), which has the support of the Department of Health and Social Security, to promote research projects and function as a 'pressure group' in preventing or reducing the smoking of cigarettes.

Elson (1972) has found that there is a difference between the carcinogenic properties of air-cured

3

and fomented tobaccos (the latter is used in cigars) and that of kiln-dried tobacco. Kiln-drying produces more sugar, which decreases nicotine emission from the cigarette; this gives less satisfaction to the smoker and hence causes him to inhale more smoke. Kiln-cured tobacco, as used in the United Kingdom, would thus appear to be more dangerous than its American and Continental 'mild' counterparts. This may explain why Britain's lung cancer rate is about twice the American rate although Americans on average smoke more cigarettes. A Government report was published in April giving tar-reading figures for all brands of cigarettes on sale in Britain.

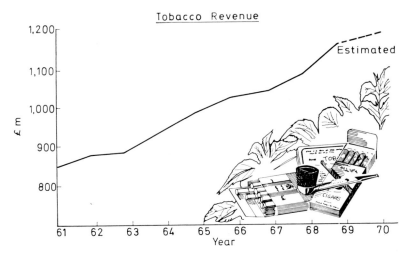

The chart shows why successive Governments are chary of clamping down on cigarette smoking despite horrifying reports like last week's from the Royal College of Physicians. Almost 90 per cent of tobacco revenue, now running at almost £1,200 million a year, comes from cigarettes.

Figure 1.3. Increasing tobacco revenue, 1961–1970

SURVIVAL RATES

Survival rates of patients with bronchogenic tumours differ to some extent from centre to centre, depending mainly on the selection of patients before they are seen in particular clinics. Christiansen and Smith (1962) found that of 462 patients referred for surgery, resection could be carried out in only 131 (35 per cent). The five-year survival rate averaged 13 per cent. Patients who had no resection showed 100 per cent mortality in the first twelve months.

A greater percentage survival has been found where the lesion is asymptomatic and confined to the lung (34 per cent by Overholt, Bougas and Woods, 1955).

Belcher and Anderson (1965), from the London Chest Hospital, studied 1,134 patients who were operated on for bronchial carcinoma between 1949 and 1963. The operative mortality was 10 per cent, the resectability rate being 79 per cent (of the patients who had a resection, 47 per cent had a lobectomy); 26 per cent of those who had a resection and survived the operation lived for at least five years, while at ten years the survival rate was 16 per cent. Of those patients in whom a resection was not possible, only 3 per cent lived longer than two years; the average length of survival after thoracotomy was nine months. Patients under the age of 45 years had a similar prognosis to the whole series, whereas those aged over 70 did extremely badly. The authors found that the incidence of the various types of tumour had changed in the later years and that the proportion of undifferentiated and oat cell carcinomas had risen at the expense of the squamous cell type. The proportion of adenocarcinomas did not alter despite the yearly increase in the total number of tumours. This was an unexpected finding, 'for if the main contributory factor in the increase of bronchial carcinoma was smoking, the proportion of adeno-carcinomas should have fallen', since Kreyberg (1962) had suggested that smoking was not related to the incidence of adenocarcinoma, though it was linked with that of the other types.

4

Similarly, Bignall, Martin and Smithers (1967) reviewed over 6,000 patients with bronchial carcinoma attending the Royal Marsden and Brompton Hospitals during the period 1944 to 1963. They found that the five-year survival rate in patients having resections (1,110 cases) was 27 per cent, and that there were a few long-term survivors among those receiving radiotherapy for inoperable tumours. Patients who had undergone a lobectomy fared better (one-year survival 73 per cent, five-year survival 35 per cent) than those who had had a pneumonectomy (54 and 22 per cent respectively). Those having radiotherapy and surgery had a five-year survival of 5 per cent compared with 1·9 per cent in those given radiotherapy alone. Bignall and his colleagues also estimated that the overall five-year survival rate in the United Kingdom was probably little more than 5 per cent, and concluded that as the prospects for a striking improvement in methods of treatment or earlier diagnosis were not encouraging, the still increasing death rate called for a more serious and energetic attempt at prevention than had yet been undertaken. The decrease in smoking that has taken place amongst doctors would seem to have reduced their mortality from the disease, while at the same time the mortality has been rising in the general public.

The better results achieved with less advanced tumours prompts further study into the radiological diagnosis and investigation of lung cancer.

2

Radiological Appearances of Bronchogenic Tumours— Historical Review and General Points

THE YEARS 1897 TO 1928

The first two chest radiographs, taken on Eastman paper and published in Great Britain, appeared in *Archives of the Roentgen Ray* in July 1897, approximately 20 months after Roentgen's discovery of x-rays. These were of a patient aged 68 years with presumptive cancer of the oesophagus and a child aged 5 years with phthisis. In 1909 Robert Knox published two cases, one a sarcoma of the chest wall and the other a pneumonia in a patient aged 20 which was very slow to clear. The same author presented a paper entitled 'The x-ray diagnosis of malignant disease of the lungs' at the seventeenth International Congress of Medicine, London, 1913, but this does not appear to have been published. He also (Knox, 1917) wrote a textbook *Radiography and Radio-therapeutics* and, in discussing the differential diagnosis in diseases of the lungs, noted the gross appearances of some lung and mediastinal tumours and their not uncommon association with tuberculosis.

Professor Wenckebach (1913) from Strasbourg also spoke at the seventeenth International Congress of Medicine. In discussing the radiology of the chest, he stated that 'tumours generally throw uniform deep shadows and are usually easy to distinguish from infiltrations by their sharp boundaries. In the case of rapidly growing malignant tumours the edges are not sharp but frayed, yet still distinguishable from the surrounding pneumonic shadow'. He also commented that 'primary tumours of the lungs, such as bronchial carcinoma, may produce fantastic x-ray pictures'.

Adler (1912) published his classical monograph in which he not only briefly summarized each of the 374 cases of malignant lung tumour which were all that he could collect from the world literature, but also gave a concise and accurate description of the pathological and clinical aspects of the disease (*see also* Postscripts, page 220). Several authors, including Adami and Nicholls (1909) and Kaufmann (1911), noted that lung tumours may cavitate and may arise either within a large bronchus or peripherally within a lobe. Woodburn Morison (1923) reported phrenic palsy secondary to lung neoplasm.

Manges (1922, 1926) showed that an inhaled foreign body might cause (1) an increased transparency of the affected lung, (2) depression and limitation of movement of the diaphragm on the affected side, (3) displacement of the heart and mediastinum away from the affected side, and (4) increased excursion of the diaphragm on the contralateral side. Golden (1925) found that similar appearances might occur with some bronchogenic tumours, and also described the effect of bronchostenosis in producing collapse. He stated that with complete obstruction there is collapse of the corresponding part of the lung because the air remaining in the alveoli is quickly absorbed by the circulating blood, whereas with incomplete obstruction the bronchi distal to it become dilated. He wrote: 'Hence in the gradually developing stenosis of a bronchial carcinoma the condition is first that of incomplete obstruction, and bronchiectasis follows with infection in its train' (*see also* page 205).

In 1928, Ralston Paterson discussed the roentgen ray treatment of primary carcinoma of the lung. References in this paper related largely to single case reports or to small series of patients. In the same year, Kirklin and Paterson published two excellent papers based on a review of the literature at this time and on the early manifestations of the disease in 55 patients who presented at the Mayo Clinic during the period 1923–27. Because of the comprehensiveness of these two papers, I shall review them in some detail.

Classification by Kirklin and Ralston Paterson

The authors divided primary malignant lesions of the lung into two main groups, *parenchymal* and *bronchial*, the pathological and clinical features differing considerably. The various roentgenological appearances allowed the same grouping.

Parenchymal tumours

Most of the parenchymal tumours were adenocarcinomas. Kirklin and Paterson stated that the clinical progress of parenchymal cancer was extraordinarily latent, with pain of an indefinable but persistent nature and loss of weight without apparent cause. Later, invasion of the pleura, erosion of a bronchus or infection produced the usual respiratory triad of cough, dyspnoea and pain in the chest. The clinical course of the disease was anything but simple, and far too often the patients were considered as tuberculous and lingered on unnecessarily in sanatoria. The authors thought that the condition was relatively rare, and considered that most other published accounts were of patients studied later in the disease or at necropsy.

These workers pointed out that the view at this time (Pfahler, 1919; Carman, 1921; Wessler and Jaches, 1923; Holmes and Ruggles, 1926) was that pulmonary carcinoma fell into two main groups on the basis of roentgenological characteristics, being (1) *hilar* or *infiltrating*, or (2) *lobar, nodular, pneumonic* or *massive*.

The *hilar* tumour was described as an infiltration centred in the hilum, most dense at the hilum and shading into healthy lung in wide strand-like processes. Assman (1914) had shown, by comparing roentgenograms taken immediately before death with the data at necropsy, that these processes were probably permeations of the lymphatic channels of the same nature as occurred with carcinoma of the breast.

[Kerley (1925) had termed the *lobar* or *nodular* tumour the *pneumonic* type and had stated that it had two main forms: (*a*) *nodular* when there was a localized area of density, roughly circular, sometimes with satellites peripherally of a much smaller size (a point also emphasized by Carman, 1921), and lacking the sharply demarcated edge of a nodular metastatic tumour; and (*b*) *lobar* when it filled a whole lobe with a dense homogeneous growth (easily mistaken for caseous tuberculous pneumonia) and was sharply limited by the interlobar septa.

A distinguishing point made by Barjon (1921) was that if the tumour was not infected it was confined to the lobe it involved, the rest of the lung being entirely clear, whereas massive tuberculosis was seldom so limited. The lobar tumour was essentially a more advanced growth and was often the later stage of either the nodular or the roentgenologically hilar (but actually parenchymal) tumour, although never of a clinically endobronchial neoplasm. To these two groups, Wessler and Jaches (1923) added another rare form in which there was a *greatly increased density of the whole ramification of the markings of the bronchial tree* but no central mass in the hilum, and assumed this to be a surface type of squamous growth which spread superficially along the bronchus and bronchioles but did not erupt through their walls. Other types of primary carcinoma had been described: miliary carcinoma or carciniasis (Assman, 1914), multiple nodular carcinoma (Holmes and Ruggles, 1926; Carman, 1921), and cavernous carcinoma (Kerley, 1925). However, Kirklin and Paterson did not think that these could be justly regarded as types of pulmonary malignant disease, since both the miliary and the multiple carcinomas were the result of local metastasis, while the cavernous carcinoma was merely a central necrosis in a nodular tumour.]

Kirklin and Paterson found that there was an extraordinary variety of possible roentgenological characteristics of parenchymal lung tumours and that it was difficult to distinguish those that might be typical of carcinoma, though early cases did fall into three groups—nodular, lobar, and hilar or infiltrating. The *nodular* type was seen, contrary to previous observers' opinions, most commonly in these writers' early cases, and they believed that all true parenchymal tumours started as definitely circumscribed nodules. They, like Rigler later, were particularly interested in this appearance, regarding it as evidence of a stage of development at which lobectomy might be of value. They stated that the nodule appeared as an irregular circular area of homogeneous density without increase of density at the margin and with edges infiltrating into the healthy parenchyma. The *lobar* tumour was much less clear-cut and appeared as a more or less complete consolidation of the whole of a lobe, less dense than fluid; it showed no mottling of any kind, nor the varied texture seen in most cases of lobar pneumonia, and it had an irregularly infiltrating edge. The *hilar* or *infiltrating* lesion was difficult to relate to typical roentgenological characteristics, although it was the commonest type. Kirklin and Paterson stated that a malignant focus situated in the lung but lying near a bronchus in the region of the hilum might appear in the roentgenogram to be a mass centred at the hilum and infiltrating through the pulmonary tissue towards the periphery, an appearance which might be produced either by actual infiltration in a peri-bronchial form or by partial atelectasis distal to a bronchus occluded from without, and that it was impossible to distinguish these two processes roentgenologically.

The above manifestations were the common roentgenological features of early malignant disease of the lung. As the disease advanced, however, secondary processes obscured the picture and it usually became impossible to distinguish 'by the roentgen ray alone' between the primary lesion and the secondary manifestations. The presence of fluid was the most important secondary and obscuring factor. In some cases the tumour would grow to involve large portions of the lung, producing a roentgenological type which was termed 'massive', an appearance often caused by widespread pneumonitis or consolidation surrounding and obscuring the growth.

Bronchial tumours

The three characteristics of early malignant disease of the bronchial type (adenocarcinoma and epithelioma in about equal numbers) were given as (1) density of the hilum, (2) atelectasis, and (3) bronchiectasis. (A hilar enlargement was usually then reported as 'indistinguishable from any other enlargement of the hilum'.) Kirklin and Paterson attempted to define the type of hilar enlargement peculiar to a bronchial tumour, but were disappointed since the enlargement could be simulated by other processes. Atelectasis was of great value in diagnosing the tumours which lay largely within the mediastinum and were thus invisible on roentgenograms of this period. Bronchiectasis, which sometimes occurred, 'must be diagnosed as bronchiectasis and the underlying malignant condition will only be discovered in an investigation for the cause of the bronchiectasis'. Pseudo-bronchiectasis (later in this book called mucocoeles—*see* page 54) was defined as a collection of fluid collected by gravity and aspiration below the lesion, the fluid-filled bronchial tree thus causing a density.* If the lesion were really an early bronchial carcinoma, 'there should be no other characters present. The unaffected lung must be perfectly clear, the upper portion of the mediastinum unthickened and there should never be an appearance as of metastasis distal to the lesion: at this early stage pleurisy is a rare manifestation'. As a bronchial tumour grew, the appearances would become concealed by secondary processes, so that there would be no real distinction between the bronchial and parenchymal types.

These secondary processes were listed as stenotic, infective, pleuritic and metastatic. The stenosis could result from a bronchial growth obliterating the lumen of a bronchus, or from a parenchymal growth occluding the lumen either by pressure from without or at a later stage by eroding the wall and fungating into the lumen. In the absence of infection such stenosis would cause complete collapse of the lung, but this was unusual since a collapsed lung usually became infected, thus producing bronchiectasis, pneumonitis or an abscess. Kirklin and Paterson regarded pleurisy as an accompaniment of tumours only in the late stages and thought that it often developed as a complication of infection. They felt that the fluid should be removed to allow 'roentgen-ray examination' of the underlying lung, and also pointed out that such an examination must be made within the following few hours as the fluid had a marked tendency to recur after tapping.

They noted that metastasis to the supraclavicular nodes might occur quite early and that 'the roentgen-ray picture may be altered by extension of the lesion to the mediastinal lymph nodes'. The lungs themselves were also a common site for metastases, and the authors observed that 'the picture of a primary carcinoma of the lung might easily be obscured by multiple metastases in the other lung or a small bronchial carcinoma may be overlooked in the picture which gives an impression of true miliary carcinosis'.

In considering the differential diagnosis of a breaking-down tumour or an infective abscess, Kirklin

---

* This sign of a bronchial neoplasm was neglected even in a recent leading article in the *British Medical Journal*—*see* Wright (1971b).

and Paterson stated that 'mottling patchiness or a lack of centring suggests abscess; homogeneous density and definite centring suggest a malignant lesion'. Moreover, abscesses often extended to involve the periphery of the lung, a feature practically never seen with malignant lesions as fluid would then obscure the picture by the time the pleura was involved.* Involvement of the periphery of the lung was also a distinguishing feature of encysted fluid or empyema.

These papers were extremely advanced for their time, and pointed out very many of the features of bronchial carcinomas which have subsequently been almost forgotten. They are seldom quoted by later writers.

THE 1930s and 1940s

Pancoast (1932) published an account of superior sulcus tumours with pain, Horner's syndrome, destruction of bone (ribs and vertebral column) and atrophy of hand muscles. This was followed by other descriptions of apical tumours by Steiner and Francis (1934) and by Browder and De Veer (1935).

Chandler (1932), discussing at the British Medical Association's centenary meeting the radiology of bronchiectasis and lung abscess by the recently introduced technique of *bronchography* using Lipiodol (*see* Sicard and Forestier, 1932), stated: 'The differential diagnosis between lung abscess and a new growth was made more difficult by the tendency of a growth to produce a secondary bronchiectasis. The distinction between abscess and a breaking down growth could be made in the early stages, when a discrete growth might be easily recognizable. Lipiodol was said to show a more conical outline at the obstruction caused by a growth and a more abrupt one when stopped by an abscess'.

At the same B.M.A. meeting, Davidson (1932), discussing intrathoracic new growths, referred to the remarkable progress in their diagnosis made by roentgen rays and the bronchoscope. He assumed that the appropriate team for diagnosis consisted of physician, radiologist and bronchoscopist. He stressed the increasing frequency of lung cancer and stated that 'the growth usually originated a short distance below the bifurcation of the main bronchus. In other cases it remained localized for a time, long before physical signs or skiagraphic abnormalities gave definite evidence of the disease'. He also briefly discussed the value of bronchography.

Korol and Scott (1934) described the value of roentgenograms taken in expiration to show *obstructive emphysema*. The effects of this condition were further discussed by Golden (1940). Also in 1934, Rabin and Neuhof showed the value of detecting well-defined peripheral lesions (later termed 'coin lesions') with no lymph node metastases.

Christie (1937), in a discussion of the diagnosis and treatment of primary cancer of the lung, observed that 'it is now the rather generally held opinion that cancer of the lung is increasing not only in total number of cases, but out of proportion to cancer in general', and described it as 'a disease with a high order of frequency and one that the physician must always have in mind as a possibility when a patient presents himself with chest symptoms'. Christie quoted Tuttle and Womack (1934), who to him offered convincing evidence that tumours arising in the peripheral portions of the lungs were more likely to involve mediastinal glands and to metastasize to distant parts at an early stage of the disease than were cancers arising in the main bronchial trunks, and that peripheral tumours often ran a more rapid course than those located in a major bronchus.

THE 1950s

During the ensuing ten to fifteen years, the main emphasis in chest radiology and in publications on the radiology of chest diseases continued to be on the diagnosis and treatment of pulmonary tuberculosis.

In 1950 Lodge, working in Sheffield, and Møller, working in Copenhagen, both emphasized the important role of diagnostic radiology in the diagnosis of bronchogenic tumours. Lodge found that the commonest tumours, as shown radiographically, were those producing collapse, a hilar or a peripheral mass; less common were those producing consolidation, infiltration or cavitation. Møller (1950)

---

* This, however, is not true, as tumours often extend to the periphery of the lung without the production of a pleural effusion.

thought that a small area of collapse or, less commonly, obstructive emphysema was the earliest sign of a bronchial tumour. He pointed out the need for routine lateral views.

At this time it was the accepted view that the majority of bronchial tumours arose in the major bronchi near the hilum. Fried (1938) had found in 152 cases that 'the tumour always originates in the main stem bronchus or in some of its smaller branches, but not in those whose diameter is about 10 mm or less'. Boyd (1950) stated: 'The hilus tumour is by far the commonest variety. Over 90 per cent of the cases fall into this group'. Willis (1948) wrote: 'At least three-quarters of the tumours demonstrably arise in the large bronchi, either the main bronchi or the lobar bronchi, in or near the hilar region'.

Schinz et al. (1953), in their well-known textbook, classified malignant primary tumours of the lung into pulmonary sarcoma, bronchial carcinoma and cancer of the alveolar epithelium. They considered that 'pulmonary sarcoma' should be suspected when there was a homogeneous extensive round or oval infiltration in a lobe without atelectasis, and thought that sarcoma differed from carcinoma in that true lobar forms of the latter were exceptional. Carcinoma of the lung was divided into bronchial or hilar carcinoma, cancer of the pulmonary parenchyma, carcinoma of the pulmonary apex (Pancoast tumour) and pulmonary cicatricial carcinoma.

Schinz and his colleagues stated that bronchial or hilar carcinoma was most common in the upper lobes and that in the early disease the roentgenograms could be negative. They also noted that in early cases 'stenotic' emphysema might be seen, whereas with progressive bronchial stenosis, segmental collapse occurred and there was often hilar enlargement. A bronchogram could be decisively diagnostic. The authors wrote that 'carcinoma growing in the bronchial wall shows up in the bronchus, the lumen becomes stenosed and the inner contour takes on an irregular aspect. In more extensive stenosis, the contrast medium passes the narrow portion irregularly or stops proximal to the narrow portion. Behind the stenosis bronchiectasis may occur, frequently accompanied by the formation of abscesses'. They thought that tomograms could not replace bronchograms, though they were useful in evaluating cavities in carcinoma with necrosis. With a carcinoma the cavity was nearly always solitary, whereas abscesses were likely to be multiple or loculated. The inner wall of a carcinomatous cavity was usually irregular, while in an abscess cavity the wall was usually smooth.

Carcinoma of the pulmonary parenchyma was defined as a neoplasm developing in the peripheral mantle of the pulmonary tissue. In the early stages a rounded shadow might be seen in the pulmonary fields, particularly in the paravertebral broncho-pulmonary segments of the upper lobes and the apical segment of the lower lobes. In such a situation the round shadow might be projected on to the mediastinum and might simulate a hilar carcinoma, though the lateral roentgenogram would rectify the error. Hilar nodes might enlarge as well. Interlobar fissures might constitute a barrier to the spread of the disease.

According to Walter and Pryce (1955), the view that the majority of lung tumours arose in the main bronchi was based mainly on post-mortem studies of the disease in its terminal stages when the tumour had, in most instances, attained a large size. By this time, direct spread and lymphatic metastases had combined to produce the familiar hilar mass involving the lung, bronchi, vessels and mediastinal structures alike. Walter and Pryce mentioned that gross involvement of the large hilar bronchi was usually present and thought that although this had previously been assumed to be the site of origin of the tumour, it was doubtful whether such an assumption was often justified. These authors found that in 207 resected lung cancers, roughly the same number of tumours arose peripherally as centrally. The most distinctive feature of the central tumours was bronchial obstruction. Peripheral tumours on the other hand often showed central scarring; bronchial involvement, when present, was due to invasion either directly by the primary growth or from secondary lymph nodes. The majority of these workers' small tumours were central, and they concluded that the central type produced early symptoms. The giant and large tumours were mainly peripheral, indicating that in this type the onset of symptoms occurred at a later stage. Of those tumours whose site of origin was located, the adenocarcinomas were always peripheral and the polygonal cell growths frequently peripheral (87 per cent). Squamous cell tumours were more often central (58 per cent) than peripheral (37 per cent), while oat cell carcinomas were equally divided between the two groups.

Rigler, working in Minneapolis and later in Los Angeles, became interested in the presentation of lung tumours at about the same time and published several papers on this subject. Two of these (Rigler, 1955, 1957b) are summarized in Tables 2.1 and 2.2.

TABLE 2.1

Appearances Suggesting a Bronchial Carcinoma

Solitary pulmonary shadow, especially if patient is past middle age
Increase in size of nodule or mass
Absence of calcification
Notching or umbilication
Hilar enlargement
Increasing infiltration of beaded or nodular type
Pneumonic lesions: Failing to resolve
                        Having a nodular appearance
                        Associated with bronchostenosis
Thick-walled cavities with irregular nodular inner walls
Segmental, lobar or unilateral emphysema
Collapse
Changes in lumen of bronchi, especially demonstration of tumour

TABLE 2.2

Roentgen Findings in the Evolution of Lung Cancer Found by Retrospective Survey

Fifty per cent show some evidence of carcinoma more than 2 years
   before symptoms
Two-thirds originate centrally; symptoms earlier
One-third originate peripherally; better for surgical resection;
   symptoms later
Bronchial obstruction may precede onset of symptoms
Obstructive emphysema of lobe or lung may be concomitant with
   segmental collapse
Cavitation may occur early in peripheral or central lesions and may
   disappear as tumour grows
Inflammatory changes may appear and disappear during life of
   tumour
Growth of tumour may show varying rapidity at various times

MORE RECENT GENERAL PAPERS, 1962–66

Garland *et al.* (1962) discussed the apparent sites of origin of carcinomas of the lung. In 150 cases the tumour appeared to arise about twice as commonly in the peripheral as in the central bronchi, and in many cases it was evident to these authors that certain of the main bronchus tumours had actually originated in adjacent pulmonary segments and had eroded into the larger bronchi to simulate a tumour arising within them. They also postulated that if a carcinogenic agent affected the whole of the bronchial tree to the same degree, one would expect many more tumours to arise peripherally, since the combined surface area of the smaller peripheral bronchi is much greater than that of the central bronchi.

In 1966, Rigler published his experiences in 'Current Cancer Concepts' in the *Journal of the American Medical Association*. He stated: 'The least expensive and simplest method for the detection of a malignant lesion in the lung when it is small, is roentgen examination. A single postero-anterior roentgenogram made in inspiration is an effective method for finding cases in their pre-symptomatic stage. An additional number of small lesions would be discovered if it were possible to add a second film so that stereoscopic or postero-anterior and lateral views were made in each case. . . . The presence of symptoms which are at all suggestive of carcinoma of the lung should lead to such a thorough investigation, to which should be added body-section roentgenography' (i.e. tomography).

Rigler further analysed the radiographs of several patients who had had chest examinations prior to the diagnosis of their carcinoma, and pointed out that the changes to be observed under these circumstances were different from those commonly seen in the patient with symptomatic cancer of the lung. These changes are of two kinds. The first type of change is caused by the growth itself which, within the contrasting areas of the air-filled lungs, may produce shadows of distinctive character. Less commonly, secondary signs in the lung, occasionally accompanied by minor symptoms, may result from the invasion of the bronchus by the tumour.

Rigler listed the following as signs of early or relatively asymptomatic tumours.

(1*a*) *A homogeneous density*, rounded and with sharply defined borders—a spheroidal nodule in the periphery of the lung.

(1*b*) *A similar nodule*, but with irregular, radiating and poorly defined borders.

(1*c*) *Linear shaped lesions* of similar size (non-homogeneous in density).

(2) *Cavitation within a solid tumour.*

(3) *A segmental, indistinct, poorly defined, dense area.*

(4) *Nodular, streaked, local infiltration* along the course of the vessels, simulating an inflammatory lesion, with the blood vessels appearing to be beaded and thickened because of the tumour process.

(5) *Segmental consolidation* resembling pneumonia.

(6) *A roughly triangular lesion* arising in the apex of the lung and extending towards the hilum. [Rigler considered that symptoms were early in superior sulcus tumours. This sign is, however, similar to that discussed in (5) before spread to the pleura and the chest wall has taken place.]

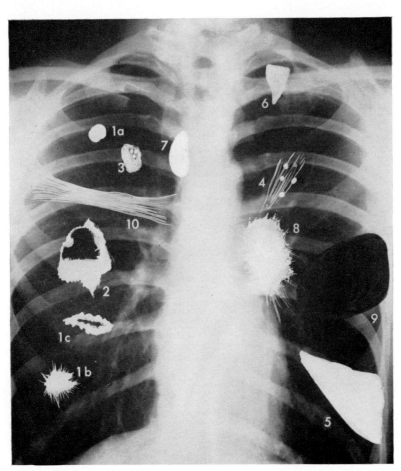

Figure 2.1. The principal roentgenographic manifestations of cancer of the lung when the lesion is small or relatively asymptomatic. The numbers refer to the descriptions in the text.

(7) *A mediastinal mass* resembling a lymphoma [this is really a late sign indicating that considerable spread of tumour has occurred through the mediastinal lymph nodes].

(8) *Enlargement of one hilum*, the shadow of the branch pulmonary artery and of the space between the artery and the mediastinum usually being obliterated—a significant and frequently overlooked finding.

Rigler added that secondary changes from bronchial obstruction usually occur somewhat later in the course of the development of carcinoma and the roentgenographic evidence is commonly accompanied by typical symptoms. Occasionally, however, the following signs may be seen in patients in whom symptoms are either absent or so indefinite that they are not considered to be of great significance.

(9) *Segmental or lobar obstructive emphysema.* Here the radiographic findings, being subtle, are best shown by fluoroscopy or on radiographs taken in expiration; however, they can occasionally be seen on views taken in inspiration but not in maximal inspiration. The affected lung shows a greater transradiancy and the vessel shadows in it are more widely spread.

(10) *Segmental atelectasis*—an area of increased density or increased size of vascular shadows, which are crowded together.

The above findings are summarized in *Figure 2.1.*

In considering the differential diagnosis of lung tumours, Rigler considered the following to be the most important points.

(1) A nodular lesion, increasing in size, in an individual aged over 45 years, without any evidence of the lesion in earlier films, is strongly suggestive of malignancy. These lesions should be examined by tomography and the morphology of the nodules should be more carefully studied. The absence of calcium or the presence of a notch (which became known as Rigler's sign) on the border of the lesion favours carcinoma, while satellite shadows favour tuberculosis.

(2) Bronchial occlusion in close association with a pathological process in the lung is strong evidence of the neoplastic nature of the lesion.

Professor Frimann-Dahl, working in Oslo with Drevvatne (Drevvatne and Frimann-Dahl, 1961), also analysed the appearances of peripheral bronchial neoplasms and in particular Rigler's sign. They took tomograms in three planes (antero-posterior, lateral and transverse axial) and found that umbilication of a 'round lesion' occurred not only in 27 out of 31 peripheral neoplasms, but also in 16 out of 22 tuberculomas. They were able to detect similar notchings in metastases of various origins, but did not encounter these with benign tumours such as hamartomas or neurinomas. They also described other signs of malignancy such as scalloping, umbilication with 'apple stalk', and radiating vessels.

Drevvatne and Frimann-Dahl considered the growth of a tumour to be very similar to the growth of an apple around its stalk. The hilum or notch of a tumour was thought to correspond with the entrance of its vascular supply. Often there was only one notch, but occasionally two or three were present, depending upon the number of vessels in the area of the lung in which the neoplasm originated. The notching was seen in tumours from 1 to 10 cm² in area and was most marked when the diameter exceeded 2·5 cm.

These authors also pointed out that the bad prognosis with central tumours occurred despite the fact that they produced symptoms earlier than the peripheral nodules. On the other hand, central tumours were often more difficult to demonstrate because they were hidden by the heart and the pulmonary vessels.

Lodge (1960) ascribed the bad prognosis in many peripheral carcinomas to their being positioned in a bed of numerous small veins, so that an invasive growth might produce early distant metastases. He reviewed the literature existing at that time and supplied further evidence regarding the distinction between central and peripheral tumours.

3

Plain Radiographic, Fluoroscopic and Some Tomographic Appearances of Lung and Mediastinal Tumours and their Differential Diagnosis

It would be of great benefit if one could distinguish tumours radiographically from benign lung lesions. To a large extent the radiographic differential diagnosis depends on a knowledge of the anatomy of the lungs, hilar regions and mediastinum, or an ability to assess the possible effects of the various pathological processes in altering the normal anatomical picture, and on a cumulative experience of anatomical variations and disease processes.

Radiological appearance		Differential diagnosis
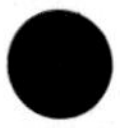	Small round focus	Carcinoma Tuberculoma Adenoma Hamartoma Metastasis Rare causes such as rheumatoid nodule, infarct
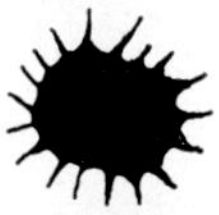	Spiculation or scalloping	Carcinoma Tuberculoma
	Notching or umbilication	Carcinoma Adenoma Hamartoma Metastasis
	Multiple notches or umbilications	Carcinoma Metastasis Hamartoma
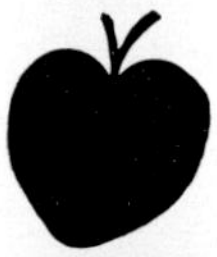	Umbilication with 'apple stalk'	Carcinoma
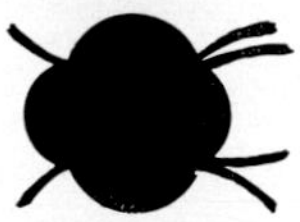	Vessels entering or radiating vessels	Carcinoma

(a)

Figure 3.1. Schematic drawing of the radiological appearances of peripheral bronchial carcinomas as seen on plain radiographs or tomograms, and their differential diagnosis

14

Radiological appearance	Differential diagnosis
Satellite sign	Carcinoma
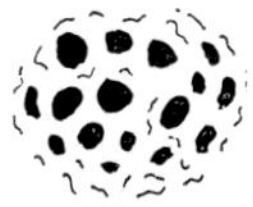 Galaxy or nebula sign	Carcinoma (distinguish from multifocal tuberculosis)
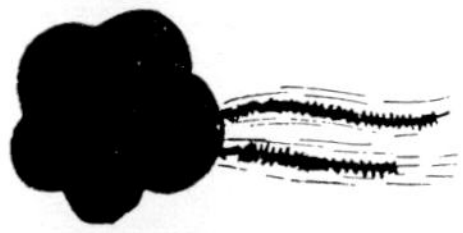 Peribronchial infiltration or 'track to hilum'	Carcinoma Infection
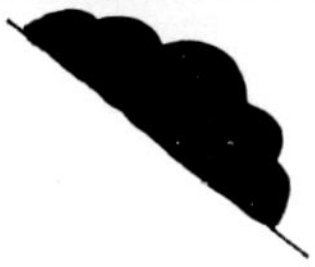 Irregular mass limited by fissure	Carcinoma
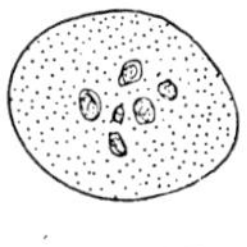 Mass with calcification	Tuberculoma Adenoma Hamartoma ('popcorn' calcification) Secondary deposit (bone sarcoma) Carcinoma unlikely unless old T.B. focus incorporated in tumour
Second mass or bronchostenosis with collapse elsewhere in lungs	May indicate more than one primary tumour
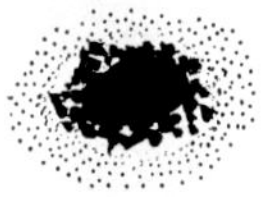 Mass with ill-defined edge	Carcinoma Fibrosis Infection Metastasis
Large round mass	Carcinoma Bronchogenic cyst Hydatid (especially if oval in shape) Secondary deposit Adenoma
Mass with eccentric cavity	Carcinoma Hodgkin's disease Fungus infection Rarely metastasis Lung abscess (if acute)
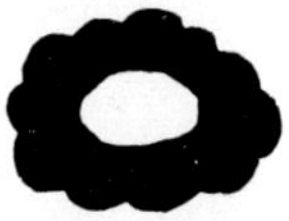 Thick-walled cavity with irregular outer border	Carcinoma
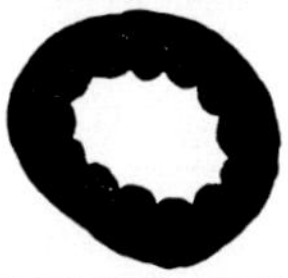 Thick-walled cavity with irregular inner border	Carcinoma Occasionally atypical mycobacteria, Wegener's granuloma
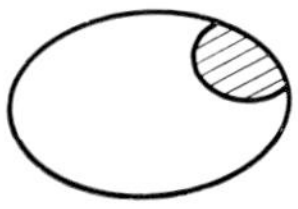 Thin-walled cavity (may have nodule on its inner wall)	Emphysematous bullae, etc. Tuberculosis Bronchial carcinoma (very occasionally), perhaps due to check valve mechanism as also occurs in staphylococcal pneumonia

Figure 3.1 (b)

Chapter 2 described how the different abnormalities produced by central and peripheral lesions came to be recognized and distinguished. The present chapter will continue this discussion, and will also consider some of the difficulties encountered in differentiating lung tumours from other conditions and in recognizing them in the presence of chronic chest diseases. In addition, an account will be given of other manifestations of bronchogenic tumours, and the radiological diagnosis of other lung, pleural and mediastinal masses will be discussed.

PERIPHERAL LUNG MASSES

The appearance of peripheral lung masses (i.e. masses in the pulmonary parenchyma) and their differential diagnosis is shown diagrammatically in *Figure 3.1*.

Small round focus or 'coin' lesion

Most of these small foci (up to 2 cm in diameter) are discovered fortuitously. They may be due to such conditions as bronchial carcinoma, adenoma, tuberculoma, solitary secondary deposit, rheumatoid nodule, pulmonary infarct, pneumoconiotic nodule or intrapulmonary lymph node (*see Figures 3.8–3.13, 3.33* and *3.46;* intrapulmonary lymph nodes causing such shadows have been discussed by Greenberg, 1961). During the past two decades the number of tuberculomas has been slowly declining,

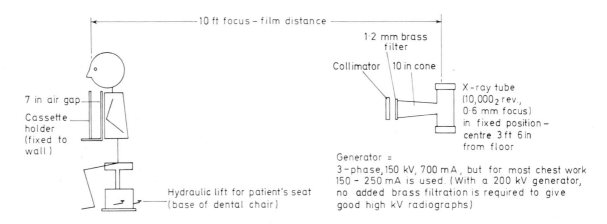

Figure 3.2. Diagram of chest radiographic installation at the Churchill Hospital, 1963 to present date. For conventional kV work, i.e. 60–120, the brass filter is removed. The cassette holder, the patient's seat adapted from an old dental chair base, and the collimator disc were made by the late Mr. A. F. Nichols in the Department of X-ray Technology, Churchill Hospital

whilst the incidence of bronchial tumours has risen. Black and Poole (1955) at the Churchill Hospital studied 124 round foci, none of which was shown to be neoplastic in origin. Garland (1958) found 25 per cent of round foci to be carcinomas, whereas Paulson (1957) stated that 50 per cent were malignant. Other series studied by Abeles and Ehrlich (1951) and by Storey, Grant and Rothman (1953) yielded figures of 27 and 17 per cent respectively. Abeles and Chaves (1952), Flavell (1954) and Good (1963) stressed the importance of calcification as indicating non-malignant disease.

If small round foci due to carcinoma could be demonstrated at an early stage, this would be of great value, since some of these tumours would not have metastasized. In *Figure 3.9*, a radiograph of a man aged 50 illustrates the chance finding of a small round shadow in the right fourth interspace. A lobectomy was carried out and the lesion was shown to be a small squamous bronchial neoplasm. The patient lived for twelve years without any sign of recurrence and died from ischaemic heart disease. In other cases a small peripheral neoplasm may be associated with gross metastatic disease. Examples of this are given in *Figures 3.10* and *10.14* (where there was gross mediastinal enlargement at the time of presentation as well as a large secondary deposit) and in *Figure 10.26* (where a small pulmonary tumour was associated with widespread bony metastases).

High kV radiographic technique

Small 'coin lesions' are not always easily detected on routine postero-anterior (P.A.) radiographs of the chest because they may be hidden by rib shadows (*see Figure 3.8*), by the heart or by the dome of the diaphragm. In an attempt to avoid these difficulties, Kjellberg (1960—personal communication) pointed out that a high kV (for example 190 kV) technique would render bony shadows, especially those of the ribs, less dense and hence allow such round shadows to be more readily seen. He installed 190 kV, 150 cycle, three-phase x-ray units in most of his x-ray rooms ('roentgen laboratories') at the Sahlgranska Hospital in Gothenberg, and favoured the use of 4 mm thick aluminium filters, stationary high ratio grids and automatic exposure timing in order to obtain high quality radiographs. A similar

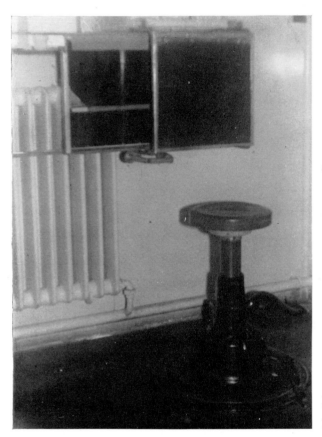

(a)

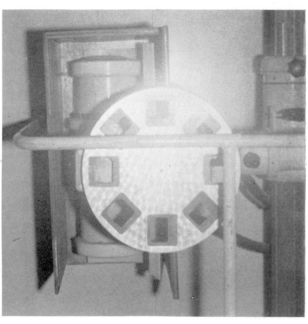

(b)

Figure 3.3. (a) Cassette holder and patient's seat. (b) X-ray tube and collimator disc. The latter contains multiple apertures suitable for each of the various cassette sizes. A guard rail surrounds the tube and its stand to prevent accidental knocks causing disalignment

technique was employed by Nordenström (1969a). Rigler (1965), having moved to Los Angeles, took radiographs with a 2 MeV linear accelerator to give an even greater high kV effect (*see Figure 3.4*). Because of the inefficiency of even thin lead intensifying screens at this energy level, this method resulted in a heavy radiation dose to the patient (0·75 rad incident skin dose per exposure). There was also the disadvantage that it was necessary to obtain the use of a linear accelerator. A long focus object distance was employed to avoid unsharpness due to the large focal spot.

I have used a 150 kV, 50 cycle, three-phase generator with high speed (10,000 rev/min) rotating anodes (foci 0·6 mm^2). The x-ray beam is heavily filtered by a 1·2 mm brass sheet so as to remove the less penetrating radiation and render the beam relatively monochromatic and homogeneous. Scatter from the brass (effectively copper) is absorbed in the air before the x-ray beam reaches the patient. If 190–200 kV is available, no heavy brass filtration is required and an even better result is obtained. Normal radiographs taken at 150 and 200 kV are illustrated in *Figure 3.5*. The apparatus and techniques used are shown in *Figures 3.2* and *3.3*. The extremely low dose rates, amounting to about one week's natural background radioactivity per exposure for each P.A. view, are given in Appendix 8.

The first use of an air gap to reduce scattered radiation was described by Watson (1958). An account of a similar chest radiographic installation using 90 kV and an air gap was published by Ardran and Crooks (1964).

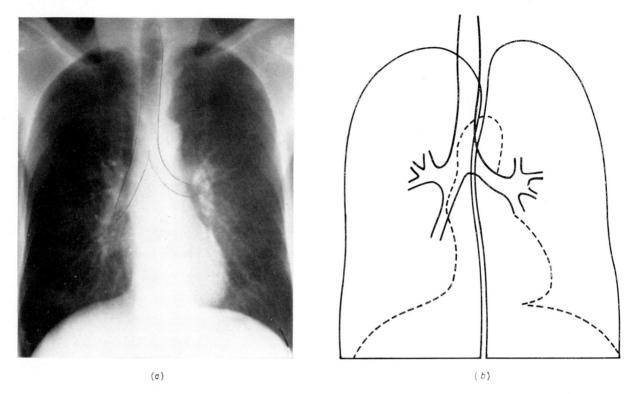

(a)   (b)

Figure 3.4. (a) Chest radiograph taken with 2 MeV linear accelerator. The tracheo-bronchial tree and the pleural boundaries are well demonstrated. (b) Diagrammatic representation of (a)

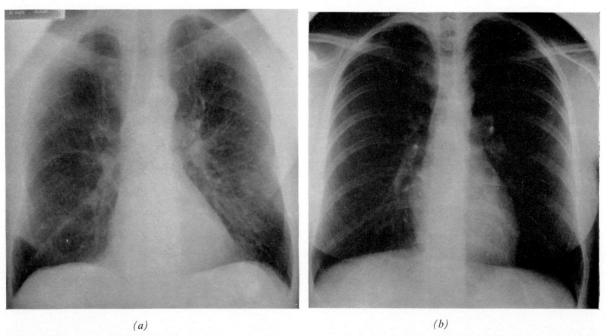

(a)   (b)

Figure 3.5. Normal high kV radiographs: (a) male at 150 kV; (b) female at 200 kV. Note penetration of mediastinum and visualization of trachea, carina and larger bronchi. The rib shadows, being less dense than on radiographs taken at a lower kV, allow the lungs to be well displayed, with the lung bases visible through the 'domes' of the diaphragm. In (a) a nipple shadow is visible at the right base and the shadows of the pectoral muscles are well seen, while in (b) the breast shadows do not obscure the lower lung fields

A high kV technique will not only show small foci in the lungs more readily; it will also give a better visualization of the structures in the mediastinum—in particular the larger air passages, the carina, and the hilar and mediastinal vascular shadows—and will show the various parts of the lungs which are often hidden by the heart, aorta, etc. For anyone used to viewing fairly contrasty low kV chest radiographs, such films may be difficult to appreciate at first, but with a little experience the rather

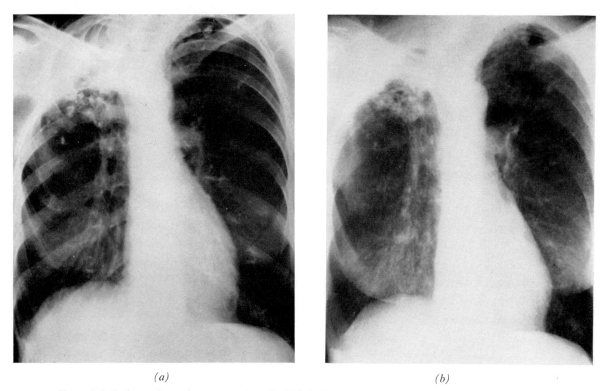

(a)   *(b)*

Figure 3.6. Radiographs to show attenuation of calcified shadows at higher voltages. (a) 80 kV. (b) 150 kV

Figure 3.7. Graph showing relationship between radiographic contrast and increasing kV for the various contrast agents and the tissues of the body. Numbers in brackets refer to atomic weights

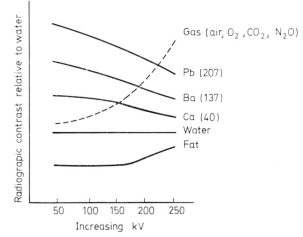

flatter or less contrasty high kV films will be found to contain much more information and will in time be preferred. Because calcification may be less readily seen, one may need to gain supplementary information by taking conventional low kV radiographs as well (*Figure 3.6*). However, for the initial detection of disease or anatomical abnormality the high kV radiograph has so many advantages that I am surprised that it is not more widely used despite the higher initial cost of such an installation. In my opinion it is quite wrong to regard as the standard chest radiograph a film displaying only about

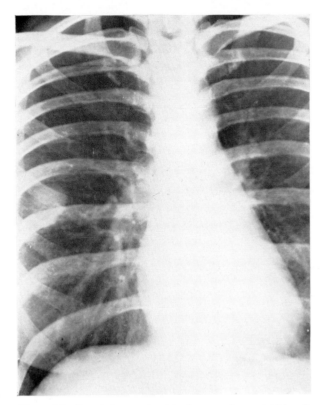

Figure 3.8. Rounded mass in right lung partly overlaid by rib shadows (bronchial neoplasm)

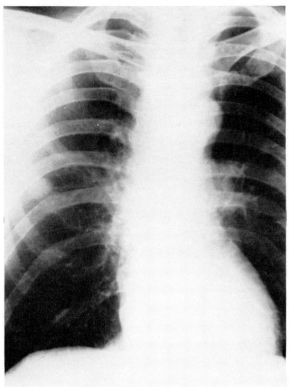

Figure 3.9. Small round peripheral mass which was resected. The patient lived for many years with no signs of recurrence (bronchial neoplasm)

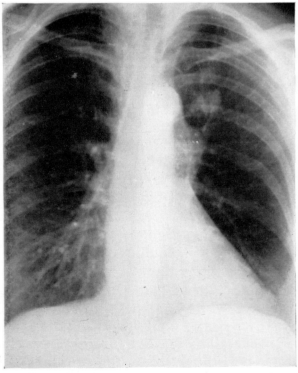

(a)

(b)

Figure 3.10. Small rounded mass in left upper lobe with enlarged left hilar nodes. (a) P.A. view. (b) Inclined frontal tomogram. (See also Figure 10.14)

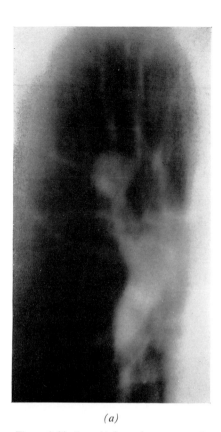
(a)

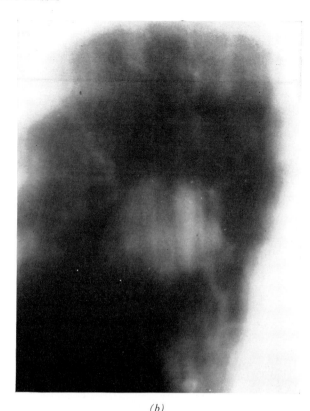
(b)

Figure 3.11. Bronchial neoplasms presenting as nodular shadows in the lungs. (a) Small round nodule, apparently with a vascular 'stalk'. (b) Larger lobulated mass

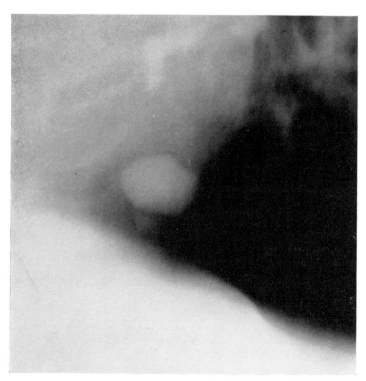

Figure 3.12. Small rounded and slightly lobulated peripheral lung tumour— a bronchial adenoma

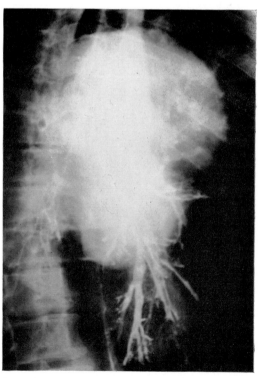

Figure 3.13. Very large and notched or lobulated bronchial adenoma. The bronchogram showed no intrinsic abnormality, only pressure deformities due to very large mass

21

two-thirds to three-quarters of the lungs. The high kV technique also results in a considerably decreased radiation dosage to the patient (*see* Appendix 8).

A graph showing the relationship between contrast and increasing kV for the common negative and positive (including air) contrast media and the tissues of the body appears in *Figure 3.7*.

A similarly well penetrated radiograph is given by photofluorography or mass miniature radiography. Here a radiograph is taken on 35, 70 or 100 mm film, using an Odelca or similar camera in which the image produced on a fluorescent screen is photographed via a paraboloid mirror. This effect has recently been discussed by Deasy (1970). It may be partly explained by the 'minification' discussed in Appendix 6.

Differential diagnosis of small round lesions

Unless there is good reason to suspect some non-malignant condition in a person over 40 years of age, a peripheral rounded lesion is best removed as soon as possible. Reasons for delay might be previous malignant disease, suspected malignancy elsewhere in the body, recent contact with open tuberculosis, adjacent soft areas of infiltration or old scarring, or the presence of calcification. However, when considering tuberculosis in the differential diagnosis one needs to be aware of the possibility of satellite shadows or other signs of local spread of bronchial tumours which may mimic tuberculosis (*see Figures 3.23, 3.24* and *3.36*). Delay in removal may allow time for considerable growth and spread of the tumour (*see Figure 3.150*). Occasionally even the presence of calcification may be misleading, since an old calcified tuberculous focus may become incorporated within a neoplasm (*see Figure 3.71*).

Calcification may be found in adenomas (*see Figures 3.108* and *3.109*) and in hamartomas (*see Figures 3.115* and *3.116*). Fine calcification may be seen in some cancers when they are examined by microradiography after operative removal, but is almost never demonstrated *in vivo* within a patient; it is also sometimes present in pulmonary metastases, especially those secondary to bone tumours, and in granulomas. It is most common in tuberculomas.

O'Keefe, Good and McDonald (1957) radiographed 207 pulmonary nodules *after resection* and found calcification in 77 (37 per cent). It occurred most frequently in the granulomas, where it was largely laminated, and was next commonest in the hamartomas. Small punctate areas of calcification, similar to those seen in some primary breast tumours at mammography, were visible in 16 per cent of primary lung tumours, in 10 per cent of pulmonary metastases and in some bronchial adenomas.

Good (1963) listed four types of calcification in peripheral nodules as seen on plain films or tomograms (*Figure 3.14*).

(*a*) A small central nidus.

(*b*) Multiple punctate foci.

(*c*) An appearance of lamination, sometimes resembling a rifle target with a bullseye.

(*d*) Conglomerate or interconnected foci giving a 'popcorn' appearance.

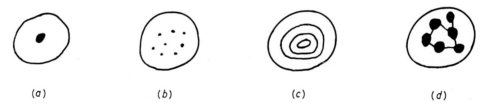

(*a*)   (*b*)   (*c*)   (*d*)

Figure 3.14. Types of calcification: (a) central nidus; (b) multiple punctate foci; (c) lamination; (d) 'popcorn' appearance

The first two types were found in granulomas or hamartomas, the third only in granulomas and the fourth in hamartomas. Good considered that the finding of calcification was a very favourable sign that the lesion was benign. He did, however, encounter one case in which a neoplasm engulfed an old Ghon focus, giving an appearance of eccentric calcification (Good and McDonald, 1956). Collins *et al.* (1972) investigated the minimum calcification which can be detected in pulmonary nodules and found that nodules containing 1·0 mg of calcium and measuring 1×2 mm could be visualized on linear tomograms.

Good and his co-workers (Good and Wilson, 1958; Good, 1963) have studied many cases of solitary pulmonary nodule and recommend that all patients with recently discovered uncalcified solitary nodules should have the mass removed and examined microscopically. However, should scrutiny of past radiographs, if available, show that such a nodule has been present for two or more years and has not enlarged during this time, the nodule may be kept under periodic review. At the Mayo Clinic, according to Good, they feel that 'it would be a very unusual cancer that would not grow, albeit slowly, in a period of two years'. He expresses the view that further investigation of such a peripheral nodule, other than by tomography, is unlikely to provide any useful information.

Visibility of small round lesions

The minimum size of rounded shadows detectable on chest radiographs is discussed in Appendix 6.

Spiculation or scalloping

An appearance very suggestive of a peripheral bronchial neoplasm is the sign first described by Wenckebach (1913) as the 'frayed' edge of rapidly growing tumours. This has also been likened to

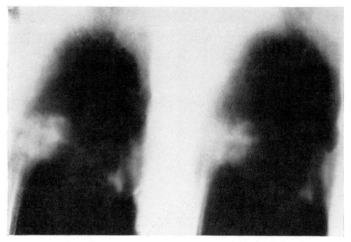

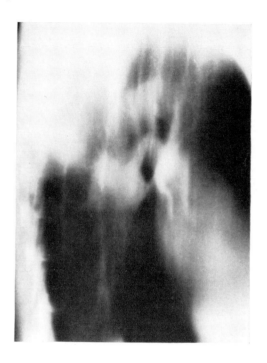

Figure 3.15 (above). Irregular peripheral tumour in right upper lobe with irregular frayed border, shown by conventional tomography. No hilar nodal enlargement demonstrated on inclined frontal tomograms or seen at operation. (Two tomographic cuts)

Figure 3.16 (right). Irregular mass in apex of right lower lobe with spread of tumour to right hilar nodes. The 'frayed' edge to the nodal shadows suggests that the tumour extends into the adjacent lung. (Lateral tomogram)

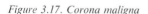

Figure 3.17. Corona maligna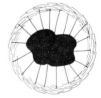

a brush ('brushed border') and somewhat resembles the spines of a hedgehog. It is occasionally seen with tuberculomas and adenomas (*Figures 3.19* and *3.31*), with scars from peripheral pulmonary infarcts, or around the edge of pneumoconiotic fibrous masses (*Figure 3.33*). The lines appear to be due to oedema in the interlobular septa, neoplastic cellular invasions of the surrounding lung tissue, distended lymphatics, tiny bronchi filled with secretions and distended small vessels.

This sign, shown in *Figure 3.17*, has been termed 'radiating line shadows' by Simon (1971) and 'corona maligna' by Nordenström (1969a). According to the latter author, 'this reliable sign of malignancy . . . is characterized by an uneven borderline of the tumour', a zone of surrounding increased

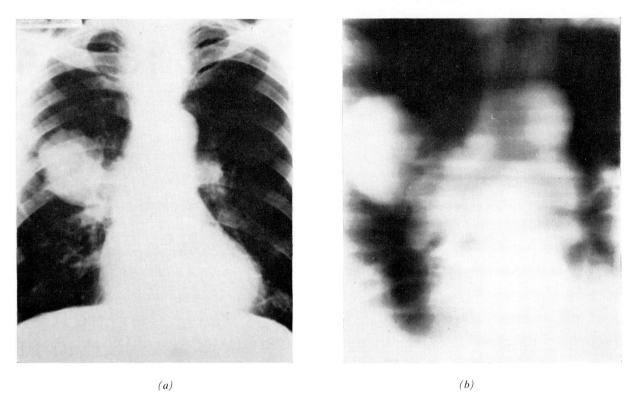

(a)   *(b)*

Figure 3.18. Fairly large bronchial carcinoma showing multiple notches on its upper lateral border. (a) Plain radiograph at conventional kV. (b) Inclined frontal tomogram shows tapering stenosis of anterior segmental bronchus of right upper lobe and marked enlargement of right hilar lymph nodes

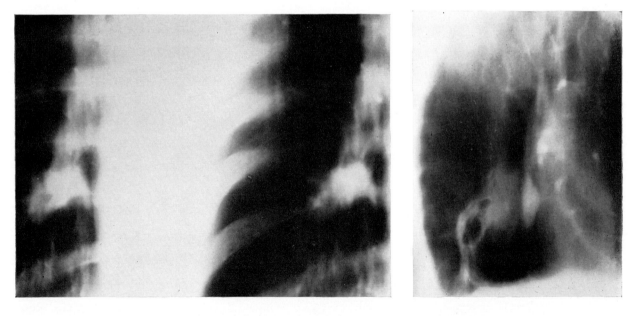

Figure 3.19 (left). Small, irregularly shaped, mainly extrabronchial adenoma in the right lower lobe in a man aged 50 years. (Two tomographic cuts)

Figure 3.20 (right). Moderately large and somewhat lobulated bronchial adenoma with distal bronchiectasis (lateral tomogram). The tumour had been present for 30 years

transradiancy, and beyond this a zone of decreased transradiancy. Through these zones, 'multiple radiating thread-like structures' extend from the tumour into the lung parenchyma, often for a distance of several centimetres.

The zones of increased and decreased transradiancy are not always present around such a mass. An irregular mass with radiating strands is one of the commonest signs of peripheral carcinoma.

Notching or umbilication and radiating vessels

My own experience agrees with that of Drevvatne and Frimann-Dahl (1961) that notching or umbilication may be seen not only with bronchogenic tumours but also with metastases, hamartomas and adenomas. Multiple notchings, on the other hand, seem to me to be most commonly associated with malignancy. The tumour may be primary or occasionally secondary. Examples are shown in *Figures 3.11, 3.18, 3.23* and *3.26*. The umbilication may be associated with radiating vessels or 'apple stalks'. As was noted by Professor Frimann-Dahl (1960—personal communication), vessels may enter and leave the tumour at the point of indentation. The tumour appears to expand outward into the lung parenchyma between these vessels (*see Figure 3.1*). Sometimes notching is seen together with spiculation, but this is more unusual. All these features are best demonstrated by tomography.

Radiating vessels have to be differentiated from pulmonary arterio-venous fistulae, which may produce a rounded 'mass lesion' with vessels passing into and out of it. These fistulae are, however, fairly typical in appearance, sometimes on plain films but more especially on tomograms or pulmonary angiograms (*see Figure 10.4*). The appearances of pulmonary varices are reviewed by Bartram and Strickland (1971).

Peribronchial infiltration

Increased shadowing alongside the bronchi or vessels passing towards a peripheral lung lesion may

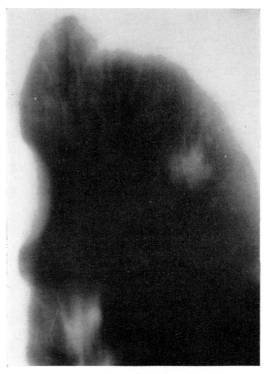

Figure 3.21. Tiny irregular multilobulated tumour in left upper lobe (conventional tomogram)

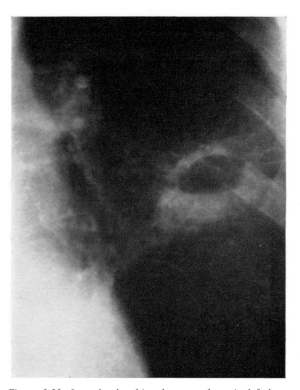

Figure 3.22. Irregular breaking-down neoplasm in left lung with peribronchial and perivenous infiltration spreading towards left hilum

be seen in malignant disease (*Figures 3.22* and *3.25*), but is occasionally also encountered in inflammatory conditions. It may be due either to inflammatory exudate or to distended small vessels or lymphatics.

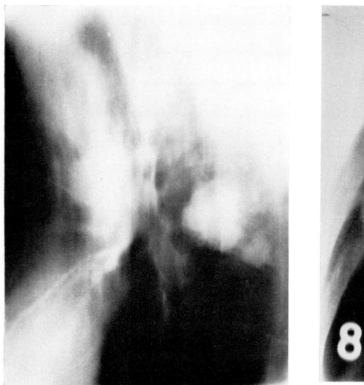 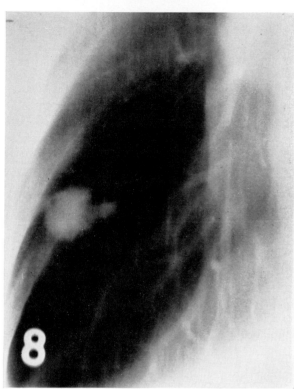

Figure 3.23 (left). Irregular notched mass in apical segment of right lower lobe, with satellite mass, as shown by lateral tomogram. There is some difficulty in determining nodal enlargement as the only visible enlargement lies anteriorly in region of right pulmonary artery; it was shown more clearly by inclined frontal tomograms

Figure 3.24 (right). Small irregular tumour in right upper lobe with small satellite shadow (conventional tomogram)

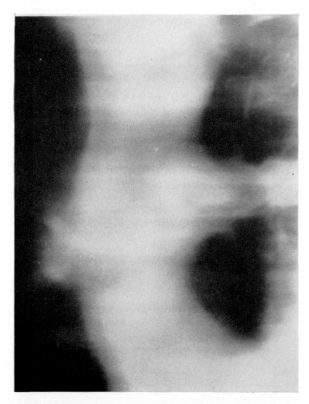 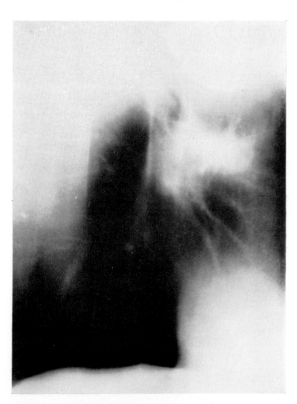

(a)   *(b)*

Figure 3.25. Irregular carcinoma in anterior segment of left upper lobe with 'frayed' edge and tiny satellite shadows (seen in (b)). There is also peribronchial infiltration spreading to the enlarged left hilum. (a) Inclined frontal tomogram. (b) Lateral tomogram

On its own this finding does not determine with certainty the presence of a neoplasm, but it should serve to direct particular attention to the hilum and mediastinum.

Mass with ill-defined edge

An ill-defined edge may be due to local macroscopic spread of the tumour into the surrounding lung, to local venous or lymphatic stasis due to involvement of these channels by the tumour, or to surrounding infection. This last cause is not uncommon even with peripheral tumours and explains the apparent partial regression of some growths following antibiotic chemotherapy. Secondary infection is, as discussed on page 55, much more frequent with central tumours causing bronchial obstruction, and where infection is present in relation to peripheral tumours, some degree of partial obstruction due to enlarged hilar or mediastinal nodes must always be considered.

Satellite sign

Local spread of a tumour into the surrounding lung may be suggested by the presence of small nodules or satellites, probably small tumours developing secondarily to interstitial permeation (*Figures 3.23, 3.24* and *3.36*). These nodules are often hidden by associated congestion or infection.

Galaxy or nebula sign

This is a particularly interesting and important sign caused by local spread of a tumour. Such a

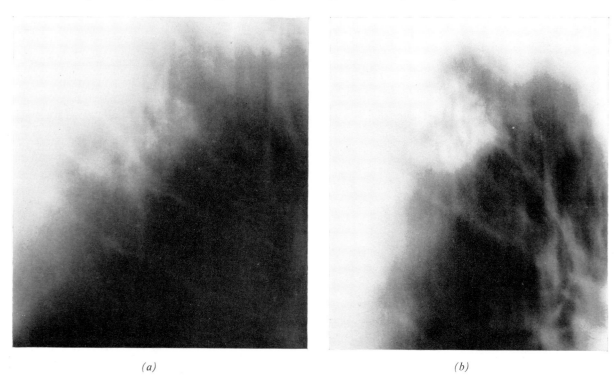

(a) (b)

Figure 3.26. 'Galaxy' or 'nebula' sign of bronchogenic tumour, caused by local diffuse spread and closely mimicking a multifocal tuberculous lesion. Tomograms (a) and (b) were taken with 9 months' interval during which the patient received anti-tuberculous chemotherapy. The true nature of the condition was recognized on tomogram (b). Lobectomy was carried out, and no evidence of spread to hilum or mediastinum was seen. A similar appearance may be given by an alveolar cell carcinoma

soft-looking multifocal lesion may easily be mistaken for pulmonary tuberculosis, as also may satellite nodules, especially when they occur in an upper lobe (*Figure 3.26*).

Carcinomatous consolidation

Local spread may become so dense as to lead to carcinomatous consolidation (*Figure 3.27*). Consolidation may also, of course, be produced by infection complicating a tumour. Ill-defined masses mimicking areas of pulmonary consolidation are sometimes produced by secondary neoplasms, for example in Hodgkin's disease or rarely in myelomatosis.

Mass limited by fissure or pleura

Interlobar fissures often constitute a temporary barrier to the spread of a tumour. Freely moving pleural surfaces appear to be less readily involved or crossed by a tumour than those which are obliterated by adhesions. Such a temporary barrier seems to be present more often in the interlobar fissures, where there is a greater degree of movement, than between the visceral and the parietal pleura. Thus a mass in the lung with an otherwise irregular outline may have an almost straight edge at the pleura, especially at an interlobar fissure (*Figures 3.28* and *3.29*). In contrast with this, an encysted collection

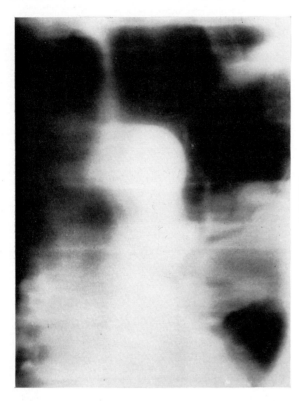

Figure 3.27. Carcinomatous consolidation with patent bronchi passing through a large neoplasm. Note.—Consolidation is more commonly produced by infection distal to a central tumour. This may sometimes be so dense as to give rise to the 'drowned' lung appearance, i.e. a lobe or part of the lung which is consolidated and larger than normal

of fluid in the fissure is typically biconvex in shape. However, a neoplasm of the right middle lobe may have a similar biconvex appearance, and a bronchogram may then be required to differentiate it from an encysted effusion (*see Figure 8.25*).

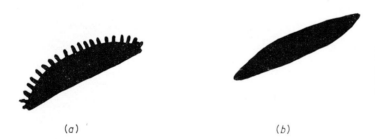

(a)   (b)

Figure 3.28. Diagram to show the difference between most tumours at an interlobar fissure and an encysted effusion. (a) Tumour with an irregular edge in the lung and a straight smooth edge at an interlobar fissure. (b) Biconvex shadow due to encysted fluid in an interlobar fissure

Other findings with pulmonary nodules

Another sign which may be associated with round nodules is a distal linear area of collapse or 'tail' (*Figure 3.31*). Simon (1956) described this as being associated with tuberculomas. I have encountered it more frequently with neoplastic masses, either primary or secondary. Simon (1971) later found that such a line shadow passing towards the pleura, especially in the axilla, was not uncommon with a circular neoplasm.

Bronchography is unlikely to provide useful information regarding small peripheral lesions (*see* Chapter 8). Bronchoscopy may allow the finding of a small endobronchial secondary deposit or an

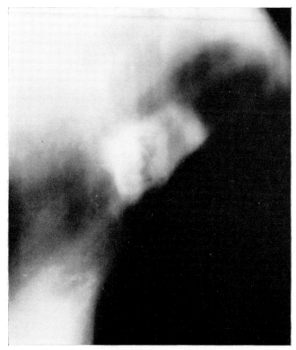

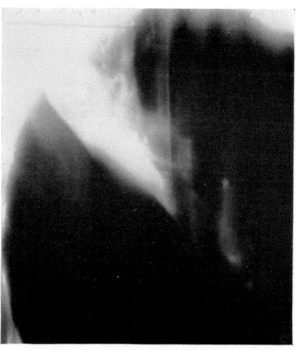

Figure 3.29. Lateral tomogram showing neoplasm with 'frayed' upper border and small central cavity. It has a well-defined lower border at the interlobar fissure

Figure 3.30. Lateral tomogram showing appearance of infective consolidation in a segment adjacent to an interlobar fissure

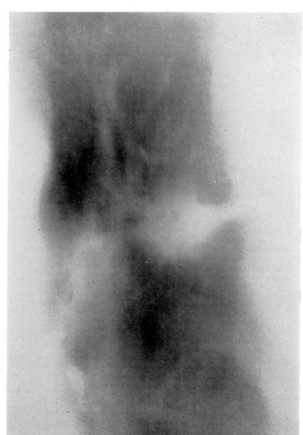

Figure 3.31. A rounded mass with regular or irregular borders may show a linear area of collapse passing towards the periphery of the lung. This is especially seen in an upper lobe, when the collapse passes towards the axilla. It may occur with primary or secondary neoplasm or with tuberculomas

unsuspected second (and endobronchial) tumour. A localized bronchiectasis in association with a small round focus might be expected to indicate previous or long-standing bronchial obstruction. The nodule associated with the segmental bronchiectasis in *Figure 3.39* was, however, a hamartoma. Occasionally tomograms will reveal a completely unsuspected finding in an apparent round focus, as in the case of the old war wound in *Figure 3.34*. Tomography may also demonstrate the irregular shape of an apparently round focus seen on plain radiographs (*see Figure 3.21*).

I have encountered a few cases where peripheral rounded and sometimes notched nodules were due to pulmonary infarction. These nodules were indistinguishable on plain films and tomograms or macroscopically at operation from a peripheral bronchial neoplasm, their true nature being revealed only by histological examination. In one patient the nodule increased to nearly double its original size over a period of fourteen months.

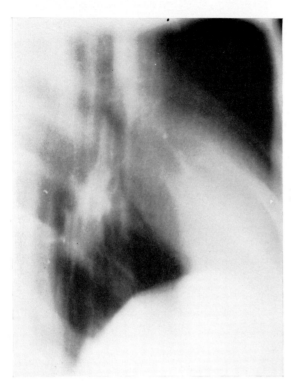

Figure 3.32. Irregular, almost dumb-bell shaped mass—a secondary deposit from an ovarian carcinoma which mimics a primary bronchogenic tumour. (Lateral tomogram)

Metastatic pulmonary lesions always have to be considered in the differential diagnosis of primary lung tumours. The majority of the former are spherical or nearly spherical in shape, but they occasionally have a lobulated or spiculated appearance which, in a solitary tumour, may suggest the presence of a primary bronchial neoplasm. Rarely they may produce a wedge-shaped area of collapse, perhaps as a result of an initial endobronchial metastasis (*see* Chapter 9). Cavitation is uncommon, as discussed below (*see* page 36).

Other multiple rounded lung shadows may be due to infected emboli (especially in patients with artificial kidneys and shunt problems), granulomatous infiltrations, collagen diseases, pneumoconiosis, or fibrotic nodules associated with retroperitoneal fibrosis. Rarely, multiple pulmonary nodules may be multiple benign tumours as shown in *Figure 3.118*. Occasionally a lung mass may contain unusual or foreign material such as the portion of rib seen in *Figure 3.34*.

Very large round or lobulated mass

Primary bronchogenic tumours may become very large, sometimes being 10 cm or more in diameter, and may have a completely smooth spherical outline. I have seen this appearance mainly in squamous cell tumours, but occasionally also in tumours of other cell types. Some of the patients were completely free from any evidence of metastasis either radiologically or at operation, and in my opinion

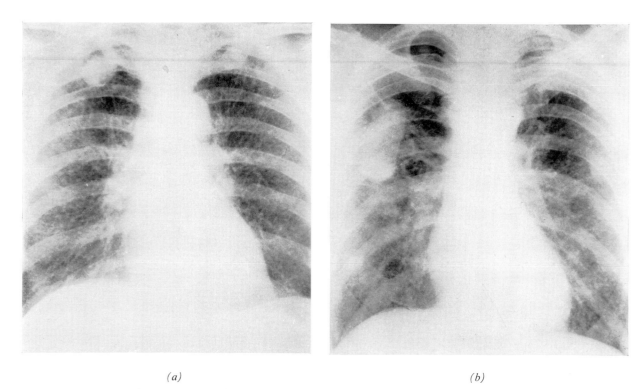

(a)   (b)

Figure 3.33. Patients with pneumoconiosis. (a) Small spherical mass at right apex, unchanged for 5 years. Patient also had multiple small nodules in both lungs, as well as rheumatoid nodules over some of his larger joints. (b) Oval mass in right upper lobe due to progressive massive fibrosis. Patient also had bullae in right upper lobe. These illustrations show the fine spiculation or radiating strands (a) and the coarser type (b) which may be seen on the borders of pneumoconiotic nodules and of some peripheral neoplasms

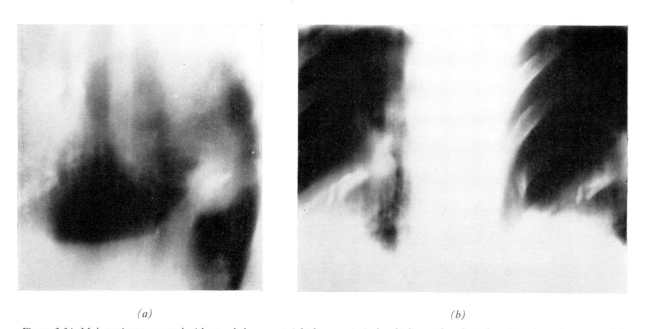

(a)   (b)

Figure 3.34. Male patient presented with rounded mass at right base posteriorly which was thought to be a bronchogenic tumour. (a) Lateral and (b) A.P. tomograms showed that it contained a bone fragment and that there was a defect in a rib (arrowed). When further questioned, the patient remembered an old war wound. He had small scars on his chest suggesting entry and exit points of a bullet

31

size alone is no bar to surgery. When the mass is very large and smooth-walled, the differential diagnosis is between carcinoma, bronchogenic cyst, hydatid cyst, hamartoma and adenoma. Large tumours with irregular outer walls not infrequently have distant metastases at the time of diagnosis (*see Figure 3.39*).

Bateson (1964), in a publication based on his M.D. thesis, analysed 100 cases of circumscribed bronchogenic carcinoma. One of the points he made was that the prognosis was better for well-defined lesions and worse for those with ill-defined borders. [For the rest of his findings, *see* Appendix 4(3).]

Rarely, a rounded lung opacity may be due to a pulmonary gumma. I have seen only one of these, and this disappeared rapidly on treatment with potassium iodide. Dziadiw, Kinkhabwala and Rabinowitz (1972) reported a single case. Gummas may also give a fibrotic or pneumonic pattern or hilar lymphadenopathy.

Cavitation of a lung tumour

Any peripheral bronchogenic tumour may outgrow its blood supply and have a necrotic centre (*Figures 3.22, 3.36, 3.37, 3.39, 3.40, 3.43, 3.53* and *3.65*). This is most typically seen with squamous cell tumours, which, when they break down, often have thick walls with irregular inner borders. However, it may also occur with the other cellular types. The cavity is frequently eccentric in position (*see*

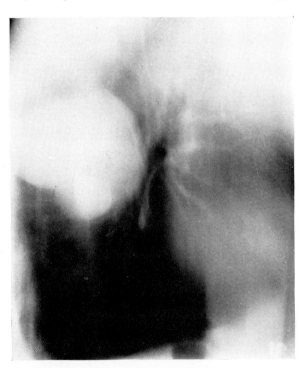

Figure 3.35. Large lobulated and notched bronchogenic tumour in the apex of the right lower lobe. Bronchogenic tumours may also present as much larger masses and, if well demarcated, may be confused with fluid-filled cysts or benign lesions

Figure 3.28), and such a position of a cavity is very suggestive of neoplasm. With a large cavitating mass, the outer border may be either smooth or irregular. The large cavitating mass with a smooth outer wall may, like its solid counterpart, be present without any evidence of distant metastases (*see Figure 3.48*).

In discussing the differential diagnosis of cavitation within a peripheral lung tumour, one has to consider other causes of lung breakdown, cavitation and cystic lesions which partially fill with air. A lung abscess or abscesses may result from infection distal to a bronchial occlusion caused for instance by a central endobronchial neoplasm, by an inhaled foreign body, or by pressure on a bronchus by enlarged nodes; it may be secondary to tuberculosis, neoplasm, etc.; or it may be due to infections which produce necrosis, such as pulmonary tuberculosis, staphylococcal pneumonia, Friedlander's (Klebsiella) pneumonia and certain fungus infections. With acute pneumonic processes there is usually adjacent pneumonic consolidation (*see Figure 3.41*). This may be present with a peripheral lung tumour, and can also be produced by local spread of tumour into the adjacent lung. A frequent problem arises in the differentiation from pulmonary tuberculosis or tuberculous scarring (*see* section on general observations, page 55). Occasionally a lung tumour, especially one that is cavitating, may present with or be complicated by a spontaneous pneumothorax (Heimlich and Rubin, 1955; Wright, 1973b).

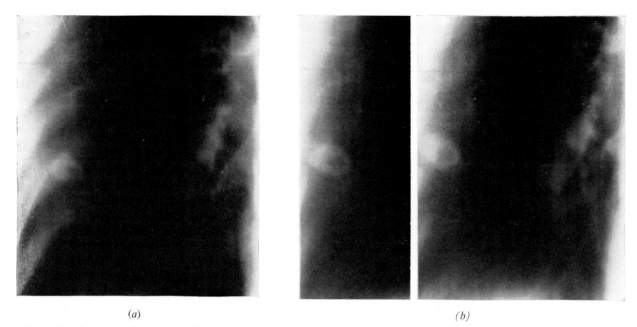

(a)   (b)

Figure 3.36. Conventional tomograms showing a small peripheral nodule with an eccentric cavity which had been diagnosed as pulmonary tuberculosis. Despite chemotherapy it was much larger 9 months later, and a neoplasm was suspected as a result of the second tomographic examination. This was confirmed at operation

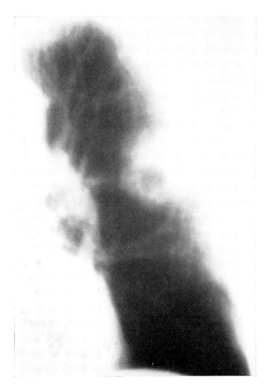

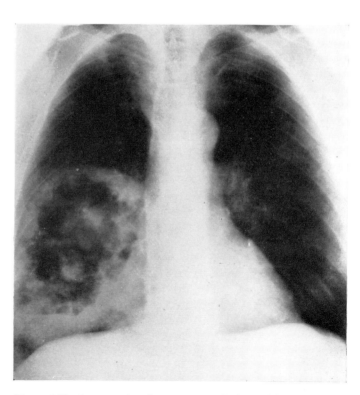

Figure 3.37. Conventional tomogram showing peripheral neoplasm with poorly defined edge and an eccentric cavity

Figure 3.38. Large cavitated tumour in right lower lobe with grossly irregular and 'knobbly' inner wall. A fluid level is present at the base of the cavity

Fungus and other chronic infections

Fungus infections producing cavitation are uncommon in Great Britain but occasionally occur. They are more common in North America—for example nocardiosis, coccidiodomycosis and blasto-mycosis. The radiological manifestations of nocardiosis were recently reviewed by Grossman, Bragg and Armstrong (1970). Pulmonary cryptococcosis mimicking carcinoma of the lung has been reported by Meighan (1972). Two cases of torulosis (cryptococcosis), complicating malignant disease and poly-cythaemia, were seen in the United Oxford Hospitals during this period. Actinomycosis of the lungs has not been seen at the Churchill Hospital in the past fifteen years. Cases occurred before this time, one with a basal cavitating pneumonia and pleurisy and with fistulae passing to the skin surface, and one with fistulae over the upper chest and neck and diffuse honeycombed cavities of the upper lobes resem-

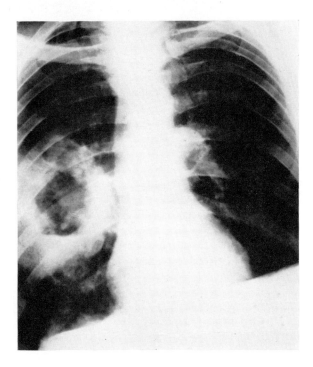

Figure 3.39. Large cavitated tumour in right lower lobe with grossly irregular inner and outer borders. Pulmonary and rib metastases are also present

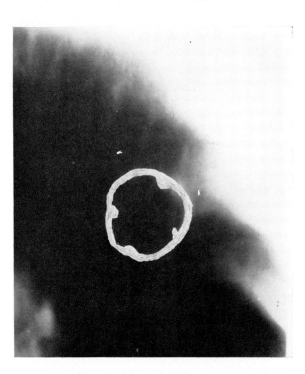

Figure 3.40. Thin-walled cavity in left upper lobe, somewhat lobulated in outline and with irregular inner walls. Squamous cell carcinoma. It has almost a 'shamrock leaf' appearance. (Retouched figure)

bling pulmonary tuberculosis. A recent review of 15 cases of thoracic actinomycosis by Flynn and Felson (1970) showed that whilst the radiological features of the disease are mostly non-specific, the extension of a pulmonary lesion through the chest wall, sometimes with wavy periostitis or rib destruc-tion, vertebral destruction or the crossing of an interlobar fissure, might suggest the diagnosis.*

The most frequent fungus infection is aspergillosis, which may complicate any pre-existing lung dis-ease. An area of lung damaged, for example, by tuberculosis, sarcoidosis, previous pneumonia causing scarring, bronchiectasis or emphysematous cysts, may have become infected with the fungus and thick-walled cavities may be produced. The most characteristic late appearance is of a mycetoma lying free within the cavity (*Figures 3.44 and 3.45*), which is best demonstrated by tomography. The fungus ball may be shown to change its position in response to gravity by radiographing the patient in the erect, supine, head down and lateral decubitus positions. Occasionally a mycetoma may develop within a slowly growing and cavitated squamous carcinoma (*Figure 3.43*). Aspergillosis in residual tuberculous cavities and histoplasmosis in Great Britain have been studied by Davies (1970) and Macleod *et al.* (1972) respectively.

* I have, however, seen similar rib destruction and sinuses caused by tuberculous abscesses of the chest wall secondary to under-lying chronic pulmonary tuberculosis.

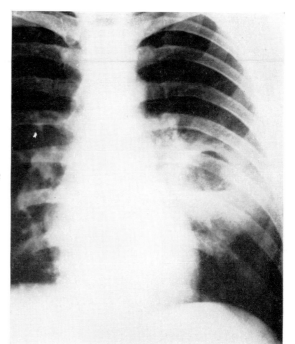

Figure 3.41. Lung abscess. Note surrounding pneumonic consolidation

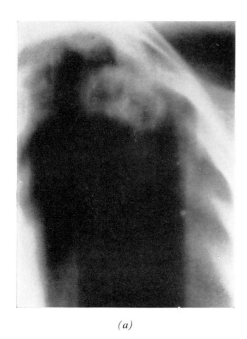

(a)

Figure 3.42. Tuberculous cavities which might be mistaken for neoplasm

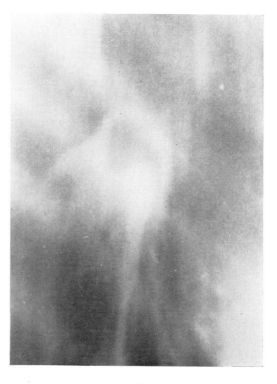

(b)

Rheumatoid or necrobiotic nodules

Cavitation may also be seen in rheumatoid nodules. These lesions tend to appear, cavitate, and then disappear leaving a small scar in the lung. One or more may be present at a time (*Figure 3.46*).

Secondary deposits

Secondary deposits occasionally cavitate, especially deposits that are rapidly growing and reach a large size such as those from soft tissue sarcomas, embryonic tumours or teratomas, but this phenomenon is fairly uncommon and seldom enters into the differential diagnosis. Cavitating deposits sometimes give rise to a severe or recurrent pneumothorax.

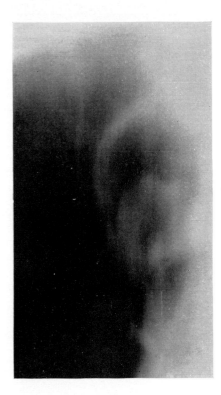

Figure 3.43. Thick-walled cavitating tumour containing a mass which was mobile and was presumably a mycetoma. The patient also had collapse of the left lower lobe due to a second bronchial neoplasm

Hydatid cysts

A hydatid cyst has a double wall, the outer layer being formed by the host and the inner layer by the parasite. Sometimes the cyst ruptures into a bronchus, so that air may pass between the two layers and give rise to a 'halo' appearance (*Figure 3.47*), or the inner layer may collapse to give a 'water lily' appearance with the cyst and daughter cysts floating in the fluid. For a review of the radiological appearances of hydatid cysts, *see* Xanthakis *et al.* (1972).

Sequestrated lung segments

Occasionally a sequestrated lung segment which has no direct connection with the bronchi and which becomes aerated by collateral air drift from adjacent lung segments in the manner first described by Van Allen, Lindskog and Richter (1930—*see also* Reich and Abouav, 1965) may be confused with a lung tumour. Part of the sequestrated segment may be relatively airless and part overdistended, appearing as a bulla or cavity within the segment and mimicking an area of breakdown or consolidation. A bronchogram shows no bronchus passing to the segment in question—*see Figure 10.9*, which also illustrates the use of aortography to demonstrate the abnormal systemic vessel supplying the sequestrated lung segment.

Carcinoma of the lung and thin-walled cysts

A thin-walled cavity (*Figure 3.40*), typically due to a cavitating squamous cell bronchogenic tumour,

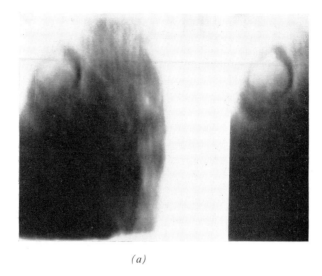

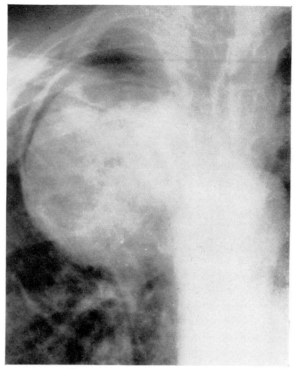

(a)

Figure 3.44. Cavities containing mycetomas (aspergillomas). One of these (b) is very large

(b)

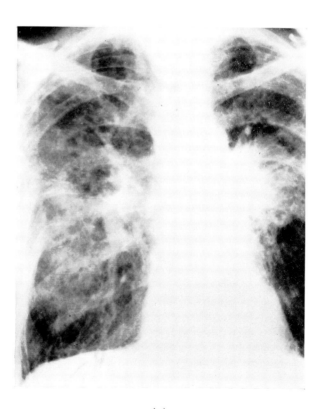

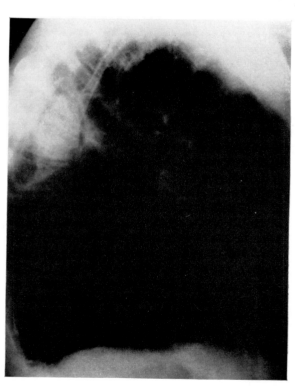

(a)

(b)

Figure 3.45. Mycetoma in apex of left lower lobe. The patient also had squamous carcinoma cells in his sputum, and the right sixth and seventh ribs were eroded posteriorly. He had no chest wall pain

37

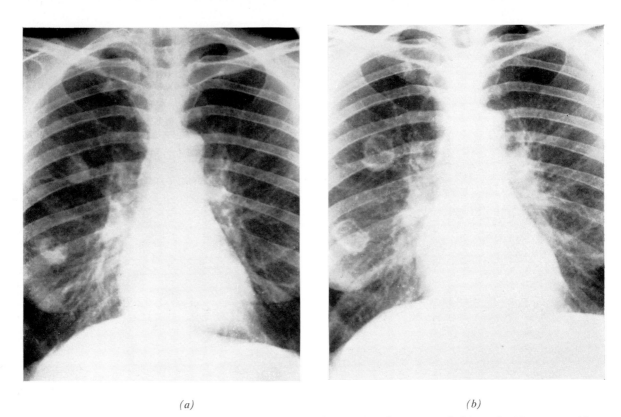

(a) *(b)*

Figure 3.46. Cavitating rheumatoid nodules. The cavitating granulomas enlarged over a period of 6 months. More appeared later and the patient was left with considerable pulmonary fibrosis. (For nodal enlargement due to rheumatoid granulomas, see Figure 7.37)

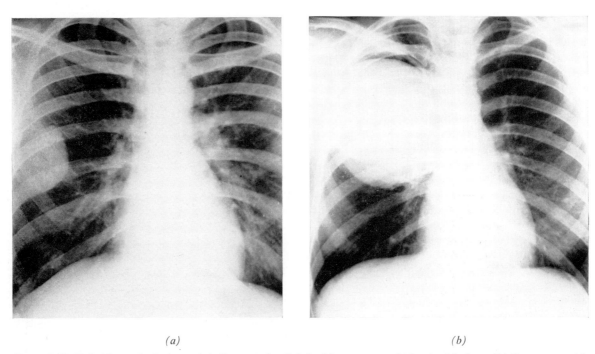

(a) *(b)*

Figure 3.47. Hydatid cysts in the lungs. (a) Almost oval well-defined homogeneous shadow in right lung. (b) Larger cyst with air between the two layers of the capsule producing the 'halo' sign. Note.—A 'water lily' sign may be produced if the inner (i.e. parasitic) wall ruptures, when air may enter the cyst. Daughter cysts may then be seen floating on the fluid in the cyst

may mimic a pneumatocoele or an emphysematous cyst. Møller (1950) and Grainger and Pierce (1969) published illustrations of very thin-walled lesions which might have passed as cysts. Peabody, Rupnik and Hanner (1957) described a thin-walled 'cyst' in the right lower lobe which increased in size, its wall becoming progressively thinner. After resection, though macroscopically benign, it proved to be an epidermoid (squamous cell) carcinoma. The tumour shown in *Figure 3.48* was also thought to be a benign cyst at operation, but the pre-operative radiological diagnosis of neoplasm was confirmed by the pathologist. Neither the 'cyst' described by Peabody and his colleagues nor those illustrated in *Figures 3.40* and *3.48* need really be confused with benign cysts, since in both instances the walls of the

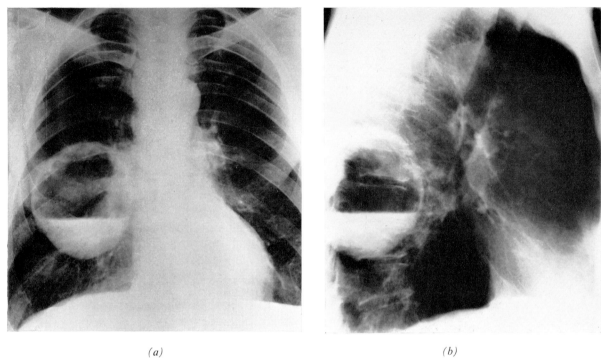

(a)   (b)

Figure 3.48. Carcinoma of bronchus (squamous cell). Large breaking-down tumour in apex of right lower lobe. This cavity has a relatively thin wall with a smooth outer edge and an irregular inner border. It contains a fluid level. No spread of tumour was found at operation

'cysts' were 2–3 mm thick. In addition, they had an irregular inner border, and one (*see Figure 3.40*) had a lobulated outer border. Simon (1971) also shows two bronchial neoplasms producing thin-walled cavitating masses.

Another example of the association of neoplastic disease with cavity formation is the occasional coexistence of carcinoma with a lung cyst (Lodge, 1960). Farinas *et al.* (1955) noted this finding in 4 out of 133 patients. Others have observed the development of a tumour in patients with lung cysts. Larkin and Phillips (1955) reviewed the literature concerning the association of cysts with neoplasm, and reported one case of a tumour within a cyst which enlarged over a period of two years. Peabody, Katz and Davis (1957) observed a cyst over a period of 33 months and watched a nodule in its lumen increase in size until it reached a diameter of 5·5 cm, at which stage it was removed and shown to be an undifferentiated carcinoma within a long-standing cyst. West and Van Schoonhoven (1957) described the chance finding of a carcinoma in the wall of a lung cyst which had been present for 16 years in a woman aged 34 years.

Position of tumours in the lungs

Schinz *et al.* (1953) stated that bronchial or hilar carcinoma was most common in the upper lobes. Kerley (1954) pointed out that tuberculomas are seldom seen in the anterior parts of the lungs or in the basic segments of the lower lobes, whereas a tumour may originate anywhere in the lungs. Garland *et al.* (1962) found not only that peripheral tumours were twice as common as those arising centrally,

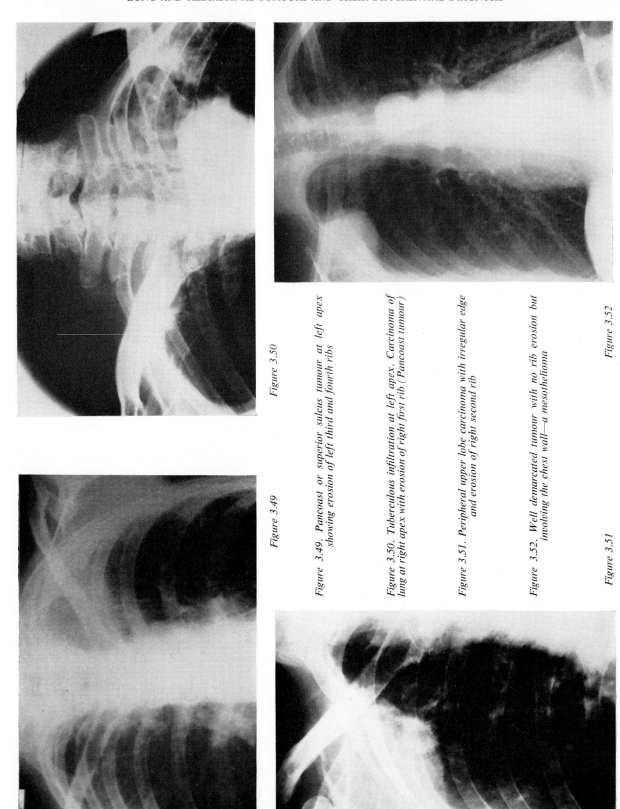

Figure 3.50

Figure 3.49

Figure 3.49. Pancoast or superior sulcus tumour at left apex showing erosion of left third and fourth ribs

Figure 3.50. Tuberculous infiltration at left apex. Carcinoma of lung at right apex with erosion of right first rib (Pancoast tumour)

Figure 3.51. Peripheral upper lobe carcinoma with irregular edge and erosion of right second rib

Figure 3.52. Well demarcated tumour with no rib erosion but involving the chest wall—a mesothelioma

Figure 3.52

Figure 3.51

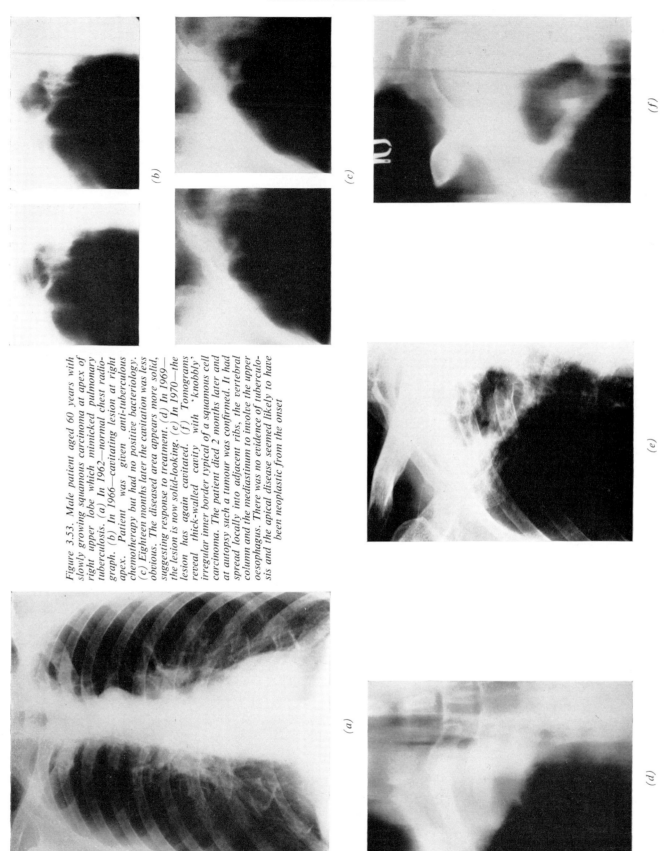

Figure 3.53. Male patient aged 60 years with slowly growing squamous carcinoma at apex of right upper lobe which mimicked pulmonary tuberculosis. (a) In 1962—normal chest radiograph. (b) In 1966—cavitating lesion at right apex. Patient was given anti-tuberculous chemotherapy but had no positive bacteriology. (c) Eighteen months later the cavitation was less obvious. The diseased area appears more solid, suggesting response to treatment. (d) In 1969— the lesion is now solid-looking. (e) In 1970—the lesion has again cavitated. (f) Tomograms reveal thick-walled cavity with 'knobbly' irregular inner border typical of a squamous cell carcinoma. The patient died 2 months later and at autopsy such a tumour was confirmed. It had spread locally into adjacent ribs, the vertebral column and the mediastinum to involve the upper oesophagus. There was no evidence of tuberculosis and the apical disease seemed likely to have been neoplastic from the onset

but that in the group of peripheral tumours in the upper lobes there was a preponderance of tumours originating in the apical and posterior segments. Others have held that the right middle lobe is virtually immune from the disease and have maintained that a lesion in this site is almost certainly not a carcinoma. My own view is that all segments of both lungs are subject to the development of lung tumours, and that the frequency with which tumours arise in any segment is roughly proportional to its volume and its bronchial surface. (An excellent paper describing middle lobe tumours is by Locke, 1953–54.)

The incidence of tumours in the various segments of the lung in 400 consecutive cases of bronchial carcinoma is shown in Appendix 4.

Pleural and chest wall involvement

Once the pleura has become involved, a pleural effusion is likely to develop, especially if there is venous or lymphatic obstruction in the underlying lung. Occasionally a '*dry*' *pleurisy* may occur (*see Figure 3.88*), or *transpleural spread* of tumour may take place with the formation of tumour plaques at places remote from the primary site of invasion. A '*knobbly pleura*' is always suggestive of malignancy, which may be secondary to a peripheral bronchial tumour, a mesothelioma, a myeloma or a secondary tumour from a distant site (*see Figures 3.89* and *3.122*).

Pleural effusions are not always due to the tumour *per se*. Many result from the secondary infection that develops especially with centrally arising tumours, which cause bronchial obstruction.

If the pleura has become obliterated or adherent, tumours may cross it without causing any significant pleural reaction and invade an adjacent lobe, the chest wall or the mediastinum. In the adjacent lung the appearance may be that of a solid tumour, of lymphatic spread or of interstitial spread with the formation of small 'miliary' satellite shadows, or the picture may be complicated by infection.

When the chest wall is involved, the patient often experiences severe pain. However, this is by no means invariable, and some patients with gross rib erosion seem to have had little or no pain (*see Figure 3.45*). Radiologically, one has to rely on the demonstration of bone erosion to diagnose chest wall invasion, though this is not always present and some tumours will infiltrate the muscle and other tissues of the chest wall without causing any bone erosion (*Figure 3.52*). When present, such erosion is best shown by means of a Bucky diaphragm. Tomography, sometimes used for this purpose, suffers from the disadvantage that the ribs curve around the chest wall and only a small portion of any one rib will be seen in each tomographic cut. Where the rib passes out of the plane of sharpness, it can no longer be seen clearly and a false impression of erosion may be given. On the other hand, where erosion is present it may be mistaken for the normal loss of definition associated with the curvature of the rib. Rarely a bronchogenic tumour involving the chest wall will cause bone sclerosis instead of bone erosion; I have myself seen this only once.

The *Pancoast* or *superior sulcus tumour* is essentially a peripheral lung tumour which has spread into the chest wall (*Figures 3.49–3.53*). One presumes that as adhesions are common at the lung apex and as pleural movement during respiration is minimal at this site, spread of tumour across the apical pleura can occur here more easily than in other places unless adhesions are present. The real problem lies in the differentiation from tuberculosis (*Figures 3.50* and *3.53*).

Direct spinal column involvement, unless gross, is often difficult to demonstrate. Localized views or tomograms, particularly in the antero-posterior projection, may show erosion of the lateral border of a vertebral body, of a transverse process or of the neck of a rib. Occasionally local spread will give rise to spinal cord compression and paraplegia.

The demonstration of chest wall involvement usually implies a poor prognosis, but I have encountered a few patients who have shown a very good response to radiotherapy, with recalcification of the eroded bone and long survival. In one case, recovery from paraparesis following laminectomy and radiotherapy lasted eight months (*see Figure 10.16*).

CENTRAL BRONCHIAL TUMOURS

Rigler (1957b) and Walter and Pryce (1955) pointed out that the symptoms of central bronchial tumours may commence earlier than those of peripheral tumours. Unfortunately, by the time most central tumours present clinically they are unresectable and have spread into the mediastinum. If lesions are to be discovered at a resectable stage, it is important that the effects of a central lesion should be fully understood, so that radiographic changes can be correctly interpreted at the earliest possible time and suspicion of neoplasm aroused in order that other investigations—including tomography, bronchography, bronchoscopy and sputum examination—may be instituted.

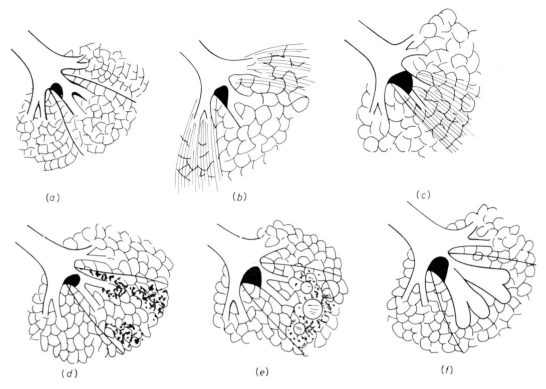

Figure 3.54. Effect of central tumours on the underlying lung. (a) No effect. (b) Obstructive emphysema (lung in expiration). (c) Collapse. (d) Pneumonia. (e) Abscess formation. (f) Mucocoeles and bronchiectasis. (Expanded from Sherman and Phillips, 1968, by courtesy of C. V. Mosby Co.) Note also that if a collapsed lobe or lung re-expands, an appearance resembling honeycomb lung may be seen (see Figure 3.69)

The early radiological presentation of a central tumour depends on the effects of partial or complete bronchial obstruction as shown in *Figure 3.54*. Central tumours are often undiagnosed for the following reasons.

(1) The obstruction has not become sufficient to cause secondary phenomena.
(2) Obstructive emphysema is not demonstrated.
(3) The partial collapse of a segment, lobe or lung is not recognized.
(4) A 'mass' lesion is unrecognized or invisible within the mediastinum or the hilar regions.

All too frequently little attention is paid to the central air passages, the trachea, the carina and the larger bronchi. As was mentioned in Chapter 1, it is unfortunate that although many patients do not have their first radiograph until the disease is far advanced, the condition often remains undiagnosed because the effects of bronchostenosis are unrecognized.

Probably the most important clinical indication of a central tumour is a wheeze over one area of the bronchial tree, noticed by the patient or heard with the stethoscope. Wheezes due to obstruction or partial obstruction of the trachea or the main bronchi may be relatively early signs of tumours developing in these air passages, but are more often late phenomena due to compression of these structures by grossly enlarged mediastinal nodes or to severe stenosis. Other early clinical signs and symptoms depend upon the development of secondary infection, with pneumonia or the expectoration of mucopurulent sputum. Frank haemoptysis is often a late symptom, but slight bloodstaining of the sputum may occur relatively early. Occasionally a slight pleurisy produced by the effects of the secondary infection may give an early presentation.

The various effects of central lesions are summarized in Table 3.1.

TABLE 3.1
Central Lesions

Obstructive emphysema
Collapse
Mucocoeles of bronchi
Infection: Pneumonia
        Abscess
        Pleurisy and effusion
        Reactivation of tuberculosis
Hilar or mediastinal mass or nodes (crossed lymphatic drainage,
   particularly from left lower lobe and right middle lobe)
Pulmonary artery invasion or thrombosis
Obstruction: Venous
          Lymphatic
Pleural involvement or effusion
Pericardial involvement or effusion
Nerve palsy: Recurrent laryngeal
          Phrenic

Obstructive emphysema

Now that it has ceased to be a routine matter to 'screen the chest' by fluoroscopy in the investigation, detection or exclusion of chest disease, obstructive emphysema and associated abnormal

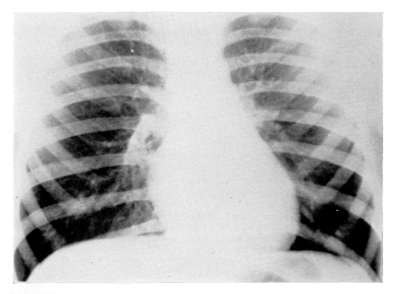

(a)

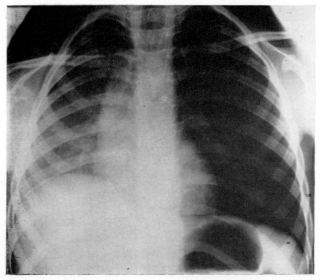

(b)

Figure 3.55. Obstructive emphysema of the left lung due to an inhaled foreign body (apple core). (a) The radiograph taken in inspiration appears normal. (b) In expiration the obstructed lung cannot deflate

mediastinal movements are rarely recognized. This is to be regretted because such phenomena often accompany resectable tumours. Obstructive emphysema is now looked for mainly in young children who may have inhaled a foreign body, by taking a radiograph in expiration as well as inspiration (*Figure 3.55*). It should be noted that the full inspiration film is usually normal.

The reasons for the neglect of this sign are the attention which has been given to maximum inspiration for almost all chest radiographs (except, for instance, where a pneumothorax might be expected); the decline in the use of chest fluoroscopy over the past 15–20 years, largely in the interests of reducing the radiation dosage to the patient; and the awareness that a radiograph provides a much better record of disease processes than a visual memory, particularly in the follow-up of chest diseases.

Where obstructive emphysema affects a main bronchus, the whole of one lung will remain distended in expiration, and the chest wall and diaphragm on the affected side will have a greatly reduced range

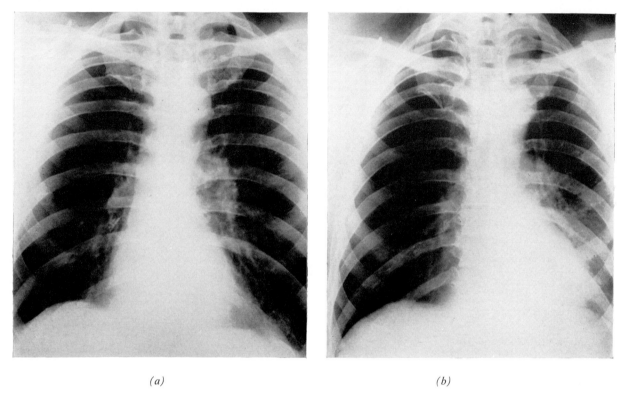

(a)   *(b)*

Figure 3.56. Obstructive emphysema of right lung due to endobronchial tumour of right main bronchus. Radiographs taken (a) in inspiration, (b) in expiration. Due to endobronchial obstruction and narrowing of bronchi in expiration, the lung distal to the obstruction cannot deflate in expiration to the normal extent. Also, the mediastinum is displaced towards the normal side in expiration

of movement. Lesser degrees of obstructive emphysema may be demonstrated in a lobe or segment. If a patient presents with blood-staining of the sputum and an audible wheeze, an expiration film should always be taken in addition to inspiration views, or a brief fluoroscopy (especially with image amplification) should be undertaken. Examples of obstructive emphysema secondary to endobronchial neoplasm are shown in *Figures 3.56 and 3.85*. The value of expiration views has also been stressed by Korol and Scott (1934), Morlock (1934), Rigler and Kelby (1947), Møller (1950) and Sherman and Phillips (1968).

Holzknecht (1899, four years after Roentgen's discovery of x-rays) described how the mediastinum moves during respiration when there is a bronchial obstruction. He found an inspiratory retraction of the mediastinum and heart into the affected side of the chest in a patient with a simple stenosis of the right main bronchus. This phenomenon was termed mediastinal jerking by Lenk (1954). Kassay (1960) further analysed mediastinal movement seen by fluoroscopy and found that in some cases valvular emphysema occurs on both sides at the same time, the mediastinum then moving during inspiration towards the side on which the greater part of the lung is affected (*Figure 3.57*).

Kassay also pointed out that the paradoxical movement of the diaphragm seen with a phrenic palsy may be differentiated from that due to obstructive emphysema or pneumothorax by observing the movement of the mediastinum during inspiration. In valvular emphysema and pneumothorax the movement is towards the abnormal side, whilst with a phrenic paralysis the mediastinum shifts towards the normal side.

Collapse

Complete collapse

Complete collapse of a segment, lobe or lung gives rise to a shadow of increased density on chest radiographs, corresponding to the anatomical distribution of the collapsed portion of the lung. The

Expiration   Inspiration

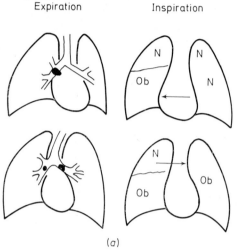

(a)

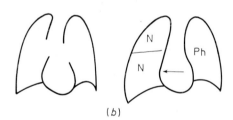

(b)

Figure 3.57. Diagram explaining the Holzknecht sign and mediastinal movements in obstructive emphysema and phrenic palsy. N=normal; Ob=obstructed lung; Ph=side of phrenic palsy. With obstructive emphysema or pneumothorax (a), the mediastinum moves towards the abnormal side in inspiration, whereas with a phrenic palsy (b) it moves towards the normal side. [(a) is after Kassay, 1960, by courtesy of McGraw-Hill Book Co., New York.] Note.—In expiration the diameter of the trachea and bronchi is less, so that an obstruction produced by an endobronchial mass is accentuated. Although Holzknecht described the movement of the mediastinum in inspiration, it is more correct to think of the mediastinal movement towards the normal side in expiration as being caused by the failure of the lung to deflate properly

patterns of lobar collapse are shown diagrammatically in *Figure 3.58* together with some notes about the pattern of collapse in each of the lobes. A summary of the signs of lung collapse is given on page 50, and radiographic illustrations of lobar collapse are shown in *Figures 3.59–3.61*. Lobar collapse in the absence of a pneumothorax or pleural effusion always causes compensatory changes in the chest secondary to the loss of lung volume, namely compensatory emphysema of the remainder of the lung, crowding of the ribs, mediastinal movement and herniation of the contralateral lung, and raising of the homolateral hemidiaphragm.

The patterns of such lobar collapse have been studied by various authors including Robbins and Hale (1945a–g), Lubert and Krause (1951, 1956, 1958, 1963), Felson (1960) and Simon (1950, 1956, 1971). Lodin (1957) studied the herniation of the mediastinum and the contralateral lung by transverse axial tomography.

Partial collapse

Partial collapse is much more difficult to visualize on radiographs and is *frequently unrecognized even when gross*. This is because partial collapse without consolidation does not itself produce an area of increased density on the radiograph. It gives rise to only secondary signs such as crowding of the ribs over the affected area, displacement of a fissure, elevation of one side (or even part of one side) of the diaphragm, movement of the mediastinum towards the affected side (sometimes with herniation of the

(a) *Usually gives well-defined shadow as illustrated, but occasionally shadow may overlie mediastinum*

Right upper lobe

(b) *Often there is a transradiant zone behind the sternum due to herniation of right lung. Shadow of collapsed left upper lobe may not be very well defined in the P.A. view. Lower lobe artery is often elevated, giving a prominent hilar shadow. Notes.—(1) A chronically collapsed upper lobe may collapse against the mediastinum—see Figure 7.19. (2) Collapse of the lingula often obliterates the shadow of the adjacent left cardiac border*

Left upper lobe

(c) *The collapsed middle lobe may not be very obvious in a P.A. view. The old-fashioned 'lordotic' view will often demonstrate it, but for exclusion of disease, P.A. and lateral views are superior*

Right middle lobe

(d) *Shadow of collapsed left lower lobe is often hidden behind heart shadow and may be visible only on penetrated or high kV views*

Right lower lobe   Left lower lobe

(e) *In lateral view, collapsed lower lobe may lie posteriorly or against the mediastinum. Where it reaches the diaphragm, this segment of the latter may be ill-defined*

Right (or left) lower lobe

(f) *Similar appearance in lateral view to left upper lobe collapse, with usually fairly obvious anterior mediastinal herniation. Due to multiple causes as there is no common bronchus. (For discussion of the problem of right upper and middle lobe collapse, see Le Roux, 1971)*

Right upper plus right middle lobe

(g) *This may mimic a raised right side of the diaphragm or a sub-pulmonary or infra-pulmonary effusion. It is a not uncommon appearance as tumours often block the intermediate bronchus*

Right middle plus right lower lobe

(h) *When a pneumothorax is present, the compensatory mechanisms for filling the space of the collapsed lobe or lung no longer operate. The lobes retract towards the hilum and become replicas of their normal inflated shapes*

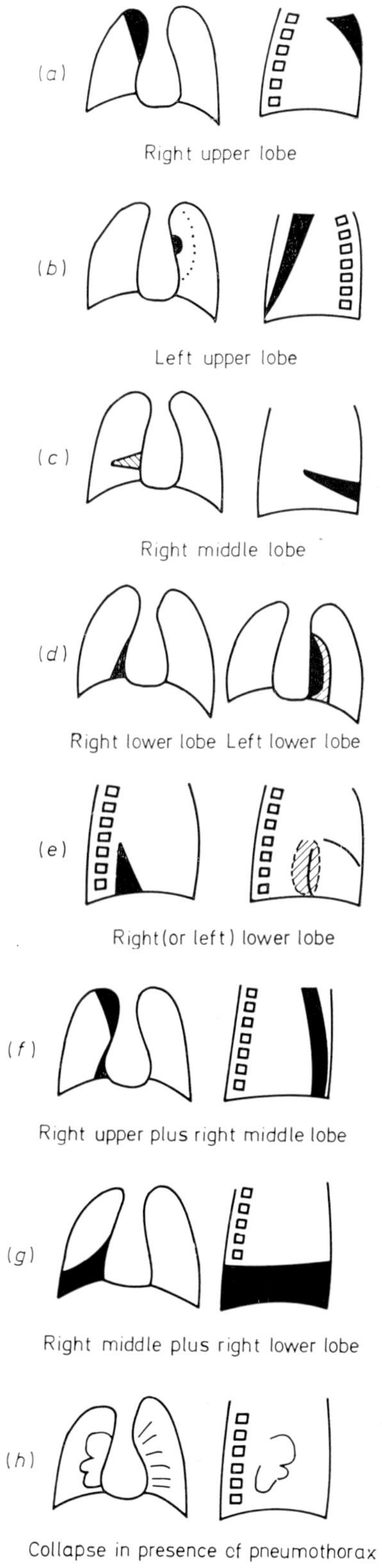

Collapse in presence of pneumothorax

Figure 3.58. (a–e) Patterns of single lobar collapse. (f–h) Patterns of complicated lobar collapse

contralateral lung), or compensatory emphysema of the remainder of the lung (*Figures 3.59–3.61*). The collapse may also be inferred from a crowding of the vascular markings in a lobe or segment or from a lack of the particular segmental or lobar vascular shadows in the lung. On fluoroscopy the affected area is recognizable because it does not inflate normally.

It is always important, when viewing a chest radiograph, to study the vascular anatomy. Crowding of the vessels may give an indication of collapse, whilst a greater than normal separation may be evidence of emphysema in that part of the lung. As stated by Cranz and Pribram (1965), the pulmonary

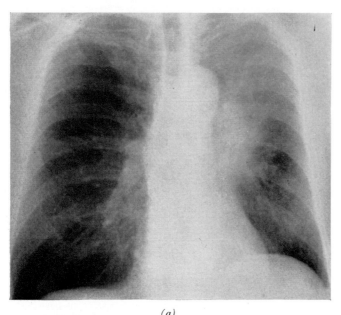

(a)

Figure 3.59. Collapsed left upper lobe. Note apparent enlargement of left hilum and triangular opacity situated retrosternally. Note also reduced volume of left lung and crowding of left upper ribs. In this example the 'tail' of the collapsed lingula does not extend very far downwards

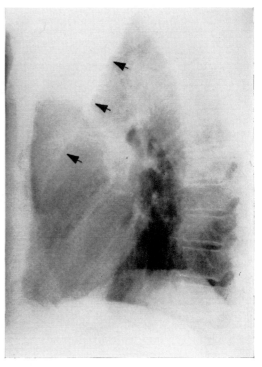

(b)

vessels can be identified and the diagnosis of pulmonary collapse may be made on this basis alone when other and better known signs are absent. Steiner (1958) wrote that 'satisfactory assessment of the radiographic pattern of the pulmonary arteries, particularly its major branches, and to a lesser extent its minor branches, is possible on adequate chest radiographs'. Simon (1962) noted the constancy of most lung vessels and stressed that the pulmonary arteries changed their position when collapse was present. The position of the pulmonary arterial and venous branches is shown in *Figure 3.64*. Bluth (1966) showed that tomograms sometimes reveal displacement of pulmonary vessels produced by peripheral tumours.

An analysis of vascular shadows is of especial value in the diagnosis of left lower lobe collapse. This condition is often difficult to recognize because of the overlying heart shadow (*Figures 3.61* and *3.66*). A collapsed right lower lobe also partly lies behind the heart shadow (*Figure 3.60*). On lateral radiographs the collapsed lower lobe may be inferred from a displaced oblique fissure, an unsharp posterior border of the heart or segment of the diaphragm posterior to the heart shadow, or increased opacity over the lower dorsal spine.

The hilar shadows may be altered in shape or position by lobar collapse, by the superadded shadows of masses, by shadows of opaque bronchi, or by consolidation distal to a bronchial occlusion.

Even experienced observers may have great difficulty in recognizing partial collapse. When reviewing the radiographs of patients referred for surgical resection, it is not at all uncommon to find films diagnostic of such collapse taken 6–12 months earlier, although at this later stage the recognition of the collapse is rendered easier by the retrospective analysis.

If the collapse is more complete, there may be a totally collapsed segment or lobe. This may be obvious on a single P.A. view, or it may be hidden behind the heart or the sternum and need well penetrated lateral views for its demonstration.

The lack of appreciation of partial collapse and the failure to see many small peripheral tumours on plain radiographs is probably the greatest problem at present in the diagnosis of lung tumours. The reading

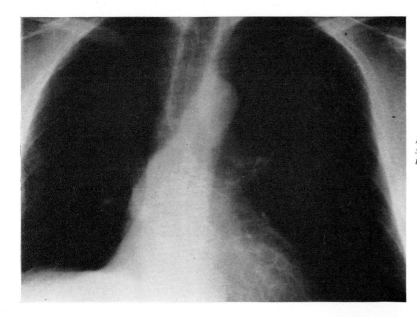

Figure 3.60. Collapsed right lower lobe shown as an almost vertical straight line and increased opacity behind right side of heart. Note reduced volume of right lung

Figure 3.61. Collapsed left lower lobe shown as a triangular opacity behind left side of heart. Note also reduced volume of the left lung and crowded ribs. The left pulmonary artery has been pulled downwards to give a 'clear' space between it and the aortic knuckle. Note.—Felson and Felson (1950) and Felson (1960) described a method of localizing an intrathoracic opacity from a single view by pointing out that where the opacity is adjacent to the border of the heart, aorta or diaphragm it will obliterate that border on the radiograph, and conversely it will not do this if it is not so adjacent. This is known as the 'silhouette sign'. It is seen in the P.A. view with an upper lobe collapse and in the lateral view with a collapsed lower lobe

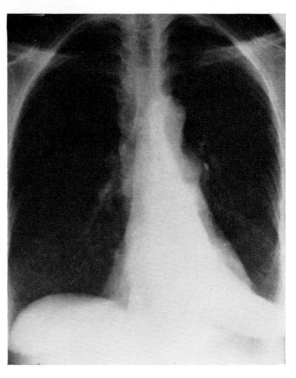

of films by two observers has been used to improve the detection of small peripheral tumours (Smith, 1965), but a greater understanding of the signs of partial collapse is required. It is a pity that many persons, clinicians and radiologists alike, do not look for signs of incomplete lung expansion when a visual inspection of chest movement and expansion is one of the first observations to be made in clinical examination of the chest (*see Figure 3.67*).

Summary of the signs of collapse

(1) Crowding of the ribs over the affected lung or lobe.

(2) Elevation of one side or part of one side of the diaphragm. This is, however, an inconsistent finding.

(3) Movement of the trachea and the mediastinum towards the side of the collapse. Herniation of the contralateral lung, especially of the right upper lobe anteriorly with left upper lobe collapse.

(4) Displacement of interlobar fissures.

    (*a*) Horizontal fissure with collapse of the right upper or middle lobe.

    (*b*) Oblique fissures with upper, middle or lower lobe collapse.

(5) Crowding of vascular markings in a partially collapsed part of a lung, and the splaying out of vessels in other parts of the lung which show compensatory emphysema (*Figure 3.62*).

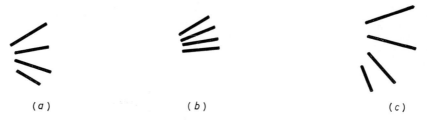

        (*a*)   (*b*)   (*c*)

Figure 3.62. (a) Normal; (b) crowded vessels (closed fan sign); (c) splayed vessels (opened-out fan sign)

(6) Changes in hilar shadows.

    (*a*) Changes due to an associated mass or enlarged nodes.

    (*b*) Changes due to alteration in pulmonary blood flow, which is reduced on the side of the collapse and increased on the opposite side (the paradoxical hilus sign).

    (*c*) Elevation of the hilum due to an upper lobe collapse.

    (*d*) Loss of normal vascular architecture, which may be seen in upper or lower lobe collapse.

(7) The pattern of collapse given by a collapsed segment or segments usually corresponds with the anatomy of the lung segments (*see Figure 8.3*). The pattern of segmental collapse is often modified by air entering the segment or segments due to collateral air drift through the pores of Kohn, so that the segment will still be aerated although the supplying bronchus is completely blocked. (For a discussion on the pores of Kohn, *see* Cordingley, 1972.)

(8) In a normal lateral chest radiograph, the radiographic density over the spine is greater in the upper than in the lower part of the chest. This is reversed with a lower lobe collapse.

(9) With a collapsed lower lobe there may be linear atelectasis in the lingula (Nordenström and Novek, 1960) or dilated lingula vessels (probably veins) running horizontally in this part of the lung.

When viewing a chest radiograph, most observers look for dense shadows in the lung fields and hence run the risk of failing to see the signs of lung collapse. It is a better plan to view the radiograph and first elicit the signs one would look for on direct inspection of the patient's chest—lung expansion and volume, equality of contralateral intercostal spaces, and so on. If this is done and other signs of possible lung collapse are seen, gross errors caused by failure to diagnose this condition will be avoided.

Anatomy of the hilar shadows

In viewing both P.A. and lateral chest radiographs, it is very important always to analyse the anatomy of the hilar shadows and their composite nature (*Figures 3.63* and *3.64*). On high kV radiographs, and to a lesser extent on those which are taken at a lower kV and are well penetrated, it is usually possible to identify separately the bronchi, the pulmonary arteries and the pulmonary veins. *Any deviation from the normal pattern should always promote further scrutiny and study in order to determine the nature of the abnormality and the possible presence of added shadows* which may indicate a mass in the hilum or in the lung in front of or behind the hilum, especially at the apex of either lower lobe.

Lavender *et al.* (1962) and Lavender and Doppman (1962) studied the vascular anatomy of the hilar

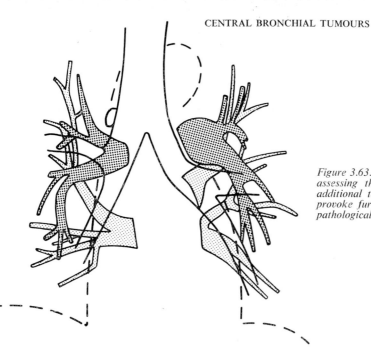

Figure 3.63. Diagram of anatomy of the hilar shadows. In assessing the normality of chest radiographs, shadows additional to those of the normal vessels should always provoke further study since they are likely to represent pathological conditions. Similarly, collapse will alter the anatomy of the vascular pattern

Pulmonary arteries

Pulmonary veins

Figure 3.64. Radiographs to show anatomy of pulmonary vasculature. (a) Arterial phase of pulmonary angiogram. The arteries tend to follow the bronchi

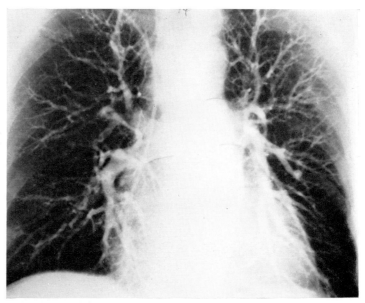

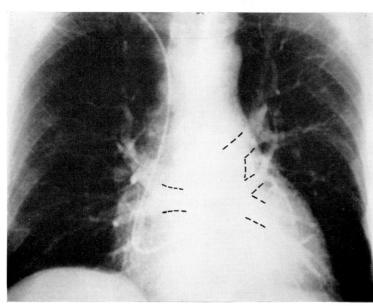

Figure 3.64 (b). Venous phase. The pulmonary veins (with the exception of those in the left upper lobe) follow a very different course to enter the posterior aspect of the left atrium at a level below the arteries and bronchi

regions by means of tomography in patients with mitral valve disease and left ventricular failure and also in normal individuals. They found that arteries could usually be differentiated from veins. They also found that there was a certain amount of anatomical variation between different subjects, but that the main vascular pattern was fairly constant. They took their tomograms in the supine position, which somewhat lessens the length of the hilar shadows; with radiographs taken in the erect position, there should be a greater separation of the hilar vascular shadows.

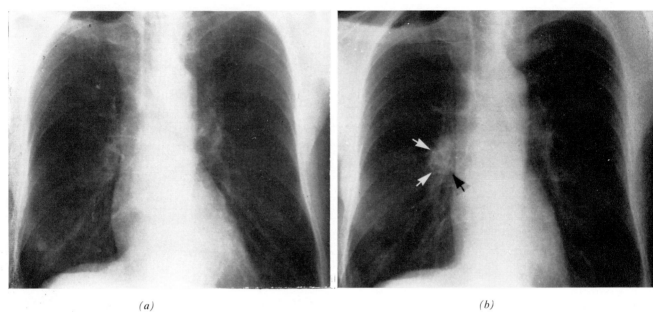

(a)   (b)

Figure 3.65. A small mass in apex of right lower lobe produces an additional shadow in the right hilar region. Radiograph (b) was taken three years after (a). On the lateral view the opacity was hidden as it overlay the spine. Fluoroscopy showed that a small mass lay posteriorly in the right side of the chest and close to the spine. This was confirmed by A.P. and lateral tomograms (c and d), which also revealed that the mass had a lobulated border with some spiculation and an eccentric cavity system [(c) shows two tomographic cuts]. No spread of the tumour was found at thoracotomy. Histological examination showed it to be a squamous cell carcinoma

(c)   (d)

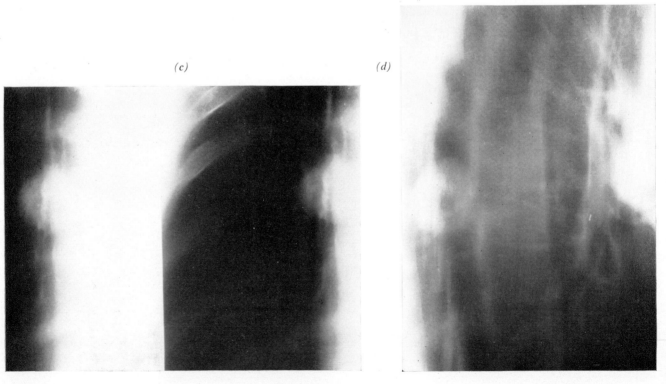

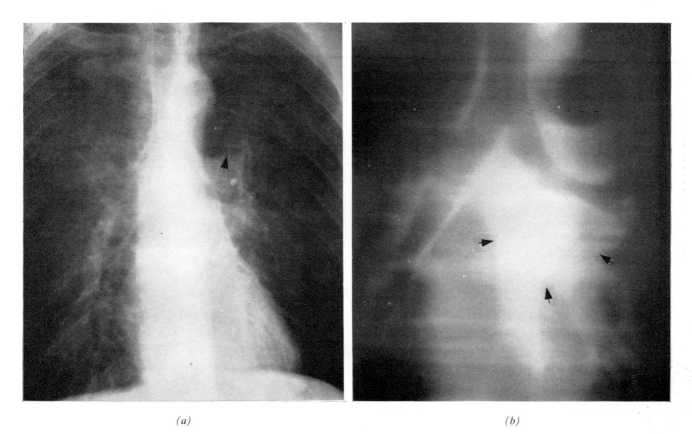

(a)   *(b)*

Figure 3.66. Patient aged 45 years with minor chest symptoms who had a routine chest radiograph. The high kV film (a) shows a mass below the left main bronchus with apparent blockage of the left lower lobe bronchus. The left hilum and left pulmonary artery shadow (arrowed) are somewhat depressed. These findings were confirmed by inclined frontal tomography (b)

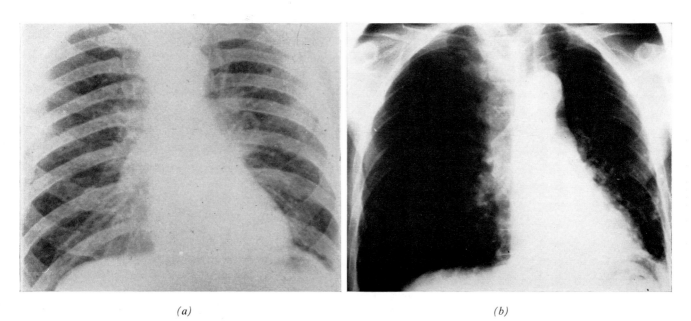

(a)   *(b)*

Figure 3.67. (a) Low kV radiograph reported as normal, but there are already signs of reduced volume of left lung, with some 'crowding' of left ribs and slight shift of heart and mediastinum to the left. (b) Nine months later, when the patient was referred for surgery, the left-sided collapse was much worse. By this time the tumour was inoperable due to extensive mediastinal involvement

53

As is demonstrated in *Figures 3.63* and *3.64*, the pulmonary arteries follow the major bronchi from the hilum to the periphery of the lung. The pulmonary veins have an independent course to the left atrium at a lower level than that of the arteries; they also run in a more horizontal direction and cross the arteries. The anatomy of each of the hilar shadows in a lateral projection is shown in *Figures 3.79* and *3.80*. Abnormalities of the anatomy of hilar shadows appear in several illustrations, including *Figures 3.81* and *3.82*.

Mucocoeles and bronchiectasis

Rees and Ruttley (1970) described the appearance of mucocoeles with bronchogenic tumours producing obstruction as a new sign, although the tendency for tumours to produce secondary bronchiectasis and cause retention of secretions had been noted by Kirklin and Paterson (1928) and Chandler (1932)

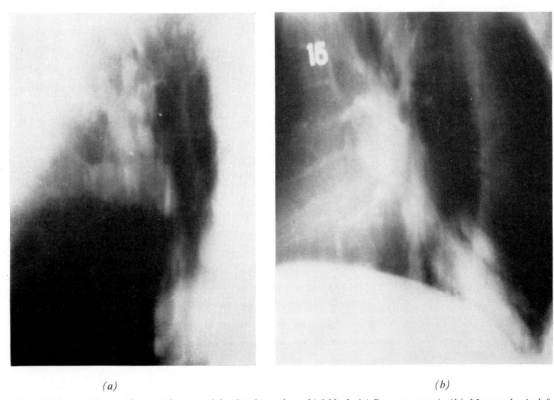

(a)   *(b)*

Figure 3.68. (a) Mucocoeles in right upper lobe distal to a bronchial block (A.P. tomograms). (b) Mucocoeles in left lower lobe distal to an endobronchial tumour (lateral tomogram). The surrounding lung remains aerated due to 'collateral air drift'

(*see* Chapter 2). It is common at bronchoscopy to find retained secretions behind an obstruction in a large bronchus, and they are also frequently seen in surgical and autopsy specimens. This is not a specific sign of bronchial neoplasm and can occur with bronchial obstruction from other causes (*see Figure 8.8*). It is particularly likely to be seen in the more dependent bronchi, but it may develop anywhere and is more often present with the more slowly growing bronchial carcinomas and adenomas. On radiographs the affected bronchi appear as enlarged, dense shadows; these may be visible on plain films or tomograms (*Figure 3.68*), or occasionally on bronchograms as the continuation of patent bronchi (*see Figure 8.8*).

Recently Lemine, Trepanier and Hebert (1970) reported six cases of mucocoeles which they termed 'bronchocele or blocked bronchiectasis'. These appeared as rounded shadows on radiographs in asymptomatic patients and mimicked lung tumours. Tomograms showed the lesions as oval or having branching patterns. These cases were thought to be caused by occlusion of a bronchus by a diaphragm across it. Talner *et al.* (1970) reported two new cases and reviewed the radiological literature on 100 cases of benign mucocoeles and on the frequent association with these of regional hyperinflation of the lung, which fails to deflate in expiration (presumably due to collateral air drift through the inter-alveolar pores of Kohn such as occurs also with sequestrated lung segments). Such bronchocoeles have to be distinguished from those produced by tumours, which are by far the commonest cause of this condition (Wright, 1971b). Sheehan and Schonfeld (1963) reported the case of a young woman in whom the shadow of the fluid-filled dilated bronchi simulated a tumour.

Effects of infection

Retained secretions distal to a partial or complete bronchial block often become infected, producing consolidation in the obstructed area of the lung, or bronchiectasis. The infection may be recurrent over a period of weeks, months, or sometimes even years (*see Figure 8.27*). The consolidation may break down to give rise to a lung abscess, or the infection may be partly responsible for the breakdown of a solid tumour. The infection may also spread to other parts of the same lung or, by aspiration, into the

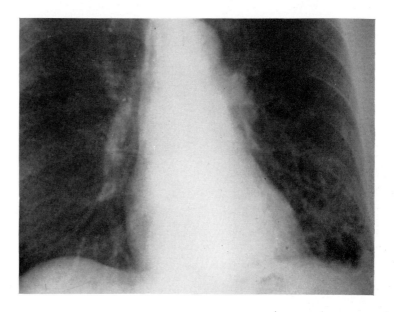

Figure 3.69. Honeycomb lung appearance in left lower lobe resulting from endobronchial tumour. Two weeks earlier, on the initial diagnostic radiograph, the left lower lobe was completely collapsed. No treatment had been given. This appearance may also be seen when a lobe re-expands after radiotherapy or tumour chemotherapy

contralateral lung. When the infection and obstruction have been present for some time and some re-aeration of the lung occurs, an appearance resembling honeycomb lung may be produced (*Figure 3.69*). The association of infection with a tumour is extremely well known and is the reason why virtually every person over the age of 40 years who has had pneumonia now has subsequent chest radiographs taken to check that resolution has occurred.

The apparent response of a tumour to antibiotic chemotherapy is dealt with in the section on the natural history of some lung tumours (*see* page 71).

GENERAL OBSERVATIONS COMMON TO BOTH PERIPHERAL AND CENTRAL TUMOURS

Bronchial carcinoma and pulmonary tuberculosis

Despite the dramatically reduced numbers of patients presenting with pulmonary tuberculosis during the past two decades, 112 new cases were treated in Oxford in 1970 and 88 in 1971, the attendance at the Chest Clinic totalling almost 12,000 in 1970 and 10,000 in 1971. These figures together with the continuously increasing incidence of bronchial carcinoma—which often develops in patients with pre-existing lung disease such as emphysema, or with scarring from pulmonary tuberculosis or other acute or chronic lung disease—mean that there is frequently a diagnostic problem regarding the causation of the disease process. Many patients with tuberculosis will not show a positive bacteriological growth of tubercle bacilli from their sputa; they will have to be treated by chemotherapy on account of the radiological appearances alone, and the lesions will most often clear.

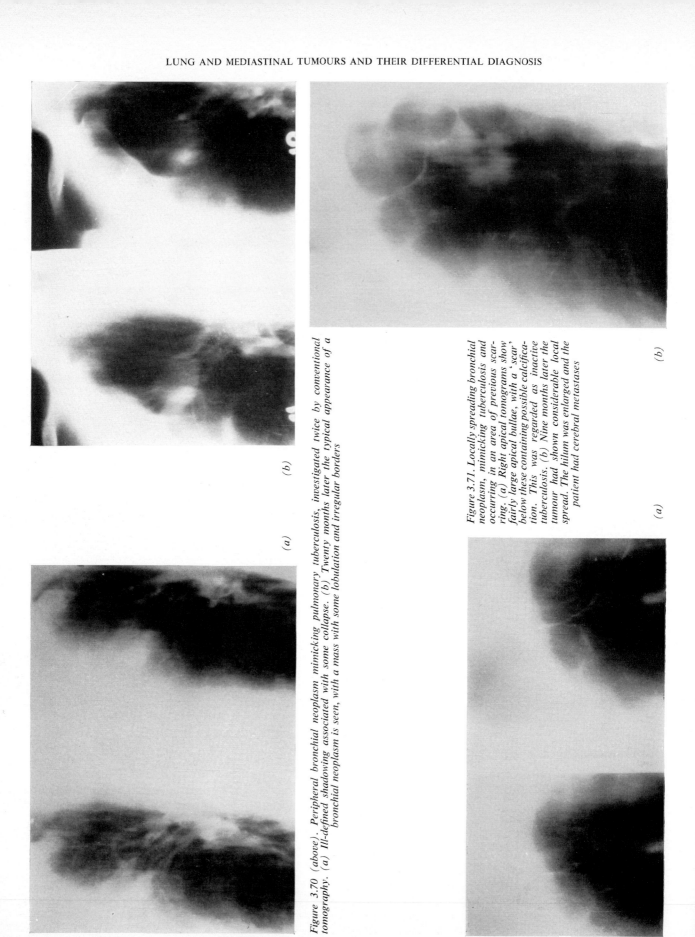

Figure 3.70 (above). Peripheral bronchial neoplasm mimicking pulmonary tuberculosis, investigated twice by conventional tomography. (a) Ill-defined shadowing associated with some collapse. (b) Twenty months later the typical appearance of a bronchial neoplasm is seen, with a mass with some lobulation and irregular borders

Figure 3.71. Locally spreading bronchial neoplasm, mimicking tuberculosis and occurring in an area of previous scarring. (a) Right apical tomograms show fairly large apical bullae, with a 'scar' below these containing possible calcification. This was regarded as inactive tuberculosis. (b) Nine months later the tumour had shown considerable local spread. The hilum was enlarged and the patient had cerebral metastases

In other cases what appeared to be tuberculous lesions (but without positive bacteriology for tuberculosis) were subsequently discovered to be bronchial neoplasms. Some of these cases are illustrated in this chapter. One had a small cavitated lesion which became apparently solid and then broke down again (*Figure 3.97*). Another showed apparent spread of infiltration on plain radiographs, although the diagnosis was recognized on the tomograms (*see Figure 3.26*). A third showed collapse, consolidation and an ill-defined mass, the true nature of the disease not being discovered for 20 months (*see Figure 3.97*), while a fourth showed progression of an apical lesion over a period of four years until its true nature was revealed shortly before the patient died (*see Figure 3.53*). Other perplexing

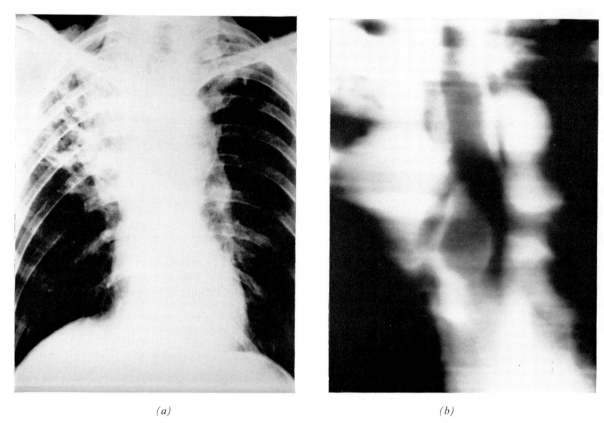

(a)   *(b)*

Figure 3.72. Pulmonary tuberculosis and bronchial carcinoma. (a) Plain film showing infiltration and cavitation in right upper lobe and infiltration at left apex. (b) Inclined frontal tomogram showing large right hilar mass with tumour extending from right upper lobe orifice into right main bronchus. The superior venacavogram of this patient is shown in Figure 10.11

problems have occurred in other cases—for example, the progressive enlargement of an almost 'dumbbell' shaped irregular tumour (*see Figure 3.32*) in a patient who had had pulmonary tuberculosis and had several small, partially calcified lesions. This tumour was found to be a secondary deposit from an ovarian neoplasm. Three of the above lesions progressed while the patients were undergoing antituberculous chemotherapy. Several other patients have received treatment for rounded lesions which have enlarged and have then been removed (*see for example Figure 3.36*).

In addition to these difficult diagnostic points regarding the diagnosis of the tumour *per se*, it must be pointed out that secondary infection distal to a bronchial obstruction may cause reactivation of pre-existing pulmonary tuberculosis (*Figure 3.72*), and that tuberculosis and cancer may be present at the same time in different parts of the lungs (*see Figure 3.50*). When a peripheral tumour develops in an area of pre-existing disease, the differentiation of the tumour from a reactivation of the tuberculosis may be extremely difficult (*see Figure 3.71*). Calcification may become incorporated within the lesion and may then create a false impression of a benign tumour. The problem of the coexistence of pulmonary tuberculosis and lung cancer was discussed by Fried (1948), Hauser and Glazer (1955), Greenberg *et al.* (1964) and Holden, Quinlan and Hiltz (1965). A bronchogenic carcinoma may cause reactivation of tuberculosis, either by eroding an encapsulated caseous focus or by reactivating dormant foci secondary to cachexia (*see* Snider and Placik, 1967).

Bronchial carcinoma, sarcoidosis and other chronic lung diseases

Goodbody and Taylor (1957) pointed out that when sarcoidosis and lung cancer coexist in the same patient, assessment of hilar enlargement may be even more difficult than in cases of tuberculosis. I have seen only one patient who had bronchial carcinoma complicating sarcoidosis, and in this case the diagnosis was not made until extremely late in the course of the disease because of the marked pre-existing lung fibrosis. Other examples of the difficulty of diagnosing lung tumours may arise where they are associated

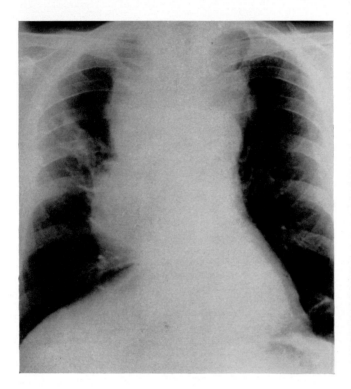

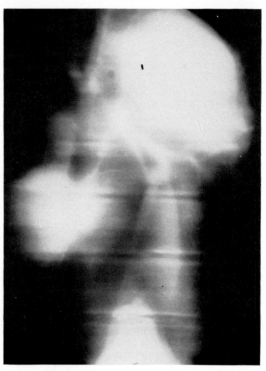

Figure 3.73. Massive right hilar and mediastinal enlargement secondary to a small neoplasm of the right upper lobe

Figure 3.74. Enlargement of lower right hilar and left upper mediastinal nodes in a patient with reticulosis (lymphoid follicular reticulosis)

with other chronic lung diseases such as pre-existing bronchiectasis or pneumoconiosis, particularly when giant massive fibrosis is present.

Hilar and mediastinal lymph node enlargement

Nodal enlargement may be seen on plain radiographs or on tomograms. Such enlargement may be gross or slight. The routine use of penetrated (or high kV) radiographs, with the oesophagus opacified by barium sulphate paste, in all cases of neoplasm will often show oesophageal displacement due to enlarged mediastinal nodes and obviate the need for any further investigation (*Figures 3.75b* and *3.76*). Lodge (1950) and Fleischner and Sachsse (1963), in assessing the spread of bronchial neoplasm by this method, took P.A. and lateral views, whilst Lenk (1954) preferred the left oblique view. This mode of assessment was also studied by Middlemass (1953).

My main experience of the demonstration of hilar and mediastinal lymph node masses by tomography will be described in Chapter 7, but the principal points are summarized below.

(1) Many hilar and mediastinal lymph node enlargements are visible on plain radiographs without any need for further investigation. Particular attention should be paid to the hilar, azygos, and superior and anterior mediastinal regions and to the retrocarinal and retrocardiac areas in assessing the radio-

graphs. Occasionally intrapulmonary nodes may be enlarged, giving rise to the appearance of a second lung mass.

(2) Views with the oesophagus opacified by barium sulphate paste or Gastrografin may show oesophageal displacement by the enlarged nodes, but one should always be aware of the normal anatomy of the oesophagus, which passes slightly to the right at the level of the aortic arch, returns to almost the midline and then passes to the left below the carina, often to be displaced by a dilated or tortuous lower descending aorta. In the lateral view the oesophagus is most often seen to be displaced by nodal enlargement in the retrocarinal area.

(3) Hilar, superior mediastinal or subcarinal nodal enlargement is best demonstrated by inclined frontal tomography or by some variant of this technique, while enlargement of nodes in the anterior or posterior parts of the hilum or in the anterior mediastinum is best shown by lateral tomography.

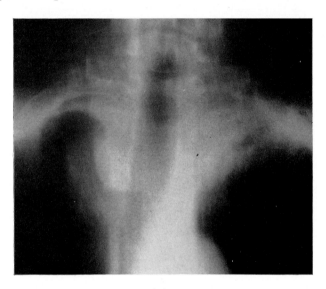

(a)

Figure 3.75. (a) Superior mediastinal spread of tumour which originated in the left lower lobe, causing bilateral Pancoast-like syndrome but without any bone erosion. (Linear tomogram.) (b) Large mass of retrocarinal nodes demonstrated by barium swallow

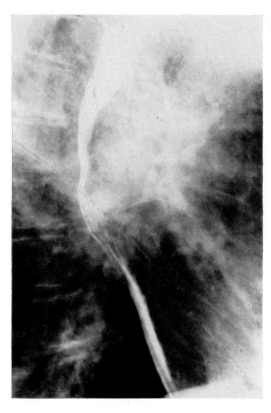

(b)

(4) Nodal enlargement must be distinguished from enlargement of vascular structures such as the pulmonary vessels in the hilum. In this connection it is important to remember that *the right pulmonary artery and most of its branches lie in front of the carina, while the left pulmonary artery and its branches lie mainly superiorly and posteriorly to the carina (Figures 3.79 and 3.80), so that if a mass or enlarged glands lie anteriorly on the left or posteriorly on the right, they are unlikely to be mimicked by enlargement of vascular structures (Figures 3.81 and 3.82)*. The pulmonary veins pass to the back of the left atrium and should be distinguished from nodal enlargements. Vix and Klatte (1970) have studied the anatomy of the hilar shadows on lateral chest radiographs and state that the left pulmonary artery lies superior and posterior to the left upper lobe bronchus and is clearly seen on lateral radiographs, while the right pulmonary artery is surrounded by structures which render it less distinct. My own view is that the lateral radiograph shows the right pulmonary artery more clearly than the left.

The azygos vein may be distended in such conditions as cardiac failure, superior mediastinal obstruction or liver disease, but if enlargement is present in the vicinity of the vein with the patient lying down and disappears with the patient sitting, it is likely to be vascular in origin. I have, however, seen one patient in whom an enlarged node, which was mobile, became visible when the patient lay down and disappeared when he sat up. A similar but smaller shadow on the left, lying adjacent to the aortic arch, which is occasionally seen on tomograms is caused by the left superior intercostal vein—termed the aortic nipple by McDonald, Castellino and Blank (1970).

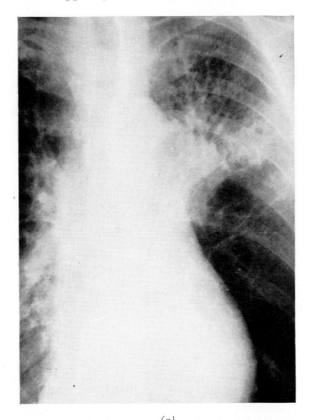

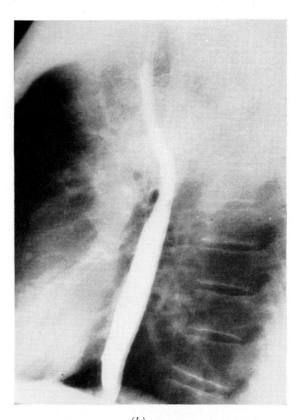

(a)   *(b)*

Figure 3.76. The barium-filled oesophagus is displaced by the enlarged mediastinal nodes at the carinal level. Note also reduction in pulmonary vasculature in left lung, particularly left lower lobe

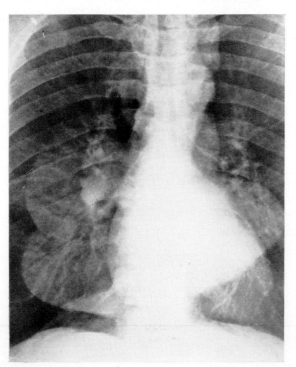

Figure 3.77. Enlarged nodes within the posterior mediastinum due to extramedullary haemopoiesis in a patient with thalassaemia. This was confirmed by biopsy. He also had coarsening of the trabecular pattern of many bones including those of the hands, ribs and skull. Similar cases have been reported by Knoblich (1960) and by Korsten et al. (1970). Note.—Similar but smaller enlargement of posterior mediastinal nodes may occasionally be found in sarcoidosis

(5) Nodal enlargement may be found with bronchial tumours in unexpected places. There may be crossed drainage from the left upper or lower lobe to the right upper mediastinum, and from the right middle lobe to the left upper mediastinum. An excellent study of the lymph node drainage of the lungs was made by McCort and Robbins (1951) (*see also* Chapter 9). Crossed drainage also explains why paradoxical neck or scalene node enlargement is not infrequently seen (Onuigbo, 1962).

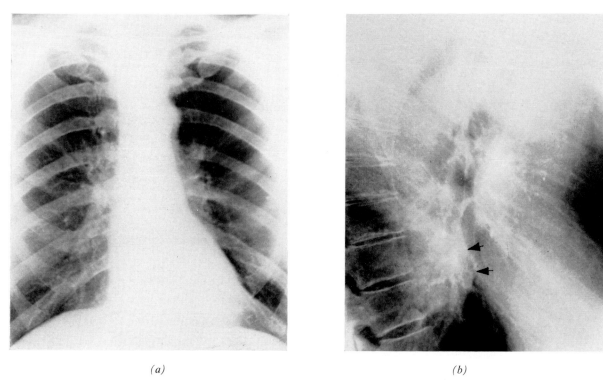

(a)   *(b)*

Figure 3.78. Enlarged mediastinal nodes, like primary tumours, may be missed if radiographs are not carefully scrutinized. In this case the opacity behind the heart, as seen on the lateral view (b), was unrecognized until it became much larger

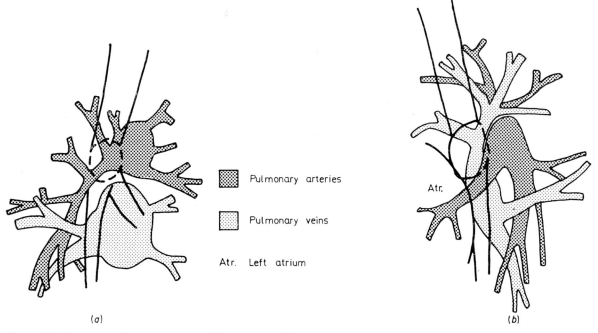

Pulmonary arteries

Pulmonary veins

Atr. Left atrium

(a)   *(b)*

Figure 3.79. Diagrammatic representations of the anatomy of the hilar regions as seen on a lateral chest radiograph or tomogram. Anterior aspects of hila face centre of diagram. (a) Right. (b) Left

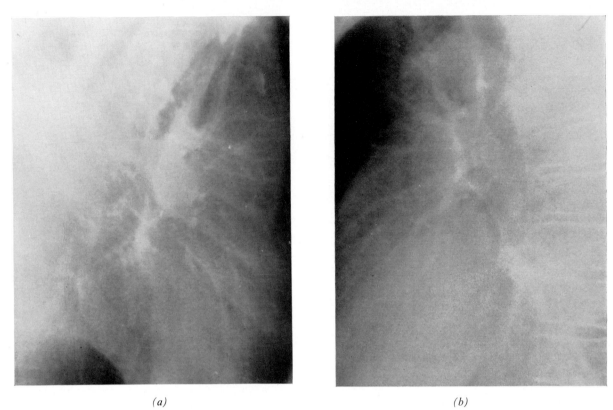

(a)   *(b)*

Figure 3.80. 'Selective' views of (a) right and (b) left hilum, the patients having previously had left and right pneumonectomies respectively. These views well demonstrate the hilar anatomy, particularly that of the arteries

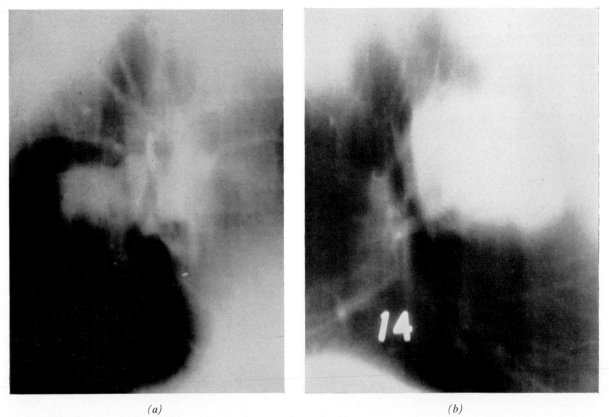

(a)   *(b)*

Figure 3.81. (a) Extensive nodal enlargement in posterior part of right hilum. (b) Large mass in posterior part of left hilum

(6) Enlargement of mediastinal nodes occurs not only in tumour, sarcoidosis, reticulosis and leukaemia, and occasionally in other blood diseases such as extramedullary haemopoiesis (*see Figure 3.77*), but may also accompany infection. Pulmonary tuberculosis can cause enlarged nodes, but pyogenic pneumonias (*see Figure 7.38*) may also cause an enlargement similar to that of the axillary or inguinal nodes following an infection in the hand or foot. Such enlargement may occasionally be massive and produce sufficient pressure on the larger bronchi to occlude them so that a tumour is simulated (*see Figure 7.39*).

(7) A 'frozen' or fixed mediastinum may be demonstrated by the fact that it remains central in position despite gross collapse of the lung or a large pleural effusion, or by its failure to move with respiration or sniffing. Such a fixed mediastinum often implies infiltration by neoplasm, but some

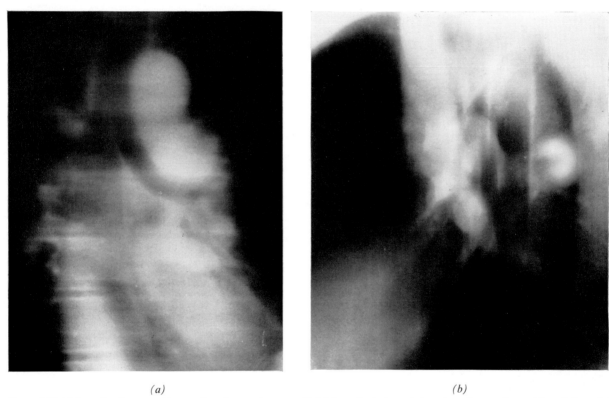

| (a) | (b) |

Figure 3.82. Enlarged nodes caused by neoplasm in anterior part of left hilum. In the lateral view alone the anterior position of the nodal enlargement clearly indicates that they are not vascular structures. (a) Inclined frontal tomogram. (b) Lateral tomogram

patients have a naturally less mobile mediastinum than others. With neoplasm there may be diffuse spread of tumour and nodal involvement (*see Figure 3.75a*). Occasionally a fixed mediastinum results from other conditions such as a diffuse fibrosis associated with retroperitoneal fibrosis, tuberculosis or syphilis ('plastic mediastinitis'—*see Figure 3.145* and page 107).

(8) Enlarged superior mediastinal nodes have to be distinguished from other structures in the superior mediastinum such as the aorta or the thymus (*see* Chapter 7), and mediastinal node enlargement may rarely be mimicked by neurofibromas (*see Figure 7.44*).

Small hilum, pulmonary artery invasion or thrombosis

A reduction in the blood supply to a lobe or lung containing a tumour is extremely common. If marked, it usually implies a considerable degree of mediastinal or hilar involvement. Lesser degrees, with a segmental or lobar distribution, may indicate only a reduced blood supply to the poorly ventilated and partly obstructed portion of the lung. Oeser, Ernst and Gerstenberg (1969) have described a unilateral reduction in the size of the hilum on the side of the lesion as the paradoxical hilus sign, and think that this may occur relatively early in the progress of a tumour due to an alveolar–vascular reflex which reduces the calibre of the pulmonary arteries on the side of the tumour (*Figures 3.83–3.86*).

For a discussion of the use of pulmonary angiography and radio-isotope lung scintiscanning in the evaluation of mediastinal metastases and the reduction of pulmonary vascularity secondary to cancer of the lung, *see* Chapter 10.

Pulmonary septal engorgement and pulmonary congestion in bronchial carcinoma, including lymphangitis carcinomatosa

Kerley (1933, 1951) described thickening of the interlobar fissures, miliary type shadows, and linear shadows termed A and B lines in patients with mitral stenosis and with pulmonary oedema due to

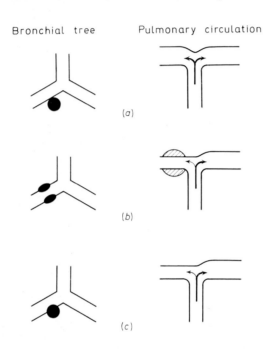

Figure 3.83. Diagram explaining the paradoxical hilus sign and illustrating reduced pulmonary circulation in the lung containing the tumour (for clinical examples of this, see Figures 3.84–3.86). (a) Extrabronchial tumour: no effect on circulation. (b) Larger hilar tumour: reduced pulmonary circulation; hilar mass. (c) Exo-endobronchial tumour: reduced pulmonary circulation in affected lung leading to a small hilum

congestive cardiac failure and to some other conditions. The B lines are horizontal lines usually 1–2 cm long, seen particularly at the lung bases, while the A lines are longer, often radiating from the hilar regions and present in the deeper parts of the lung. Kerley suggested that these lines might be due to dilated lymphatics. However, Grainger (1958), in a very clear account of their nature and causation, and Trapnell (1963, 1967, 1970) have shown that both A and B lines are caused by dilated connective tissue septa, the B lines being due to dilated superficial interlobular septa. Both the latter authors suggested that they should be called septal and not lymphatic lines.

These septal lines may be visible when they are abnormally thick, as in pulmonary oedema from any cause such as left ventricular failure secondary to myocardial infarction, renal failure, lymphangitis carcinomatosa (Trapnell, 1964b), infection, sarcoidosis (Trapnell, 1964d), or deposition of abnormally opaque material in or beside them as in pneumoconiosis (Trapnell, 1964c) or haemosiderosis (Fleischner and Reiner, 1964). When these lines are seen in patients with bronchial carcinoma, this finding is usually secondary to hilar obstruction of veins and/or lymphatics or to diffuse permeation of the lung by tumour. With localized septal or lymphatic permeation, there may occasionally be a fine nodularity in the lung due to multiple small tumour deposits. Dilated septal lines are commonly associated with small or larger pleural effusions. Occasionally a patient with no other signs of bronchial neoplasm will present with 'congestion' or dilated septal lines in one or both lungs which may mimic sarcoidosis, infection or left ventricular failure. *Figure 3.87* illustrates examples of bilateral and unilateral septal engorgement secondary to diffuse spread of tumour into the pulmonary lymphatics (lymphangitis carcinomatosa).

For details of the lymphatics of the lung and mediastinum, *see* Chapter 9.

Figure 3.84. Reduced vascularity in right upper lobe (a), present six months before tumour was recognized (b)

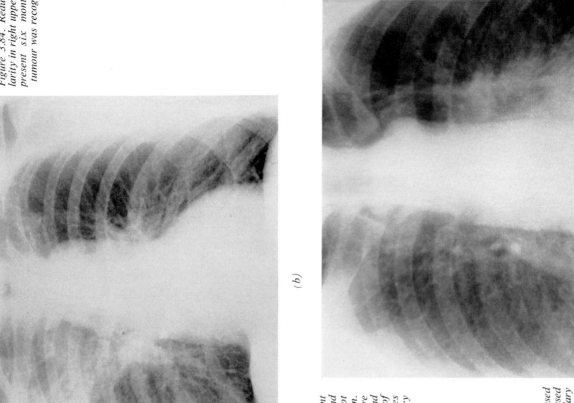

(b)

(a)

Figure 3.85 (left). Patient with cancer of the larynx and bronchial neoplasm, a not very uncommon association. In this example there are right hilar enlargement and obstructive emphysema of right middle and lower lobes as well as reduced pulmonary vascularity

Figure 3.86 (right). Increased transradiancy of left lung caused by reduced vascularity secondary to small tumour in left main bronchus which is just visible on the original radiograph (see also Chapter 9)

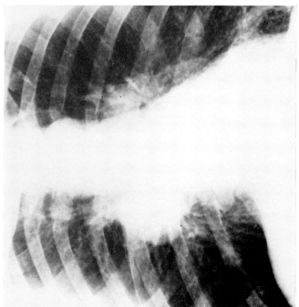

Pleural involvement

This is most commonly shown by a pleural effusion, but a 'knobbly pleura' (*see Figures 3.89* and *3.122*), or a fixed mediastinum in association with pleural thickening or effusion, is always suggestive of malignancy. A knobbly pleura may also be seen with mesotheliomas, secondary neoplasms or myelomatosis.

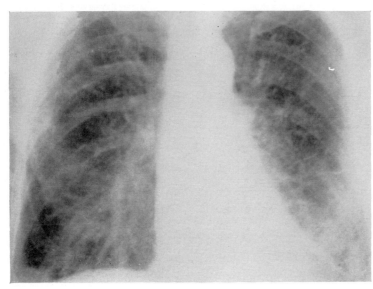

Figure 3.87. Examples of lymphangitis carcinomatosa. (a) Bilateral pulmonary septal engorgement (interstitial and interlobular) in a patient with bronchial carcinoma. He also developed pericardial thickening on the left side (see Figure 9.1). The diagnosis was established by biopsy at thoracotomy

(a)

Figure 3.87 (b). Unilateral pulmonary septal engorgement secondary to bronchial neoplasm. Cells typical of squamous cell carcinoma were found in the sputum

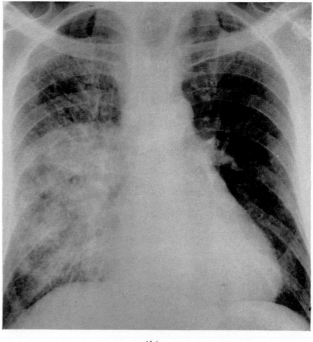

(b)

Pericardial involvement and effusion

The development of a complicating pericardial effusion may be suspected from an enlarging heart shadow and reduced cardiac pulsation seen on fluoroscopy (*Figure 3.90*). Further confirmation can be obtained by the use of ultrasound, heart scintiscanning, or negative or positive contrast angiocardiography (*see* Chapter 10). For reviews of these methods, *see* Bates (1970) and Wright (1971b).

Occasionally angiocardiography has been carried out to show whether the pericardium or the mediastinum is involved (*see* Chapter 10), but pericardial involvement is usually diagnosed only at thoracotomy. A mass alongside the pericardium demonstrated by tomography (*Figure 3.91*), which may be associated with a phrenic palsy, is highly suggestive of spread of tumour on to or into the pericardium.

Nerve involvement

The recurrent laryngeal and phrenic nerves may both be involved by tumours within the thorax. Recurrent laryngeal nerve palsy due to this cause is commoner on the left than on the right (*Figures 3.93* and *3.94*) because of the lower anatomical course of the left recurrent laryngeal nerve, which passes

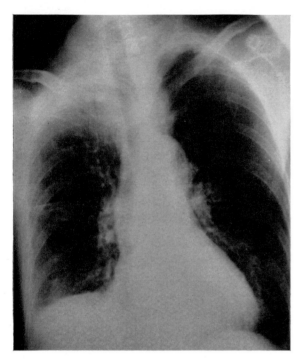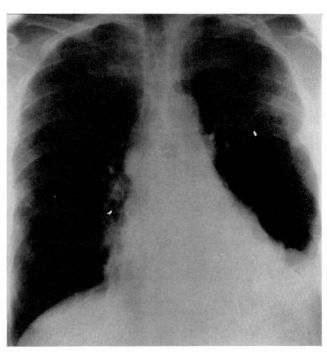

Figure 3.88 (left). Patient with severe pain in right side of chest due to 'dry pleurisy', a diffuse spread of tumour in the pleura without any significant effusion. Note grossly diminished volume of right lung. Even at autopsy 6 months later, no significant fluid was present in the pleura

Figure 3.89 (right). 'Knobbly pleura' due to secondary spread of bronchial tumour into the pleura. Small pleural effusion at left base

around the aortic arch. Recurrent laryngeal nerve involvement is nearly always a contra-indication to surgery, whereas phrenic nerve involvement may not indicate inoperability and incurability if the tumour in the mediastinum or on the pericardium can be resected (Grimshaw, 1970—personal communication). In some cases there is no definite direct relationship between the paralysis and the tumour. Virus infections, which may complicate the tumour, are sometimes the cause of various nerve palsies, and a phrenic nerve paralysis is not uncommon in such cases. In some patients the nerve palsy may have been present before the development of the tumour. Eventrations and partial degrees of impaired movement, as well as masses below the diaphragm such as an enlarged liver, have to be distinguished from phrenic palsy (*Figures 3.92, 3.131* and *3.133*).

Sherman and Phillips (1968), from the Memorial Hospital, New York, pointed out that during fluoroscopy radiologists should study the movements of both the diaphragm and the *vocal cords*—a practice which is also carried out on the Continent of Europe but almost never in the United Kingdom.

Figure 3.94 shows the radiographs of a patient in whom the occasional inhalation of food or fluid, produced by a recurrent laryngeal nerve palsy secondary to bronchial neoplasm, caused her to present with a swallowing difficulty.

Alexander (1966) discussed some of the difficulties in the diagnosis of phrenic palsy. He found that

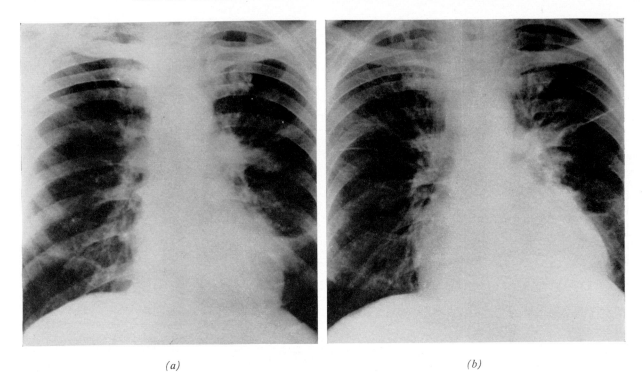

(a)   (b)

Figure 3.90. Patient with carcinoma of left lower lobe who developed a pericardial effusion. Radiograph (b) was taken one month after (a). (See also Figure 10.2)

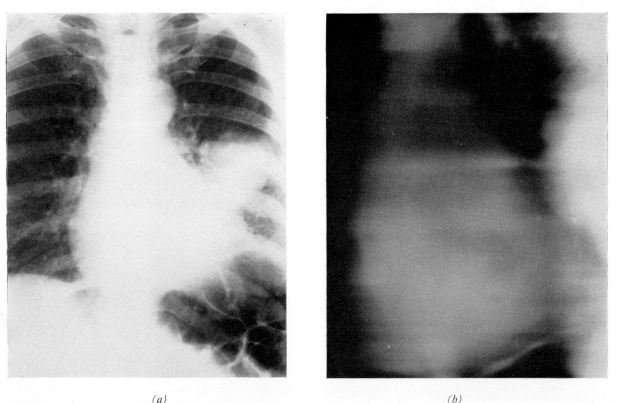

(a)   (b)

Figure 3.91. Bronchial neoplasm invading the pericardium. (a) P.A. view. (b) Inclined frontal tomogram showing the tumour abutting on to the pericardium

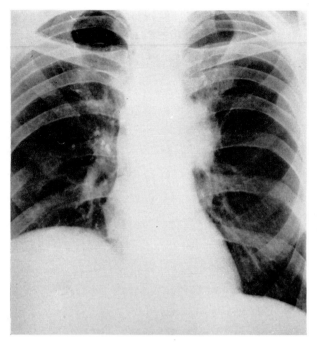 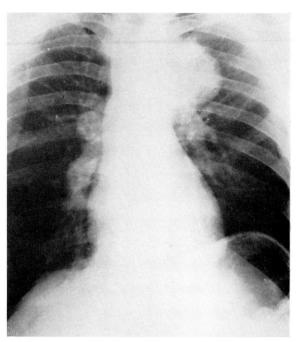

Figure 3.92. Left hilar mass, metastases in right eighth and left third ribs, and raised right side of diaphragm due to liver metastases. (The raised diaphragm could equally have been due to a phrenic palsy)

Figure 3.93. Large mass in upper left hilum in region of aortic arch. The trachea is displaced to the right. Left side of diaphragm is raised due to phrenic nerve palsy. The patient presented to the E.N.T. department with hoarseness secondary to left recurrent laryngeal nerve involvement

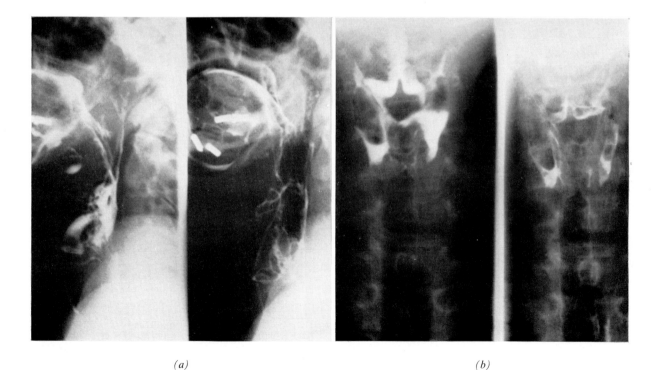

(a)   *(b)*

Figure 3.94. A female patient with a bronchial carcinoma presented with a swallowing difficulty caused by left recurrent laryngeal nerve palsy. She could swallow at times without any abnormal symptoms but could not entirely clear the lower pharynx of barium or secretions. When she inhaled some of this material she was unable to swallow until coughing had cleared the larynx of barium. The left vocal cord was paralysed. (a) and (b) Barium swallow showing paralysed left vocal cord, retained secretions in lower pharynx and some inhalation of barium into larynx

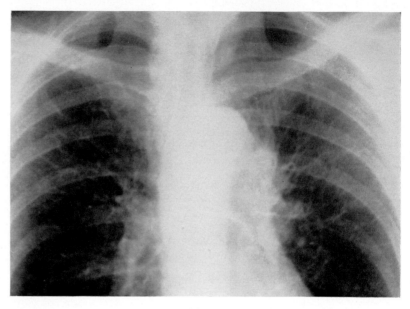

(c)

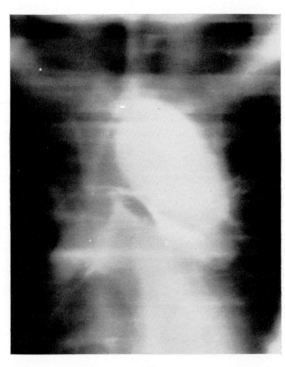

Figure 3.94 (c) and (d). Chest radiograph and inclined frontal tomogram revealing large mass on lower aspect of aortic arch, the trachea and left main bronchus being displaced to the right and downwards

(d)

one side of the diaphragm was usually dominant, left dominance being twice as common as right, and that the sniffing test was not always a reliable guide. Young and Simon (1972) have shown that inequality in movement of the two domes of the diaphragm is frequently present; in young adult males, the greater range of movement is more usual on the right.

Pulmonary secondary deposits from lung tumours

Pulmonary secondary deposits are not uncommon with primary malignant tumours of the lung. They may vary in size from multiple small miliary shadows (*Figure 3.106*) to single or multiple rounded deposits. The deposits may at times be so numerous as to mimic consolidation due to pneumonia on clinical examination at the time of presentation (*Figures 3.95* and *3.96*). Pulmonary deposits may occur on their own or together with other distant metastases to bone, brain, liver, and so on. Pulmonary metastases are probably explained by spread of tumour into the bronchial veins.

Natural history of some bronchial tumours and their apparent response to antibiotic chemotherapy

Antibiotic chemotherapy may cause apparent regression of a tumour by controlling and reducing the secondary infection so that as this surrounding infection clears, the tumour appears to decrease in size. The filling in of a cavitated lesion should not necessarily be regarded as a direct response to antibiotics in tuberculous and other infections, or even as an indication that such an infection was the cause of the disease process, if a trial of treatment has been undertaken without positive bacteriology. A tumour

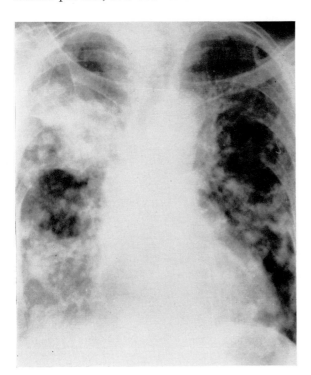 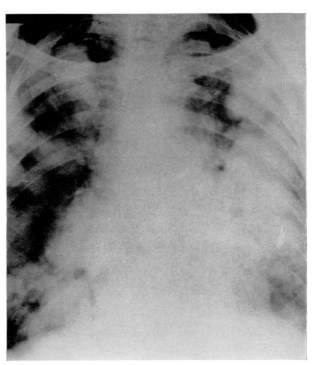

Figure 3.95 (left). Multiple small pulmonary secondary deposits from carcinoma of right upper lobe
Figure 3.96 (right). Large pulmonary secondary deposits, in a young man, from bronchial (oat cell) carcinoma which gave rise to clinical signs suggesting pneumonic consolidation of left lung

may break down to form a necrotic cavitated centre and may then become solid again. Such breakdown and filling up of a cavity in a tumour may occur several times during its growth (*Figure 3.97*).

Presence of more than one primary lung tumour

Figure 3.1b illustrates in diagrammatic form the concept of looking for more than one primary lung tumour. With metaplasia of the bronchial epithelium secondary to cigarette smoking and other carcinogens, it would not be surprising if multiple tumours were to develop either at any one time (synchronous) or at intervals of time (metachronous). Many such cases of apparent multiple primary lung tumours have been reported in the literature (Warren and Gates, 1932; Robinson and Jackson, 1958; Britt, Christoforidis and Andrews, 1960; Hughes and Blades, 1961; Le Gal and Bauer, 1961; Langston and Sherrick, 1962; Payne, Clagett and Harrison, 1962; Peterson, Pirogov and Smulevich, 1963; Cliffton, Das Gupta and Pool, 1964; Glennie, Harvey and Salama, 1964; Shields, Drake and Sherrick, 1964; Watson, Cameron and Percy, 1964; Leafstedt *et al.*, 1968; Ott and Titscher, 1969; Chaudhuri, 1971).

Abbey Smith (1966) followed up 269 patients who had undergone previous lobectomy. Of these, 19 appeared to develop second pulmonary tumours. It is, of course, difficult to prove that the second tumour was not a metastasis from the first. However, as many primary tumours have a fairly characteristic peripheral or endobronchial appearance, whereas pulmonary secondary deposits are usually spherical,

Figure 3.97. Male patient aged 42 who had a small peripheral tumour which twice showed cavitation, with subsequent closure of the cavity. (a) Small peripheral cavitating lesion in right upper lobe. (b) Three months later, during anti-tuberculous chemotherapy, the cavity closed and the lesion became smaller. (c) Eight months later, and while continuing with chemotherapy, the lesion had again cavitated. (d) A month later a bronchogram showed no abnormality, but this was to be expected with a very peripheral lesion. (e) A tomogram following the bronchogram showed that the lesion was again no longer cavitated. The patient had a thoracotomy and a resection of the right upper lobe. Histology revealed a squamous cell carcinoma. Nine months later he was found to have mediastinal node enlargement

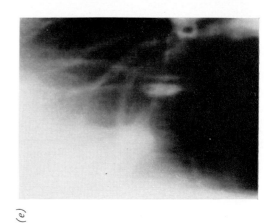

(e)

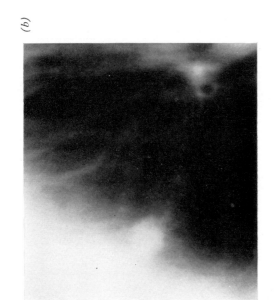

(b)

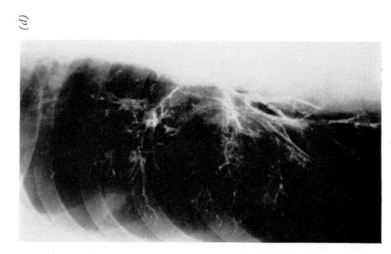

(d)

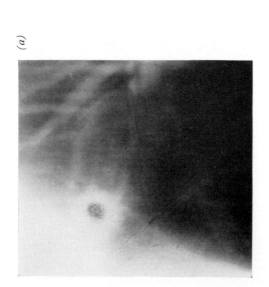

(a)

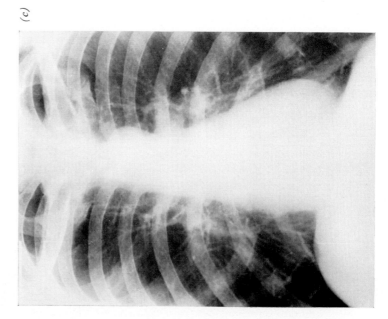

(c)

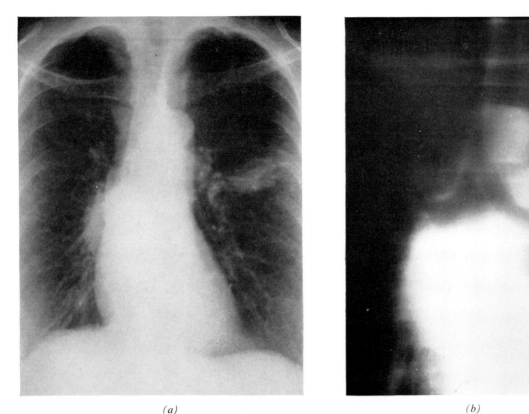

(a)   *(b)*

Figure 3.98. Synchronous bilateral bronchial neoplasms. (a) P.A. view shows peripheral mass in left upper lobe. (b) Inclined frontal tomogram shows a large mass behind right side of heart, situated in right lower lobe and extending into mediastinum

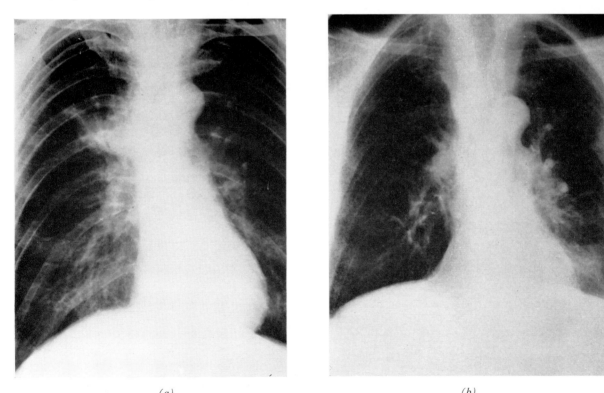

(a)   *(b)*

Figure 3.99. Metachronous bronchial carcinoma (the second tumour arising in the contralateral lung). (a) In 1958—collapse of anterior segment of right upper lobe; this was resected and the patient remained well until he developed his second tumour in 1965. (b) Collapse of left lower lobe due to the second tumour

the radiological appearances of two characteristic lesions are in favour of two primary tumours. In other cases with a metachronous appearance, the long interval—often several years—between the appearance of the tumours suggests the development of a fresh tumour (but *see* the discussion in Appendix 5 on the 'doubling time' of tumours, which could explain why metastases sometimes take a long time to become apparent). In some cases the demonstration of different histological types also supports the theory of multiple development of bronchial tumours, but this on its own is not absolute proof, since Willis (1953) found a heterogeneous or variable microscopic structure in 23 per cent of necropsy

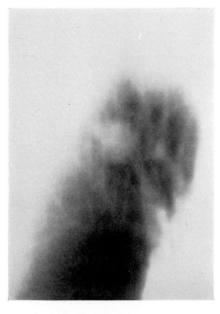

Figure 3.100. Metachronous primary bronchial carcinomas occurring in the same lung. (a) Small irregular peripheral tumour. The patient had a right upper lobectomy. (b) Five years later she had peripheral shadowing in the right middle lobe, but the significance of the bronchial occlusion seen on the bronchogram was not recognized. (c) Almost two years later an inclined frontal tomogram showed an obvious cavitating neoplasm. Note.—In the 400 consecutive cases listed in Appendix 4, there were 6 patients with probable double synchronous primary tumours and 3 with metachronous tumours. The author has also seen patients with three or more apparently primary lung tumours

(a)

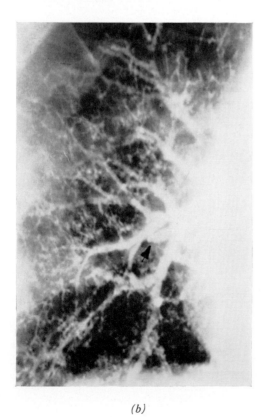

(b)

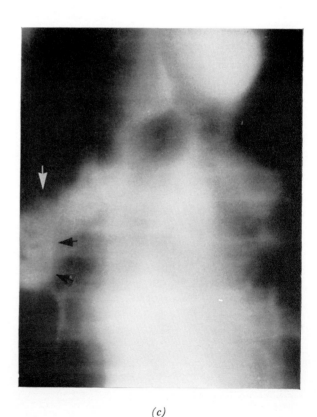

(c)

74

specimens. Examples of synchronous lung tumours appear in *Figure 3.98* and of metachronous tumours in *Figures 3.99* and *3.100*. Other cases with more than one primary lung tumour are shown in *Figures 3.43* and *8.28* (*see also* footnote to table A.3, page 224).

Metabolic effects and unusual presentation of bronchogenic tumours

Bronchial neoplasms may become manifest due to the primary tumour, to the presence of metastases, or to metabolic effects or degenerative changes in remote organs. Craig (1937) pointed out that hypertrophic pulmonary osteo-arthropathy*, often accompanied by finger or toe clubbing, is sometimes present at a relatively early stage of tumour growth (*Figure 3.101*). The periosteal reaction may be seen along the lower shafts of the radius and ulna, the femora, the tibia and fibula, and along the shafts of the

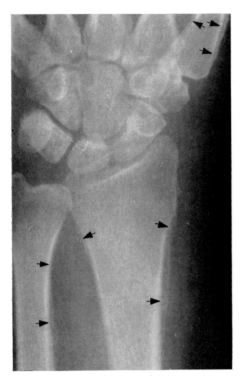
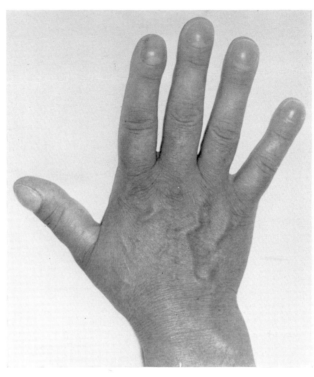

(a)   (b)

Figure 3.101. Patient with bronchiolar carcinoma who presented with finger clubbing (Hippocratic nails) and hypertrophic pulmonary osteo-arthropathy (Marie–Bamberger syndrome). See Figure 10.7 for other radiographs and a scintiscan of this patient. Hypertrophic pulmonary osteo-arthropathy may also be demonstrated at the ends of other long bones, e.g. femora, tibiae and fibulae

metacarpals and metatarsals. This, the Pierre Marie–Bamberger syndrome (Marie, 1890; Bamberger, 1890), may be accompanied by painful gynaecomastia (Court *et al.*, 1964) or by acromegalic features (Fried, 1948). An intrathoracic fibroma may also give rise to similar syndromes.

Other patients experience general malaise, loss of weight, neurological manifestations caused by cerebellar degeneration, peripheral motor, sensory or mixed neuropathy, or progressive myopathy. Other endocrine and metabolic disorders may also occur in association with bronchial carcinomas, such as hypercalcaemia, nocturia and Cushing's disease (Barden, 1967; Azzopardi, Freeman and Poole, 1970; Doyle, 1970) (*Figure 3.102*). Munro and Crompton (1972) have shown that the administration of intravenous cyclophosphamide may potentiate the secretion of anti-diuretic hormone and the loss of body sodium in patients with bronchial neoplasm.

* Hippocrates, c. 460–357 B.C., was probably the first to describe pulmonary osteo-arthropathy (οἱ ὄνυχες τῶν χειρῶν γρυπτοῦνται —the finger nails become bent), which he described in association with empyemas. Later such nails were considered to be pathognomonic of tuberculosis, but in the nineteenth century the specificity of 'Hippocratic nails' for tuberculosis was challenged and it became recognized that the phenomenon occurred in patients with cachexia and with circulatory and respiratory disturbances.

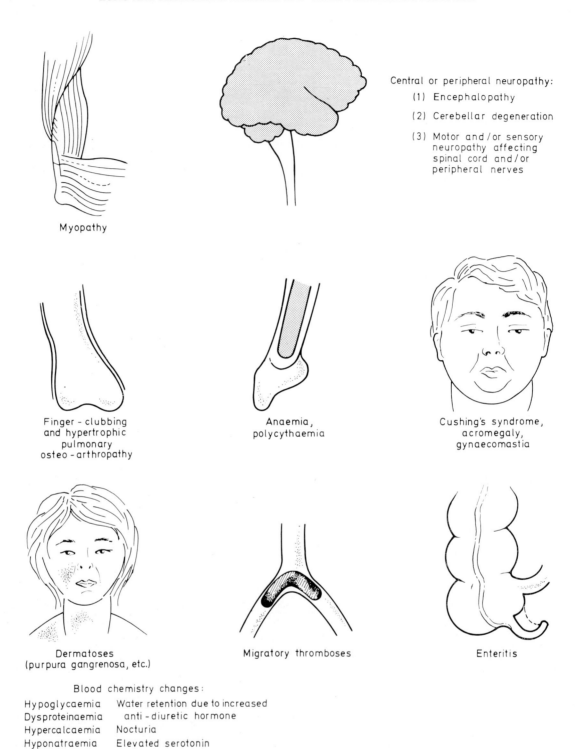

Myopathy

Central or peripheral neuropathy:

(1) Encephalopathy

(2) Cerebellar degeneration

(3) Motor and/or sensory neuropathy affecting spinal cord and/or peripheral nerves

Finger - clubbing and hypertrophic pulmonary osteo - arthropathy

Anaemia, polycythaemia

Cushing's syndrome, acromegaly, gynaecomastia

Dermatoses (purpura gangrenosa, etc.)

Migratory thromboses

Enteritis

Blood chemistry changes:

Hypoglycaemia	Water retention due to increased
Dysproteinaemia	anti-diuretic hormone
Hypercalcaemia	Nocturia
Hyponatraemia	Elevated serotonin

Figure 3.102. Some of the endocrine-like syndromes which may occur with bronchial carcinoma. Such effects may be produced by localized tumours which were not metastasized

For a discussion of various abdominal presentations of bronchogenic tumour, *see* Chapter 9, page 187.

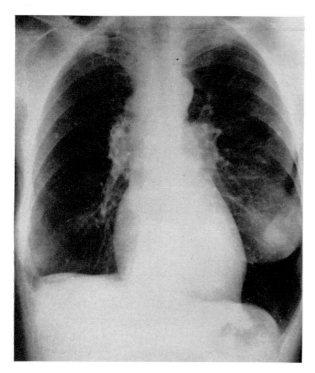

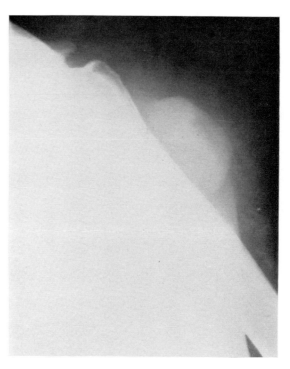

Figure 3.103. Small primary bronchogenic tumour in apex of right upper lobe which was clearly seen only on tomograms. There is enlargement of the azygos nodes and an elevated left breast caused by local extension of tumour into the breast from a rib metastasis. (Radiograph taken at 200 kV)

Figure 3.104. Soft tissue secondary deposit in region of subdeltoid bursa

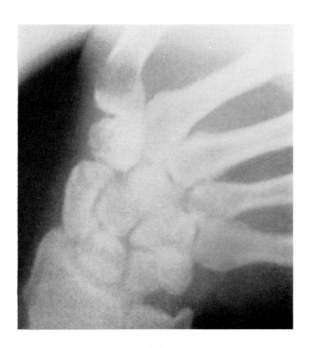

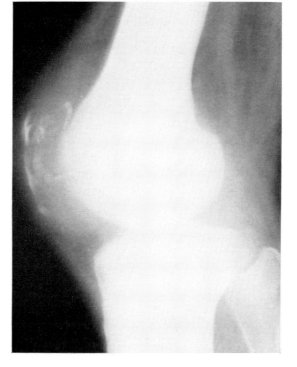

(a)

(b)

Figure 3.105. Bone metastases in unusual sites. (a) Metastasis in base of first metacarpal with pathological fracture. (b) Extensive metastasis in the patella

Abnormal superficial soft tissue shadows are sometimes produced by metastases (*Figures 3.103* and *3.104*), and metastases are occasionally the presenting feature in unusual bony sites such as the bones of the hand or the patella (*Figure 3.105*).

Can radiology predict the histological type of bronchogenic tumour?

Sometimes the histological type of a bronchial carcinoma may be suggested by its gross radiographic appearance. A squamous tumour tends to grow more slowly and to show cavitation with a large irregular cavity, often having a fairly well-defined outer wall, whereas anaplastic tumours frequently give rise to early lymph node involvement. Adenocarcinomas may also attain a large size and present as large spherical masses with well-defined smooth borders. However, there is a considerable overlap in the morphological appearance of all three types, and all may exhibit cavitation. Liebow (1955) tried to relate the pathology of such tumours to the 'roentgen shadow'. Although his classification has considerable merit, the problems are that (1) each of the cellular types may arise either centrally or peripherally; (2) all types may show cavitation; and (3) all types may give rise to nodal or other metastases and have varying rates of growth.

LESS COMMON LUNG AND PLEURAL TUMOURS

Bronchiolar or alveolar cell carcinoma

The radiological appearances of this tumour have been reviewed by Howells (1964) and Berkman (1969). This condition accounts for about 1–5 per cent of malignant lung tumours, the variation in the estimated incidence depending on the strictness of the diagnostic criteria. The sex incidence is about equal, compared with an average of five men to one woman in the case of bronchial carcinoma (*see* Appendix 2). In one form of the disease the patient may have copious gelatinous sputum, haemoptysis or dyspnoea.

The morphological resemblance of pulmonary adenomatosis, an epizootic disease of sheep (Jaagsiekte), to this condition has been discussed by Bonne (1939), Wood and Pierson (1945) and Fried (1948).

Woodruff, Ottman and Isaac (1958) pointed out that the lesion may be radiologically invisible when symptoms start. Spread occurs locally, giving rise to satellite nodules, infiltrates or a mass, and generally presenting a picture of wide dissemination throughout the lungs.

Some patients have an irregular, slowly growing nodule which may cavitate (Wormer, 1969). Others have a large area of infiltration or consolidation. Both these types of case may be suitable for surgical resection. A bronchogram may show a thin elongated bronchus with a 'leafless tree' appearance due to few side branches being filled (*see Figure 10.7*). Ciné and TV fluoroscopic studies will show that the bronchus does not alter in calibre with respiration—a non-specific appearance seen in other infiltrative conditions such as reticulosis and sarcoma (Zheutlin, Lasser and Rigler, 1954). Tomograms may show an air bronchogram within the lesion. Disseminated lesions may give rise to small, medium-sized or large nodules throughout the lungs. Lymphatic and pleural spread also occurs.

Figures 3.101, 3.106, 3.107 and *10.7* illustrate alveolar cell tumours.

Cylindromas and bronchial adenomas

These are a group of tumours originating in the tracheo-bronchial tree. They may be carcinoid, muco-epidermoid or adenocystic (cylindromatous) in type. They display slow local growth with later local spread to adjacent tissues and occasionally distant metastases. The adenocystic or cylindromatous type tends to be more common in the trachea and the larger bronchi.

In a series of 40 cases of bronchial adenoma reported by Zellos (1962), 26 patients had endobronchial tumours with secondary lung collapse and 14 had rounded peripheral lung opacities. In 13 patients there was spread of tumour to mediastinal nodes, and 2 had distant metastases in the liver. One patient exhibited the carcinoid syndrome. Twenty-three of the patients were women and 17 were men. Their ages ranged from 16 to 70 years (average 40 years). The 40 adenomas were encountered over a 12-year period during which 3,000 bronchial carcinomas were seen, representing an incidence of bronchial adenoma of 1·3 per cent. Other reports comparing the incidence of bronchial adenoma with that of bronchial carcinoma have varied from 8 per cent (Naclerio and Langer, 1948) to 2 per cent (Thomas, 1954). The latter found on reviewing the literature that the ratio of men to women was one to four, whereas his own figures gave only a slight female preponderance.

About half the patients with bronchial adenomas present with haemoptysis (Price Thomas gives 53 per cent). Dyspnoea may result from bronchial obstruction, or from bronchospasm either secondary to the tumour or due to associated endobronchial infection. Often patients are able to locate the tumour by the wheeze. Many have repeated attacks of infection which may lead to severe bronchial or lung damage

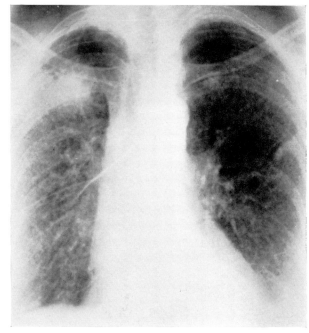

Figure 3.106 (right). Alveolar cell carcinoma. An irregular mass is present in the right upper lobe and there has been a miliary type of spread of tumour to both lungs. (Similar spread may occur with the more common bronchogenic carcinomas)

Figure 3.107 (below). Consolidating type of alveolar cell carcinoma. Radiograph (b) was taken three months later than (a)

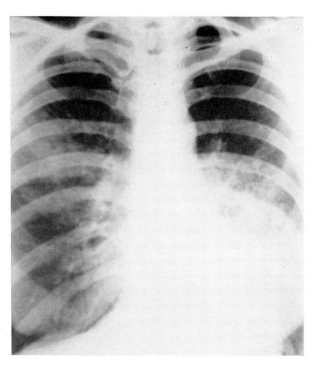

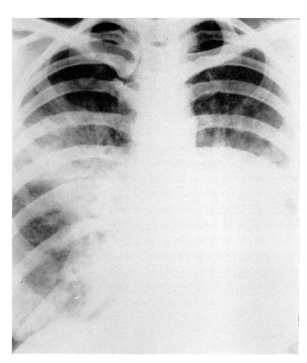

(a)　　　　　　　　　　　　　　　(b)

(McBurney, Claggett and McDonald, 1952). Peripheral adenomas themselves usually cause no symptoms.

In the various published series the right lung was affected twice as often as the left. The most common site was the right lower lobe. In Zellos' series, eight tumours arose in the right middle lobe.

The first diagnosis of an adenoma during life appears to have been by Kramer (1930), although the condition had been identified in autopsy specimens by Müller (1882), Heine (1927) and Reisner (1928). Kramer recognized that the tumour might undergo malignant change and that the patient might give a long history of his illness, a fact which he correlated with the slow growth of the tumour. A similar view was taken by Goldman (1949) and by Clerf and Crawford (1936). Fried (1947) described the tumour as benign and arising from the mucous glands of the bronchi. Hamperl (1937) distinguished two varieties of bronchial adenoma, the cylindroid and carcinoid types, and stated that the carcinoid type of bronchial adenoma, unlike the carcinoid tumour of the appendix, did not contain argentaffin cells. Holley (1946), Feyrter (1959) and Williams and Azzopardi (1960) have shown that this view is incorrect and that the carcinoid type of bronchial adenoma is a carcinoid tumour arising in a bronchus, little different from carcinoid tumours elsewhere in the body and capable of giving rise to the carcinoid syndrome. Holley divided his 38 cases into polypoid and carcinoid types; several showed features of malignancy, with local invasion and nodal or hepatic metastases. Occasionally a metastasizing bronchial adenoma associated with the carcinoid syndrome will give rise to osteoblastic metastases in bone, as reported by Pollard *et al.* (1962). Burcharth and Axelsson (1972) presented a series of 26 cases of adenomas and stated that these should be regarded as malignant tumours with a slower rate of growth and slower development of metastases than bronchogenic carcinomas.

At bronchoscopy the appearance of these tumours is often different from that of a bronchial carcinoma. The tumour may be sessile or pedunculated, or may be only partially endobronchial with a large portion of the tumour outside the bronchus (like the larger part of an iceberg lying invisible under the surface of the sea). The cylindromatous type of tumour may have a smoother surface and a paler colour and may bleed less readily than the carcinoid type. Like bronchial carcinomas, these tumours may be multiple in the lungs. The endobronchial adenomas commonly cause distal bronchiectasis.

Pulmonary adenomas are shown in *Figures 3.12*, *3.19*, *3.20*, *3.108–3.110*, *7.26*, *8.6* and *8.7*, and cylindromas in *Figures 3.112–3.114*. A very large lobulated adenoma is shown in *Figure 3.13*.

Hamartomas

A hamartoma was defined by Albrecht (1904) as a tumour-like formation in which there is an abnormal arrangement of the normal components of the organ from which it arises. The abnormality may take the form of a change in the quantity, in the arrangement or in the degree of differentiation of cell types, or may be a mixture of all three. Hamartomas are found in almost any organ of the body. In the lungs there are two types (Hochberg and Schachter, 1955)—the adult and the infant or newborn type. The adult type may appear as a small or large peripheral lung mass, or occasionally as an endobronchial lesion similar to an adenoma (*see Figure 3.115*, which shows a small hamartoma associated with segmental bronchiectasis). The newborn type is a massive diffuse process often occupying a lobe or even an entire lung.

Hamartomas are typically solitary, sharply delineated masses without any demonstrable change in the surrounding lung. They may be spherical or ovoid and are occasionally notched (Rigler's sign), giving an appearance similar to that of a peripheral bronchial carcinoma.

Calcification is relatively common in lung hamartomas, probably due to the large amount of cartilaginous tissue within them—a finding seldom encountered in other hamartomas such as those of the kidney, which usually contain muscular, vascular and fatty tissue elements (Wright *et al.*, 1973). Lung hamartomas may, like renal hamartomas, be very vascular and may show hypervascularity and a well marked blush when examined by bronchial arteriography (Botenga, 1970). Hickey and Simpson (1926) reported that when calcification was present in the 'popcorn' form it was usually diagnostic of a hamartoma (*see Figure 3.111*). The incidence of calcification has varied in reported series of these masses. Lemon and Good (1950) studied 17 hamartomas removed surgically at the Mayo Clinic and found calcification in 11 (65 per cent), although only 2 had the typical 'popcorn' appearance and only 6 showed calcification on plain films. In a further study of these masses at the Mayo Clinic (O'Keefe, Good and McDonald, 1957), again without tomograms, 11 out of 32 hamartomas showed calcification;

in 4 cases it was of the 'popcorn' type, and in 7 others there were small scattered areas of calcification. Bleyer and Marks (1957) found calcification in 15 per cent of cases. These authors also reported that 4 of their hamartomas had been present as round lesions in the lungs of patients with malignant disease. In 2 patients the same lobe contained both a bronchogenic carcinoma and a hamartoma, in a third case

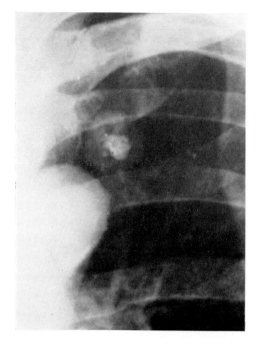

Figure 3.108 (left). Small rounded adenoma with calcified central area

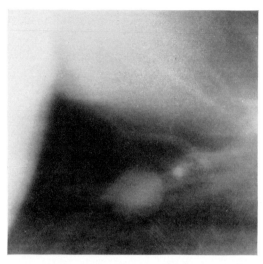

Figure 3.109. Small almost spherical tumour in left lower lobe, not containing any calcification, due to bronchial adenoma. (Bronchogram showed small smooth crescentic convex mass in posterior basic bronchus)

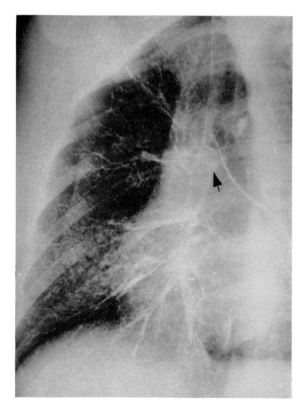

Figure 3.110. Small rounded adenoma in right main bronchus, not causing any bronchial obstruction

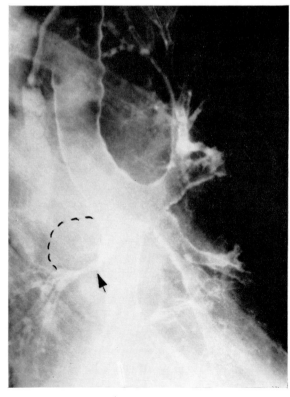

Figure 3.111. Extrinsic pressure on apical segmental bronchus of left lower lobe by rounded, almost completely extrabronchial adenoma

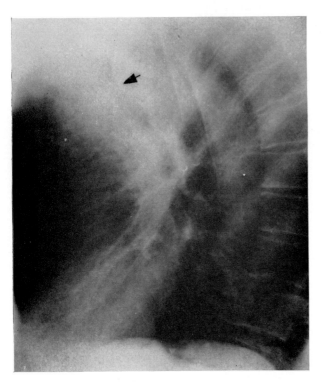 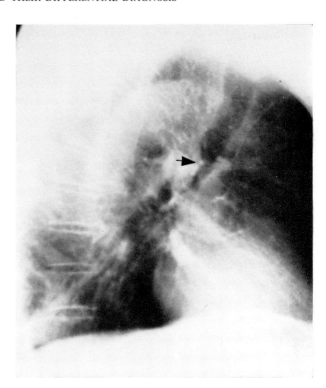

Figure 3.112 (left). Carcinoma of trachea. The patient had had three previous radiographic examinations which were regarded as normal. The trachea is narrowed and bowed anteriorly by a fairly large soft tissue mass formed by extension of tumour posteriorly into superior mediastinum. P.A. view appeared normal

Figure 3.113 (right). Small tumour of lower trachea, seen as small mass projecting into airway in lateral view at level of carina. P.A. view appeared normal

Note.—Very careful scrutiny of a radiograph is required to detect such lesions

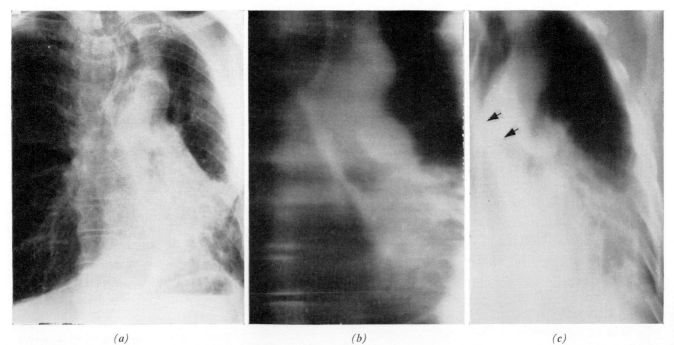

| (a) | (b) | (c) |

Figure 3.114. Cylindroma of left main bronchus with collapse of left lower lobe and lingula. Tomograms, (b) inclined frontal and (c) conventional longitudinal, show large rounded mass in the left main bronchus arising from its upper wall. There was no evidence of any soft tissue mass outside the bronchus. The patient had a sleeve resection of the left main bronchus, and the left lung showed good re-expansion

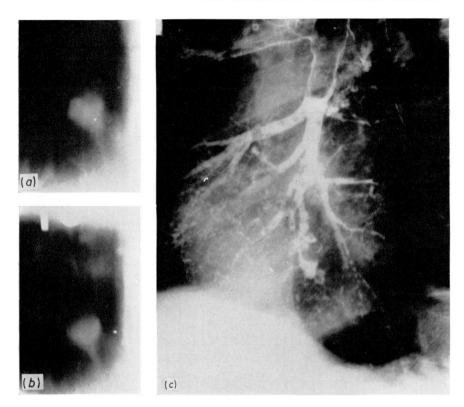

Figure 3.115. Small hamartoma containing a little calcification in medial basic segment of right lower lobe, associated with localized bronchiectasis in this segment. (a) and (b) Conventional tomograms. (c) Bronchogram

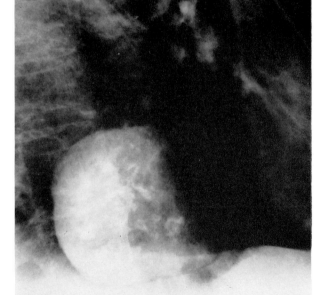

Figure 3.116. 'Popcorn' type of calcification in a fairly large hamartoma

the same lobe contained both a metastatic tumour and a hamartoma, whilst in the fourth patient a carcinoma of the oesophagus was accompanied by a hamartoma in the left lower lobe.

As with hamartomas elsewhere in the body, malignant change may occasionally ensue (*Figure 3.117*). A similar case was described by Barnard (1952), who termed it an embryoma of the lung*. Another

* Spencer (1968), however, classified an embryoma as a separate entity.

patient in my series, a man aged 30, initially had no more than a small round focus. This was thought to be a tuberculoma, but the patient developed an enlarged hilum and other nodules in the lung. Pathology revealed a malignant mesenchymoma. Malignant change in lung hamartomas is, however, unusual, most authors stating that these growths are always benign.

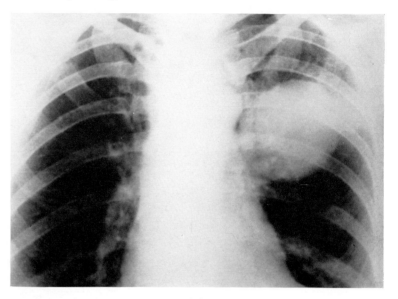

(a)

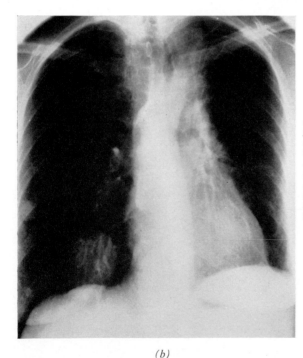

(b)

Figure 3.117. Pulmonary mesenchymoma or embryoma of lung. The patient, a woman aged 42, had a left upper lobectomy for a rounded tumour in the left upper lobe (a). At this time the smaller mass in the right lower lobe had not been recognized. The tumour showed cystic spaces lined by columnar epithelium, lying on a rather primitive-looking stroma. Four years later there were three masses in the right lung (b). Six years after this (1971) she remained well apart from eye trouble due to glaucoma, and had refused to have her chest radiographed since 1965. It is uncertain whether the masses in the right lung are metastases or multiple primary tumours. (See also Barnard, 1952)

Hamartomas of the lung have been variously reported as papillomas, fibro-adenomas, mixed tumours, chondromas, adenochondromas and lipochondromas (Stein and Poppel, 1955). Ramchand and Baskerville (1969) reported the presence of multiple hamartomas in the same lung. Multiple small hamartomas may produce a coarse miliary pattern in about 5 per cent of patients with tuberose sclerosis.

Chondromas, lipomas, chemodectomas, neurofibromas and myomas

These are uncommon tumours of the lung, giving rise to mass lesions in the lungs or bronchi. Some of them, particularly leiomyomas and leiomyosarcomas, may like the 'chondromas' really be hamartomas derived from the bronchial wall. They may be single or multiple and may show expansive growth. When they are large, their centres may undergo necrosis and cavitate. All masses which contain cartilaginous tissue tend to show calcification, and this is particularly true of pulmonary hamartomas.

Benign lung tumours have been studied by Randall and Blades (1946) and by Freireich, Bloomberg and Langs (1951). Sherman and Malone (1950) described a patient presenting with multiple asymptomatic round leiomyomatous masses throughout the lungs, and Sargent, Barnes and Schwinn (1970) found seven other cases in the literature and reported another of their own. These all occurred in women aged between 35 and 60 years. A similar case is shown in *Figure 3.118*. Robbins (1954) also discussed the radiographic appearances of benign lung tumours. A chemodectoma of the pulmonary artery is shown in *Figure 7.45*, and a chemodectoma of the aorta in *Figure 7.18*. Both tumours probably arose from chemoreceptive tissues.

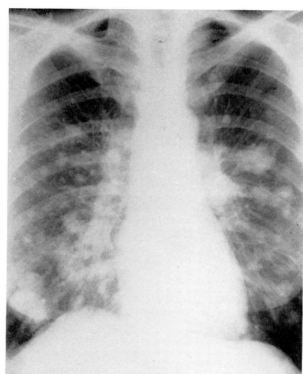

Figure 3.118. Multiple tumours in both lungs which were found on biopsy to be benign myomas

Reticulosis

A lymphosarcoma may appear as an area of consolidation or infiltration with rigid though patent bronchi (Baron and Whitehouse, 1961). Secondary reticulosis (for example, Hodgkin's disease) of the lung may show a similar appearance or may produce rounded shadows resembling other metastases. Dahlgren and Overfors (1969) reported a primary malignant lymphoma of the lung which had a ten-year course. There was a rounded, poorly delineated infiltration which later broke down to give a cystic appearance.

Figure 8.31 shows a patient who had a lobectomy for a lymphosarcoma of the right upper lobe and has survived for ten years without any sign of recurrence. Another example of a primary lung reticulosis appears in *Figure 10.32*. The author has also seen a pulmonary reticulosis presenting as a 2 cm 'coin' lesion.

Pleural tumours

The most common pleural tumour is a metastasis, and the most usual source of such a metastasis is a primary tumour of the lung. Le Roux (1962) thought not only that primary pleural tumours were rare but that their origin from the pleura could be disputed. He assessed 3,000 patients investigated in Edinburgh over a ten-year period and found that 220 of these were shown at thoracoscopy, thoracotomy or necropsy to have pleural metastases, as distinct from pleural invasion in continuity with either the primary tumour or mediastinal glandular metastases. Of the 220 patients with pleural metastases from bronchial carcinoma, 80 per cent died within six months of the diagnosis having been established and none survived for twelve months. In the same ten-year period, Le Roux found 16 patients with what he termed 'so-called primary pleural tumours'. In 9 of these patients the radiographic abnormality was a

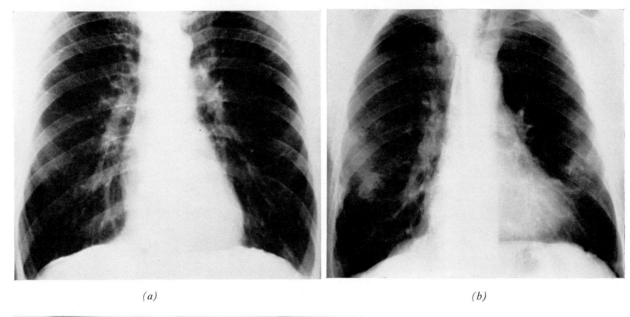

(a)   *(b)*

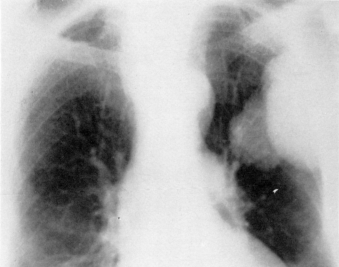

Figure 3.119 (above). Pleural calcification secondary to asbestosis. (a) Bilateral basal pleural calcification. (b) Multiple areas of pleural calcification in both mid zones and at left base. Notes.—(1) Localized oblique views may also be taken to show such plaques to advantage. (2) Asbestosis may also cause pulmonary fibrosis, which may be severe. The author has seen this in wives who have been washing, and presumably shaking, their husbands' overalls and in persons who have lived close to an asbestos factory

Figure 3.120 (left). Fairly large left-sided mesothelioma which mimics a bronchogenic tumour. The patient had been exposed to asbestos in the lagging of railway engines. Asbestos bodies were found in the lung. Asbestos may also be a predisposing factor in the development of a bronchogenic tumour

pleural shadow suggestive of a pleural effusion, and in all these cases the diagnosis of a mesothelioma was made on histological grounds, a diagnosis of fibrosarcoma being offered as an alternative in one case. In the remaining 7 cases the radiographic abnormality was a single, well circumscribed peripheral opacity; 3 of these were fibrosarcomas and 4 were fibromas.

Two types of primary pleural tumour—a fibromatous type and a group described as mesothelioma—were recognized by Klemperer and Rabin (1931) and by Clagett, McDonald and Schmidt (1952), who considered that the two groups were distinguishable by the circumscription of the one and the diffuseness of the other. Stout and Murray (1942) thought that an intrathoracic fibroma was a localized form of pleural mesothelioma. This tumour as well as bronchial neoplasm may be associated with hypertrophic pulmonary osteo-arthropathy.

Radiologically the tumours may present as localized masses, either small or large, within the pleura (overlying the lung) or in an interlobar fissure. The masses may be accompanied by a pleural effusion.

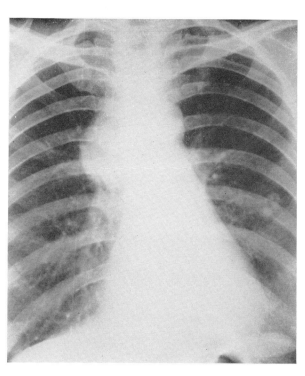

Figure 3.121. Female patient with meso-thelioma which appeared on medial side of right lung. Calcification can be seen in a pleural plaque in left mid zone. The patient's sister also developed a mesothelioma, but of the peritoneum. Both sisters had asbestosis from making asbestos table and oven mats. Radiograph (b) was taken 9 months after (a). Note.—'Blue' asbestos (crocidolite) appears to be much more pathogenic than 'white' (chrysolite or amosite)

(a)

(b)

In many cases they are associated with asbestosis and pulmonary fibrosis. Plaques of pleural thickening and calcification may also be present and may precede the tumour by many years (*Figure 3.119*).

A radiological review of diseases and tumours of serosal surfaces was carried out by Samuel (1969), who thought that more mesotheliomas had been misdiagnosed as bronchial carcinomas than vice versa. The association of asbestosis with serosal malignancy was noted by Gloyne (1933), who was the first to publish two reports of pleural and peritoneal mesotheliomas complicating asbestosis. Keal (1960) reported a series of 26 female patients with asbestosis: in 4 of them the disease was complicated by lung cancer, in 9 by intra-abdominal neoplasms and in 4 by peritoneal metastases of ovarian cancer. Wagner, Sleggs and Marchland (1960) collected a series of 120 patients who had had diffuse mesotheliomas of the pleura and had all been exposed to asbestos. In this series there were also some peritoneal mesotheliomas.

Examples of pleural tumours are given in *Figures 3.52* and *3.120–122*.

At present the incidence of mesothelioma appears to be increasing, as is the annual industrial consumption of asbestos (Lawther, 1971; Wagner *et al.*, 1971). The interval between exposure and the development of a tumour may be very long, in some cases up to 40 years. Asbestosis not only occurs in

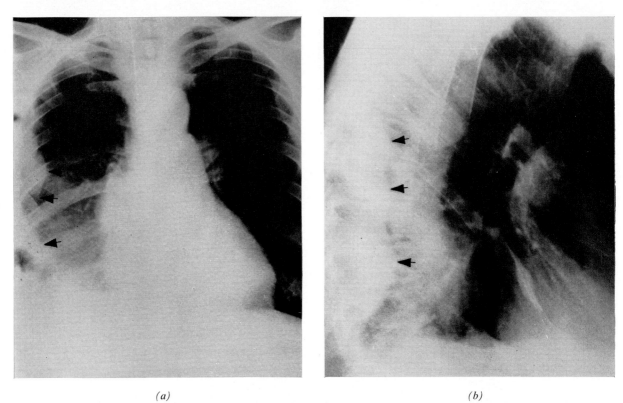

(a)   *(b)*

Figure 3.122. '*Knobbly' pleural thickening on right side of chest, extending into lower part of oblique fissure caused by a mesothelioma*

those who actually work with asbestos or its products but may affect others working near them and even people living near asbestos factories, due to the escape of asbestos particles into the atmosphere.

MEDIASTINAL MASSES AND TUMOURS OF THE CHEST WALL

MEDIASTINAL MASSES

Mediastinal masses may arise from any of the various types of tissue within the mediastinum. They may be tumours *per se*, cystic swellings or dilated vascular structures; they may be due to a hernia, to a dilated oesophagus, or to an abscess or other fluid collection, or they may be secondary to a neoplasm arising either within the chest or outside it. As Grainger and Pierce (1969) point out, the relative incidence of the different mediastinal masses is difficult to determine because many of the reported large series do not include inflammatory and parasitic masses, aneurysms, mediastinal goitres or metastatic tumours. Excluding these conditions, a series of 1,200 patients gave the following approximate incidence: neurogenic tumours 30 per cent, thymic tumours 20 per cent, lymphomas 10 per cent, teratodermoid cysts 10 per cent and endodermal cysts 10 per cent, the remaining 20 per cent consisting of a few examples each of many unusual tumours.

The mediastinum is defined as the space which lies between the medial surfaces of the parietal pleura of the two lungs, extending from the sternum anteriorly to the dorsal spine behind. Anatomists divide it into (1) the superior mediastinum, lying above a plane through the manubrio-sternal joint and the fifth dorsal vertebra, and (2) the inferior mediastinum, which is subdivided into the narrow anterior mediastinum (anterior to the pericardium), the posterior mediastinum (behind the posterior pericardial surface) and the middle mediastinum containing the heart, great vessels, lower trachea and main bronchi. From the radiological diagnostic point of view, however, the location of a mass within the mediastinum is of prime importance in the differential diagnosis. A classification on this basis is given in Table 3.2, where superior mediastinal masses are included in the anterior, middle or posterior mediastinum according to their position in the sagittal plane of the chest.

TABLE 3.2

Masses and Tumours of the Mediastinum

Site	Lesion
Anterior mediastinum Superiorly	Retrosternal thyroid Parathyroid tumour Thymic tumour or cyst Enlarged lymph nodes in reticulosis Neurogenic tumour Aneurysm of internal mammary artery
In middle portion	Dermoid cyst Teratoma
Inferiorly	Pericardial fat pad Pericardial cyst Hernia of liver, omentum, colon, stomach or small bowel through foramen of Morgagni

Middle mediastinum	Mediastinal or hilar lymphadenopathy due to various
	  causes including tuberculosis, reticulosis, sarcoidosis and
	  secondary neoplasm
	Mediastinal abscess or blood collection
	Aneurysm of arch of aorta
	Bronchogenic cyst
	Tumour of oesophagus
	Neuro-enteric cyst
	Neurogenic tumour

Posterior mediastinum	Dilated oesophagus, especially due to achalasia of cardia Oesophageal diverticulum Oesophageal tumour Mediastinal abscess or fluid collection Hiatus hernia or neuro-enteric cyst Enlarged para-oesophageal lymph nodes Hernia through foramen of Bochdalek Aneurysm of descending aorta Neurogenic tumour Paravertebral swelling Lateral thoracic meningocoele

Anterior mediastinal masses

These tumours may lie within the anterior mediastinum proper or in the anterior portion of the superior compartment. When small in size, such masses may be hidden on a postero-anterior radiograph, and will be more readily seen on lateral views in the position of the normal increased retrosternal transradiancy. With large tumours there may be blurring of the definition of the anterior border of the heart as well as displacement, bowing and narrowing of the trachea and occasionally bulging of the sternum.

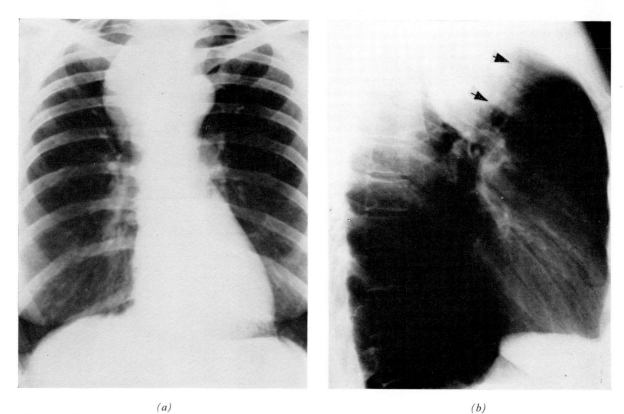

(a)   *(b)*

Figure 3.123. Large superior mediastinal goitre. In approximately one-third of cases the goitre lies behind the trachea (arrowed) as it does in this patient

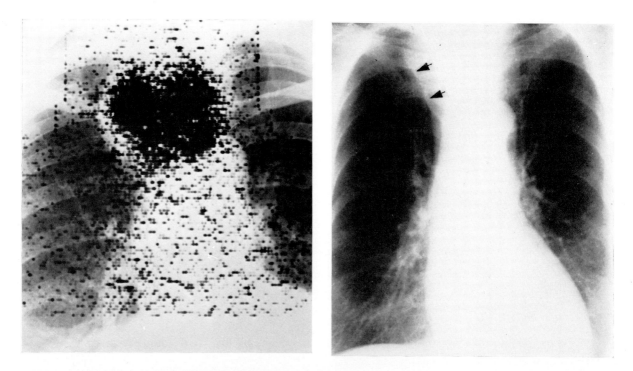

Figure 3.124 (left). Retromanubrial goitre. In this instance the mass has taken up a radioactive isotope ($^{99}TcO_4$, which has similar properties to halogens) and is a functioning goitre. More often a retrosternal goitre is non-functioning and does not take up the isotope, a normal thyroid usually being present in the neck

Figure 3.125 (right). Retrosternal parathyroid mass.

Retrosternal goitre

A retrosternal goitre is a common upper anterior mediastinal mass (*Figures 3.123* and *3.124*). It usually lies anterior to the trachea, frequently displacing and narrowing it. It may contain calcification. Occasionally it lies posterior to the trachea in the middle mediastinum. If not fixed because of its size, it may move upwards on swallowing. Unfortunately many retrosternal goitres are not hormonally active and a scintiscan is often unremarkable, showing a normal thyroid in the neck and no uptake in the tumour (using ^{131}I, ^{132}I or ^{99m}Tc as TcO_4, which behaves as a halogen). Angiography is sometimes of value in demonstrating an enlarged inferior thyroid artery in association with an enlarged avascular mass (Feldman *et al.*, 1969; Rossi, Tracht and Ruzicka, 1971).

Retrosternal parathyroid tumours

A parathyroid tumour may rarely give a similar appearance (*Figure 3.125*) and may take up increased amounts of ^{75}Se-labelled selenomethionine. The problem with this technique is that the affinity of the tumour for selenomethionine is not great and the adjacent bony tissues, such as the sternum, may take up more isotope than the parathyroid mass. Fewer than 10 per cent of parathyroid tumours in the neck can be reliably identified by using selenomethionine.

Dudley (1971) has shown that parathyroids and parathyroid tumours in the neck are readily found at exploratory operations by giving the patient a blue dye such as methylene blue pre-operatively. The parathyroids and their tumours selectively take up the blue dye and are easily recognized. Such dyes, as well as Evans blue and toluidine blue, contain a sulphur atom, but this is in an SH grouping, and as both the colour and the specificity of the uptake seem to depend on this SH group, the replacement of S by ^{75}Se may make the dye inactive. The Radiochemical Centre has not yet been successful in the substitution of ^{75}Se for S in this dye, but Yeh, de la Hay and Kriss (1968) have managed to label the dye with ^{99m}Tc and have used it for liver scanning. Further work on these lines is proceeding.

Angiography may also be helpful in the demonstration of parathyroid masses, usually adenomas but also carcinomas, which mostly show as vascular structures with a well marked vascular blush (Seldinger, 1954; Doppman *et al.*, 1969; Rossi, Tracht and Ruzicka, 1971). Shimkin *et al.* (1972) used retrograde thyroid venography in the demonstration of parathyroid adenomas. Samuels, Dowdy and Lecky (1972) have found thermography (detecting infra-red heat radiations) extremely valuable in the location of parathyroid tumours.

Thymic masses

Thymic masses may be of three types.

(1) The normal infant thymus. This often shows as an extensive well-defined opacity in the anterior and superior mediastinum—which may be incorrectly interpreted as an abnormal mass (the 'sail-like' shadow described by Kemp, Morely and Emrys-Roberts, 1948). This opacity may be more prominent in expiration, since in young babies the relative size of the lungs will then be decreased, also causing the well-known spurious cardiac enlargement seen only in expiration. The opacity may also be more prominent on a lordotic view or on slight rotation of the child.

(2) Thymic cysts or tumours. The latter are often associated with myasthenia gravis, about 20 per cent of patients with this condition having a thymic tumour.

(3) Enlarged lymph nodes in the region of the thymus (internal mammary nodes) due to reticulosis (*Figures 3.126* and *7.43*), sarcoidosis, secondary neoplasm or occasionally leukaemia. A cystic hygroma of the neck or arm may be associated with a lymphatic cyst of the mediastinum, or the latter may occur on its own. Such a cyst may be very large, with convex or lobulated borders which change in shape with respiration. They may also be associated with chylous pleural effusions.

As already mentioned, small anterior mediastinal masses, particularly those arising in the thymus, may be invisible on postero-anterior radiographs of the chest, and oblique or lateral views and oblique or lateral tomograms will often demonstrate them best (*Figures 3.127* and *3.128*). A large lobulated tumour is well shown by inclined frontal tomograms in *Figure 3.129*, and examples of transverse axial tomograms are given in *Figures 7.8* and *7.9*. Gas mediastinography (*see* Chapter 10 and *Figures 10.21* and *10.22*) may be used to demonstrate these tumours.

A thymic mass may lie at any vertical level in the superior or anterior mediastinum, but is most commonly situated behind the upper sternum. It may be spherical, ovoid, lobulated, triangular or plaque-like in shape. Occasionally faint linear or nodular calcification may be seen. A mass with a peripheral rim of calcification is more likely to be a dermoid cyst. If the mass is sufficiently large, it will project beyond the lateral borders of the normal mediastinum and show as a rounded or lobulated mass on the postero-anterior film. Sometimes angiography will help in defining a thymic tumour (*Figure 7.8*). Selective thymic venography (Kreel, 1967; Yune and Klatte, 1970) has also been employed for the diagnosis of thymic tumours. Yune and Klatte used a transfemoral approach to reach the thymic vein of Keynes and stated that this procedure can be performed safely even in patients with severe myasthenia gravis, in contrast to pneumo-mediastinography which often aggravates the patient's respiratory difficulty.

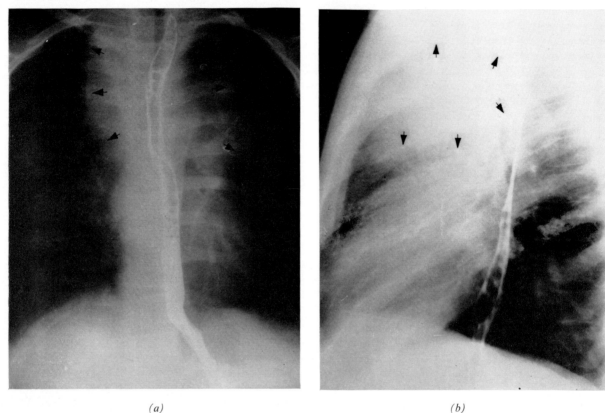

(a)   (b)

Figure 3.126. Marked enlargement of anterior mediastinal lymph nodes in region of thymus in a child, caused by reticulosis (Hodgkin's disease)

Dermoid cysts and teratomas

Dermoid cysts and teratomas, including seminomas of the mediastinum, should be considered as a single group, since all these tumours are derived from multipotential embryonic cells. In the dermoid, ectodermal (or skin) tissues predominate, but mesodermal and endodermal tissues are also present. The dermoid cysts tend to be well demarcated and often contain a peripheral rim of calcification (*Figure 3.130*), whilst the teratomas or seminomas may not have a capsule. These latter in particular may spread through the mediastinum. These lesions may be malignant, may become infected, and may rupture into the pleura, pericardium, mediastinum or lung.

These tumours usually cause no symptoms. They may rarely display a tooth or bone element within them or be relatively radiolucent due to their fat or cholesterol content, such features being more commonly seen in dermoid tumours of the ovary.

Pericardial cysts

Pericardial ('spring-water') cysts may be true independent cysts or diverticula of the pericardium. They most frequently occur in the anterior cardio-phrenic angles and are usually ovoid or spherical,

92

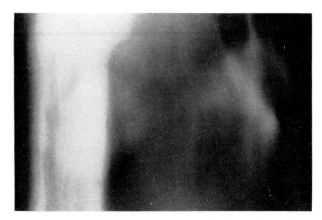

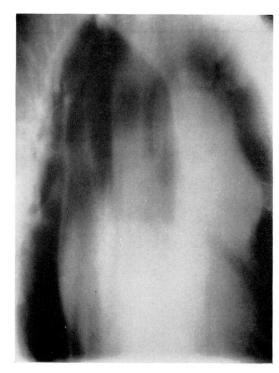

Figure 3.127 (above). Lateral tomogram showing a fairly small, somewhat lobulated thymoma in a patient with myasthenia gravis. (The tumour lies anteriorly and to the left)

Figure 3.128 (right). Fairly large thymic tumour with smooth outline. Tomogram taken in oblique projection

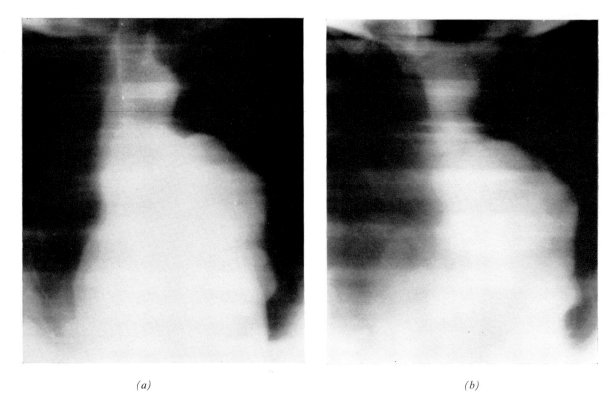

(a)   (b)

Figure 3.129. Inclined frontal tomograms showing very large and lobulated thymoma. The tomograms demonstrated that the mass extended to the midline and not beyond it, so that it was possible to remove the tumour through a left-sided thoracotomy

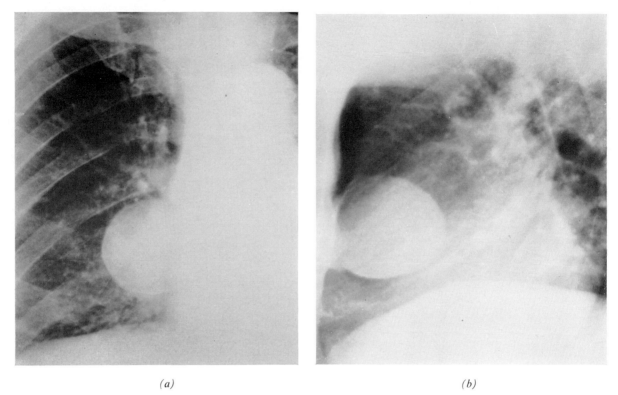

(a)   *(b)*

Figure 3.130. Dermoid cyst in anterior mediastinum alongside the heart. The cyst has a thin line of calcium in its wall

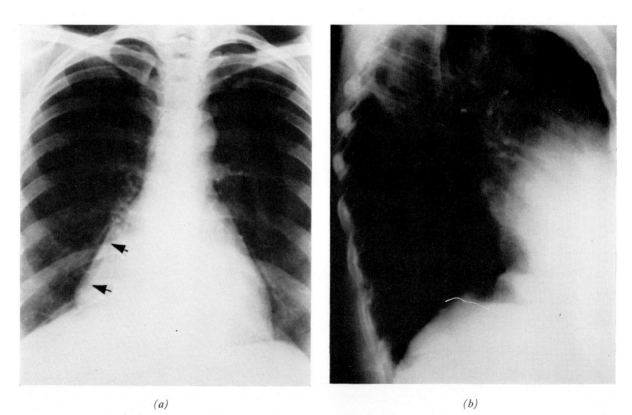

(a)   *(b)*

Figure 3.131. Large pericardial fat pad at right base. A similar appearance is found in some patients with reticulosis producing a para-cardiac mass

though this shape may change with respiration or be altered by the patient's posture. Rarely a small area of fat may be present between the cyst and the pericardium. Pericardial cysts are shown in *Figures 7.6* and *10.22*. (Edwards and Ahmed, 1972, described and reviewed intrapericardial cysts.)

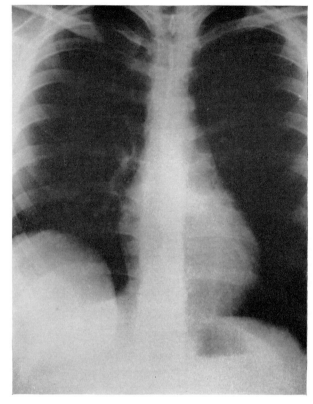

Figure 3.132. Large right-sided and anterior herniation or eventration of the diaphragm. Liver and spleen scan was carried out using ^{113m} *In colloid*

(a)

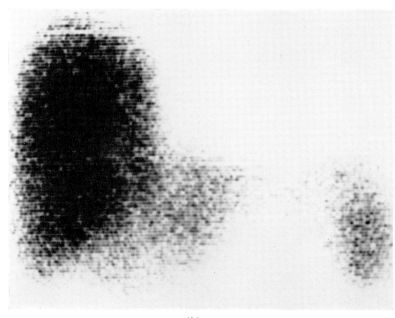

(b)

95

Fatty masses

Fatty masses are often seen in obese patients in the form of triangular pericardial fat pads in the anterior cardio-phrenic angles. Usually these are so characteristic in appearance that their nature is obvious (*Figure 3.131*), but errors sometimes occur when the fat pads are more readily seen in the lateral view and are mistaken for lung or mediastinal tumours. When they are present in thin patients, the more transradiant fatty tissue (compared with the water density of the heart) may occasionally be noted. Gramiak and Koerner (1966) pointed out that fatty tumours are often pliable and may change their shape with respiration. Rarely, true lipomas or liposarcomas may occur, particularly on the diaphragm or in the anterior mediastinum, and these may become very large.

Several authors, including Koerner and Sun (1966), Price and Rigler (1970) and Taetes (1970), have described abnormal fat collections in the mediastinum and mediastinal widening following steroid therapy. Fayos and Lampre (1971) have shown that a fat pad over the apex of the heart is sometimes mimicked by masses caused by Hodgkin's disease.

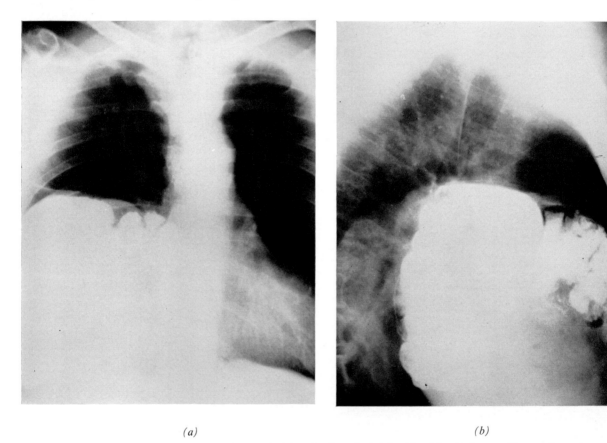

(a)   *(b)*

Figure 3.133. Patient with a large Morgagni hernia which simulated a raised right side of the diaphragm. These radiographs were taken about 6 hours after a barium meal and show the colon opacified by the barium

Transdiaphragmatic hernias

A Morgagni hernia takes place through the defect between the septum transversum and the costal portion of the diaphragm. It may contain bowel, omentum or liver. If bowel is present, gas may be seen in the loop, or barium after a barium meal or enema. Omentum or liver may simulate an intrathoracic mass, in which case a liver scan may demonstrate the liver herniation (*Figure 3.132*).

Similar considerations apply to other hernias through the diaphragm—for example, a post-traumatic hernia, or a Bochdalek hernia (*see also* page 103) occurring posteriorly through an unobliterated pleuroperitoneal canal. On the left side the spleen may herniate into the chest and the nature of this mass may be recognized by scintiscanning, using erythrocytes damaged by heat or an organic mercurial (benzyl-mercuri-hydroxypropane), labelled with [57]Cr or preferably [197]Hg.

Tumours of the retrosternal premediastinal space

Pfister, Oh and Ferrucci (1970) have pointed out that between the sternum and the parietal pleura lies a distinct group of anatomical structures—the 'transverse thoracic muscle', the internal mammary arteries, veins and lymphatics, the intercostal nerve fibres and connective tissues—and that masses or vascular dilations may arise from any of these. Scheff and Laforet (1966) and Shopfner, Jansen and O'Kell (1968) discussed the significance of the shadow produced on a lateral radiograph by the transverse thoracic muscle, especially if the radiograph is slightly 'off lateral', and felt that this shadow should not be diagnosed as abnormal (*Figure 3.134*). Similar shadows due to the intercostal muscles are sometimes seen in relation to the ribs.

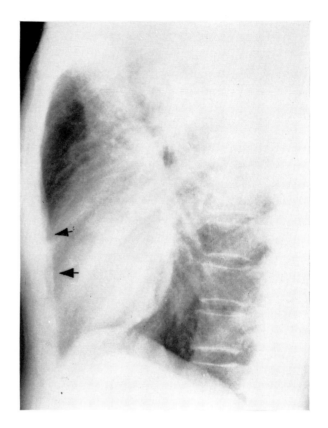

Figure 3.134. Vertical retrosternal shadow caused by transverse thoracic muscle

Neurofibromas may arise from nerve fibres, and a bizarre appearance may be given by dilations (sometimes calcified) of the intercostal arteries in association with coarctation of the aorta (*see* Stern, Richardson and Wolfe, 1970, and *Figure 10.10*).

Middle mediastinal masses

Enlarged lymph nodes

The most frequent abnormal masses in the middle mediastinum are enlarged paratracheal, tracheo-bronchial, hilar, retrocarinal or subcarinal lymph nodes. The enlargement may be caused by *neoplasm* (particularly bronchogenic neoplasm), reticulosis, inflammatory disease, sarcoidosis, or occasionally leukaemia or extramedullary haemopoiesis. This mediastinal enlargement may be seen on plain radiographs, especially those which are well penetrated and taken with high kV (*see* section on peripheral lung masses, page 16); it is better demonstrated on tomograms (*see* Chapter 7); or it may be inferred from displacement of the oesophagus as shown by barium swallow (or air—*see* Chapter 7) or from displacement of the opacified superior vena cava (*see* Chapter 10).

In enlargements due to *reticulosis*, the paratracheal nodes are the most frequently involved and their enlargement may be the sole apparent abnormality. On the right the paratracheal or azygos nodes may project as a well-defined shadow from the right border of the superior mediastinum (*see Figures 3.103* and *7.30*), whilst on the left the enlarged paratracheal nodes cause a convex opacity above the aortic knuckle with which the latter may appear to be continuous (*see Figure 7.31*). When massively enlarged, these nodes project with convex, straight or lobulated lateral margins to form a wide superior mediastinal shadow, and this enlargement may spread forward into the thymic region so that the normal retrosternal transradiancy becomes lost. In reticuloses the tracheo-bronchial and hilar lymph nodes tend to be affected later than the paratracheal group.

Sarcoidosis and erythema nodosum are common causes of mediastinal lymphadenopathy, and here the hilar enlargement is more often bilateral. Such enlarged hilar nodes tend to produce a bulky hilum with a well-defined convex or lobulated border which does not continue into the pulmonary vessels (*see Figures 7.34–7.37*).

Bacterial pneumonia may give rise to enlarged hilar nodes as shown in *Figure 7.38* and *7.39*, although

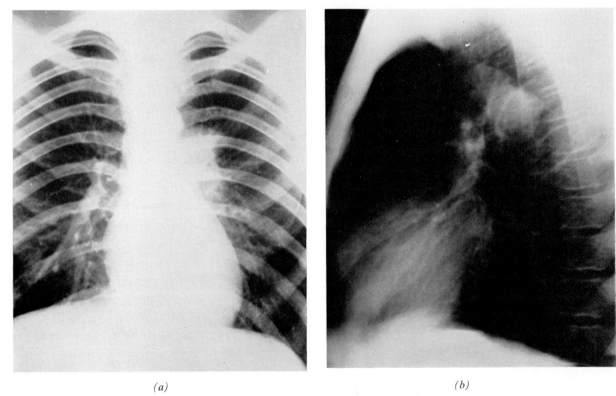

(a)   (b)

Figure 3.135. Small bronchogenic cyst overlying the arch of the aorta in lateral view (compare with Figure 7.17). Note.—Occasionally a bronchogenic cyst may rupture and then contain air

this cause of nodal enlargement is frequently not appreciated. *Tuberculosis* may produce mediastinal enlargement in children and in some adults because of either enlarged glands or an associated abscess. Similarly, glandular fever and other virus infections may result in hilar and mediastinal lymphadeno-pathy.

Vascular structures

Aneurysms of the aorta or its branches may give rise to mediastinal masses which closely resemble mediastinal tumours. The difficulty of distinguishing between these conditions is illustrated in Chapter 7 (*see Figures 7.11–7.19*). An *aneurysm of a sinus of Valsalva* may produce a mediastinal opacity. The *azygos vein* is usually seen as a rounded opacity on the right side of the superior mediastinum opposite the aortic arch and, when dilated, may cause confusion with the diagnosis of nodal enlargement. *Pulmonary artery dilation* and its differentiation from enlarged hilar nodes and masses is discussed in Chapters 7 and 10. A tumour may rarely develop in the aortic wall or in that of the pulmonary artery as shown in *Figures 7.18* and *7.45*. A previous description of a chemodectoma of the mediastinum was given by Mapp *et al.*, 1969.

High quality, adequately exposed radiographs are required to demonstrate aortic swellings due to aneurysms of the lower descending aorta behind the heart (*see* Chapter 7). The left lateral border of the descending aorta is more easily demonstrated than the medial and right border, the latter being shown only by the position of the medial border of the right pleural cavity which normally lies just to the left of the midline. In addition, mediastinal haematomas may be seen by displacing the medial borders of the pleural cavities where they overlie the spine and the descending aorta.

A recent review of the appearances of thoracic aortic aneurysms on plain radiographs and aortograms but not on tomograms has been carried out in 40 African patients by Le Roux, Rogers and Gotsman (1971).

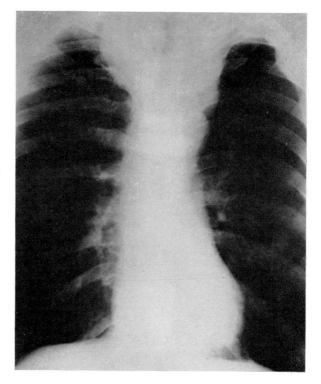

Figure 3.136. Neurofibromatosis: multiple left intercostal and superior mediastinal masses. (For neurofibromatosis of the vagi, see Figure 7.44)

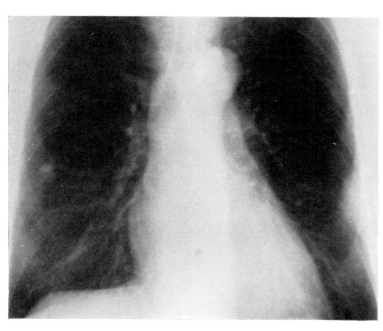

Figure 3.137. Multiple neurofibromas of the chest wall. (For multiple nodular shadows in the chest wall caused by aneurysms secondary to coarctation of the aorta, see Figure 9.12)

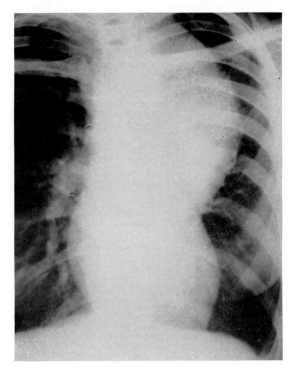

Figure 3.138. Very large posteriorly situated neurogenic tumour (schwannoma). It contained some calcification and caused pressure deformities of posterior parts of left third to seventh ribs

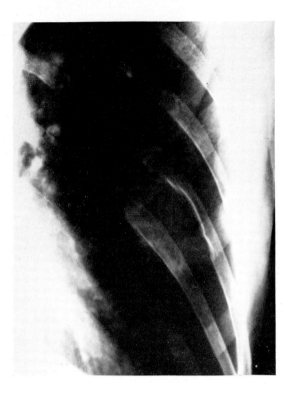

Figure 3.139. Pressure erosion of lower border of a rib due to neurofibroma

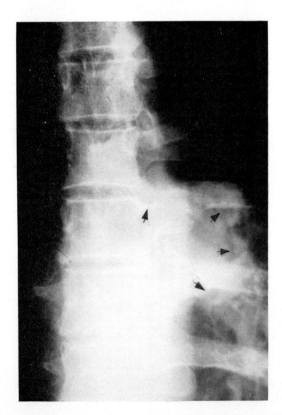

Figure 3.140. Neurofibroma (arrowed) elevating a pedicle and enlarging an intervertebral foramen

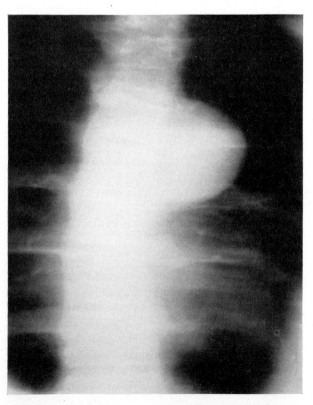

Figure 3.141. Rounded neurofibroma lying paravertebrally as shown by inclined frontal tomogram

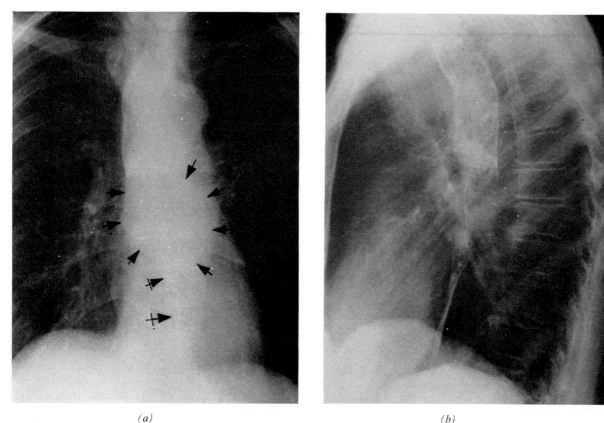

(a)   *(b)*

Figure 3.142. Soft tissue shadow of oesophageal tumour is readily seen within the mediastinum. A little barium is present in the dilated oesophagus above the tumour. Plain arrows mark outer border of mass, and hatched arrows show medial border of right pleural cavity

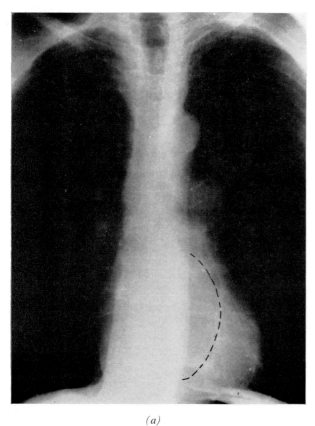

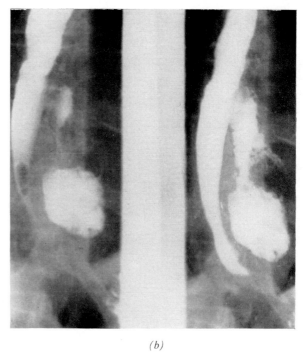

Figure 3.143. Para-oesophageal mediastinal abscess secondary to perforation of oesophagus. The soft tissue shadow of the abscess was just visible on original radiograph. Such an oeso-phageal or para-oesophageal mass will displace lower oeso-phageal–pleural stripe and medial pleural border of right lung

(a)   *(b)*

Bronchogenic cysts

Bronchogenic cysts are of developmental origin and usually arise close to the larger bronchi. Their walls are formed by respiratory epithelium with cartilage, muscle and mucous glands, and the fluid content is usually clear. These cysts are mostly smooth, well-defined spherical shadows and never contain calcification. They may be small or large and tend to be found in symptomless young people. A large cyst lying close to the shadow of the descending aorta is illustrated in *Figure 7.17*, while a smaller cyst appears in *Figure 3.135*.

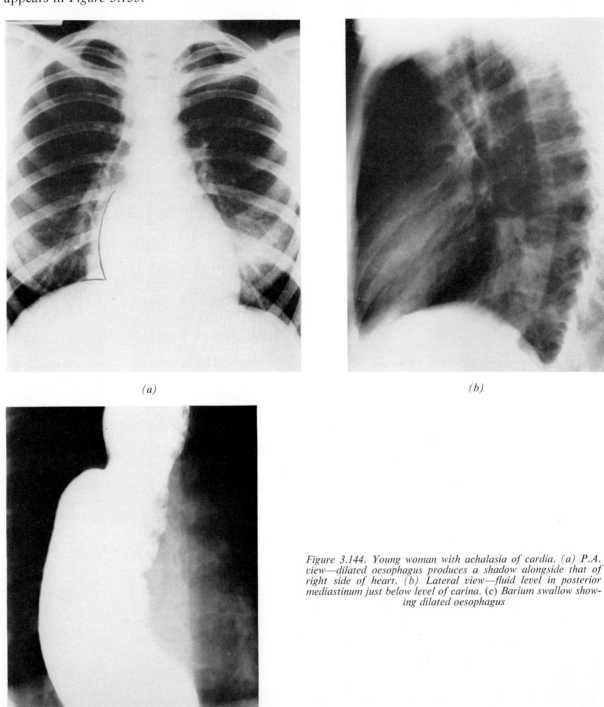

(a)

(b)

(c)

Figure 3.144. Young woman with achalasia of cardia. (a) P.A. view—dilated oesophagus produces a shadow alongside that of right side of heart. (b) Lateral view—fluid level in posterior mediastinum just below level of carina. (c) Barium swallow showing dilated oesophagus

Posterior mediastinal masses

Neurogenic tumours

Neurogenic tumours (including several types of neurofibroma, neurilemmoma, schwannoma and ganglioneuroma) may arise from any of the nerves which pass through the thorax, namely the intercostal nerves, the sympathetic chain, the vagi and the phrenic nerves, but are most commonly seen arising from the two first mentioned (*Figures 3.136* and *3.137*). They have to be distinguished from other lesions arising in the mediastinum. The tumours are usually well-defined homogeneous, spherical or ovoid, non-lobulated masses. Those arising from the sympathetic chain lie in the posterior costo-vertebral gutter and extend laterally to displace the mediastinal pleura. Calcification may be present in the malignant variety of neurogenic tumour and also in those which are benign (*Figure 3.138*). An example of neuro-fibromatosis of the vagi is shown in *Figure 7.44*.

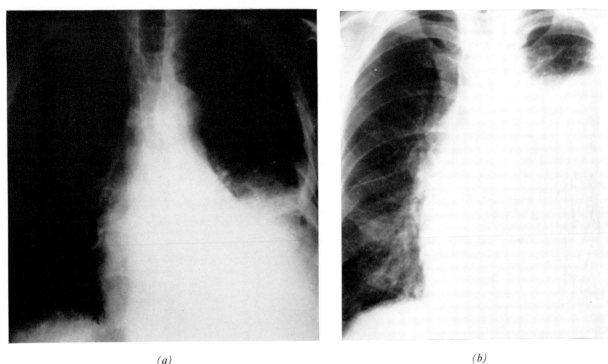

(a)   *(b)*

Figure 3.145. 'Plastic' or fibrous mediastinitis due to syphilis causing oedema with septal engorgement in left lung and increasing left pleural effusion. The patient was thought to have a bronchial neoplasm, but the true nature of the disease process was discovered at autopsy

Posterior mediastinal neurogenic tumours are nearly always in contact with bone, the posterior ribs or the vertebral column or both (*Figure 3.141*), and secondary bone changes are of great help in the differential diagnosis. The ribs may be displaced or may show pressure erosions on their upper or lower margins (*Figure 3.139*). With multiple tumours as in neurofibromatosis, the ribs may display multiple notchings. The vertebral appendages—such as the transverse processes, the pedicles or the vertebral bodies themselves—may be eroded or be displaced by the tumours, and a dumb-bell tumour which is partly in the spinal canal and partly in the thoracic cavity may enlarge the intervertebral foramen and displace a pedicle (*Figure 3.140*) or may present an extradural mass demonstrable on myelography. A mass passing through an intervertebral foramen can be distinguished from a *lateral thoracic meningo-coele* by gas or positive contrast myelography, when contrast medium will be seen to enter it.

Neuro-enteric cysts, dilated oesophagus, oesophageal tumours and diverticula, hiatus and Bochdalek hernias

These may all give rise to mediastinal masses. The most common is a hiatus hernia. A tumour of the oesophagus usually has a considerable soft tissue extension outside it (*Figure 3.142*).

Radiographs are unfortunately not as a rule sufficiently penetrated to show the soft tissue shadow of an oesophageal tumour, as has already been discussed in the case of mediastinal masses secondary to bronchial tumours, but if high kV radiographs are taken of sufficient quality to display the mediastinum properly, it is sometimes possible to detect an oesophageal tumour before the patient has experienced symptoms from it. Gladnikoff (1948), Cimmino (1961) and Ormond, Jaconette and Templeton (1963) have studied the value of the oesophageal pleural stripe, i.e. the relationship of the oesophagus to the medial margin of the lung, in the diagnosis of oesophageal disease (*Figure 3.143*). This stripe may also be seen on well penetrated or high kV radiographs or on tomograms.

An air and fluid filled oesophagus such as may be seen in *achalasia*, or rarely in scleroderma and dystrophia myotonica, projects to the right side of the mediastinum more commonly than to the left. It may be a central cucumber-shaped opacity rather than marrow-like, and occasionally gives a very bizarre appearance (*Figure 3.144*). Such an opacity together with absence of gas in the fundus of the stomach should always prompt a barium swallow for confirmation of the diagnosis, as should low-lying shadows

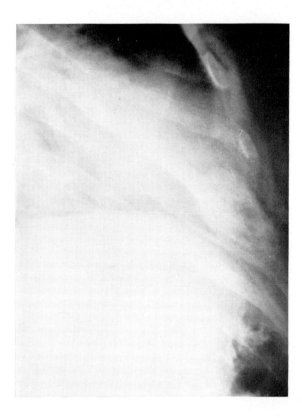

Figure 3.146. Patient suspected of having a lung tumour because of marked finger clubbing and possible lung masses seen on a rather underpenetrated radiograph. Bucky view of ribs shows marked decalcification and expanded areas in the ribs suggesting 'brown tumours' and hyperparathyroidism. She had hypercalcaemia, and a parathyroid tumour was removed

in the mediastinum, which may be due to stomach or bowel passing into the thorax through a hiatus or Bochdalek hernia. The gas content of these will often show on plain films.

Neuro-enteric (or enterogenous) cysts and diverticula appear on radiographs as rounded or elongated and vertically orientated mediastinal swellings, usually behind the heart in the posterior mediastinum or in the retrocarinal area. Occasionally these cysts have a connection with the spinal canal.

Paravertebral masses

Paravertebral masses may be abscesses, secondary deposits of neoplasm or myeloma, or rarely masses of erythropoietic tissue in patients with extramedullary haemopoiesis. The associated vertebral or disc lesions or the clinical features will assist in determining their aetiology.

Other mediastinal masses

Other mediastinal masses include haematomas, which may occur in the anterior or posterior mediastinum (*see Figure 7.7*); fibromas and fibrosarcomas; vascular tumours such as angiomas, haemangiomas and endotheliomas; and rare conditions such as thoracic duct cysts or intrathoracic hygromas.

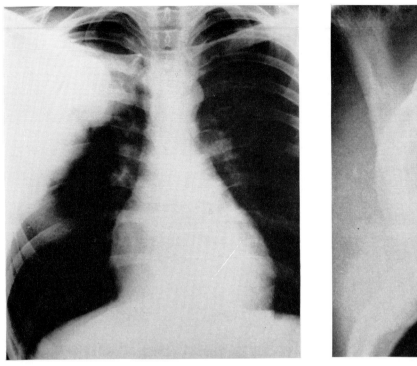
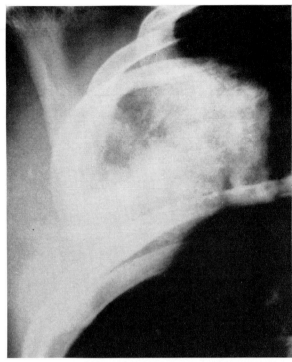

(a)   *(b)*

Figure 3.147. Young male adult with osteochondrosarcoma of right fifth rib. View taken with Bucky diaphragm clearly shows the extent of the large soft tissue mass, the calcification within it and the rib destruction. The patient had previously had several attempted pleural paracenteses for a supposed loculated pleural effusion

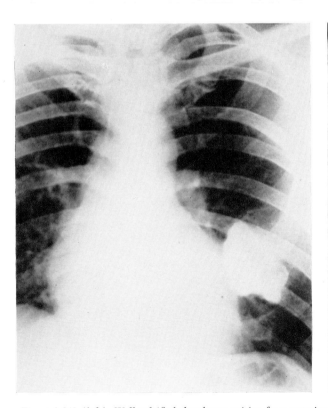
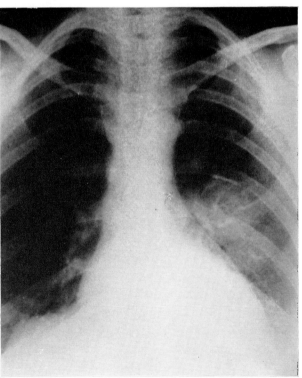

Figure 3.148 (left). Well calcified chondroma arising from anterior end of left fourth rib

Figure 3.149 (right). A chondroma without any calcification within it arising from anterior end of left third rib. Diagnostic pneumo-thorax was used to show that the tumour was situated in the chest wall and did not arise in the lung (see Figure 10.18b)

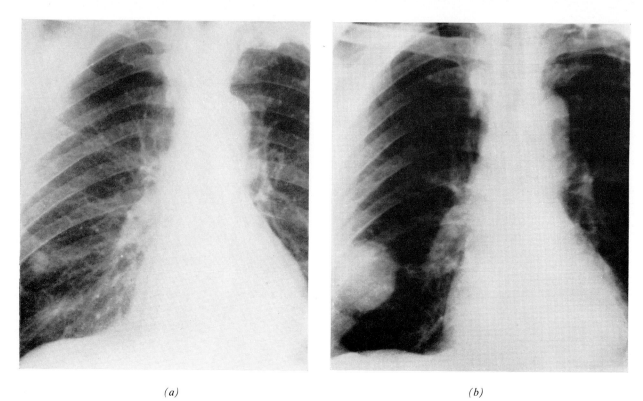

(a)   (b)

Figure 3.150. A shadow at the right base which had been ignored, presumably as a nipple shadow, had enlarged 18 months later into a large unresectable tumour. Doubtful nipple shadows should always be checked by markers placed on the nipples, oblique views, fluoroscopy or tomography. This patient also had tuberculous infiltration at the left apex and was undergoing treatment for a tuberculous knee

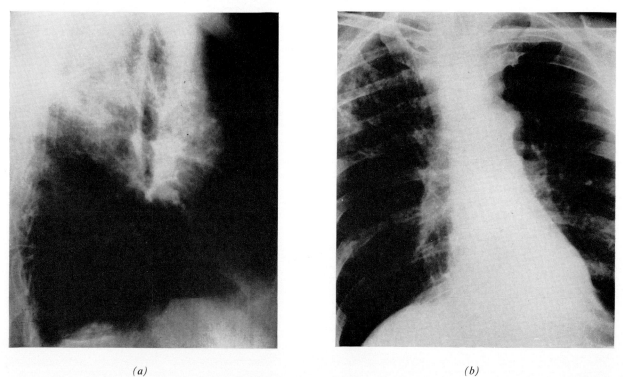

(a)   (b)

Figure 3.151. Large mass seen on lateral view apparently in the superior mediastinum. This shadow was caused by the stump of an amputated arm which could not easily be elevated. The patient also had partial collapse of the right upper lobe due to an endobronchial tumour

GENERALIZED MEDIASTINAL DISEASE

Mediastinitis

An acute or chronic mediastinitis may result in mediastinal widening. An acute infection most commonly follows a perforation of the oesophagus or the pharynx. Such perforation may be secondary to neoplasm, to peptic ulceration, to perforation by a swallowed foreign body, or to bouginage, oesophagoscopy or other surgical procedures. Spontaneous perforation occasionally occurs from vomiting (Mallory–Weiss syndrome—*see* Carr, 1973). Mediastinitis may also be secondary to diseases of the lungs or the larger air passages, or may be seen in patients with long-standing tracheostomies. The mediastinum will often be widened and a gas/fluid level may be present. Barium or iodine contrast swallow may demonstrate the oesophageal displacement or a perforation. If the trachea is suspected as the origin of the condition, tomography may demonstrate it more clearly.

A patient with chronic mediastinitis will tend to develop a fixed mediastinum, as was discussed under the heading of general observations (*see* page 63), and may develop venous obstruction, enlarged mediastinal nodes or a pleural effusion (*Figure 3.145*). Mediastinal fibrosis may also be associated with retroperitoneal fibrosis, biliary cirrhosis and fibrosis of the pancreas or salivary glands as part of a widespread disease complex.

Tumours of the chest wall

Chest wall tumours also have to be considered in the differential diagnosis of lung tumours. Neurogenic tumours have already been discussed. Others may arise in soft tissue or from bone or cartilage. Bone and cartilage tumours may be benign or malignant and include such entities as osteochondromas, bone cysts, 'brown tumours' in hyperparathyroidism, chondrosarcomas, osteogenic sarcomas, myelomas and metastatic lesions. The lesions may expand out of the bone and involve the pleura, lung or mediastinum. Bony lesions of the ribs are best demonstrated by straight or oblique views taken with the aid of a Bucky diaphragm (*Figures 3.51, 3.139, 3.146* and *3.147*). Sternal lesions may be shown by lateral views or by tomograms (McKinlay and Wright, 1967), while lesions arising from the spine may be shown by Bucky views, tomography or myelography. Tumours arising from the anterior ends of the ribs may contain calcification (*Figure 3.148*). When this is not present, a diagnostic pneumothorax will sometimes help in differentiating the mass from an intrathoracic tumour (*Figures 3.149, 10.18* and *10.19*).

SPURIOUS LUNG AND MEDIASTINAL TUMOURS

These spurious tumours are shadows projected on to the lungs or mediastinum on postero-anterior or lateral radiographs. They may be caused by film or processing artefacts, by clothing worn by the patient, or by anatomical structures.

The most common confusing shadow is created by the male nipples which, projecting out into air, produce a rounded density on a postero-anterior chest radiograph (*Figure 3.150*). They are usually symmetrical in position. If there is any doubt as to the nature of the shadows, the nipples may be marked with an opaque marker and further postero-anterior and oblique radiographs taken. Fluoroscopy will also be of value in verification, but tomography will sometimes be required to prove that no shadow is present in the lung. The nipples of adult females are more variable in position. In women with large and pendulous breasts, the nipples do not cause any difficulty since they will hang below the level of the dome of the diaphragm when the patient is in the erect position. Females with tiny breasts may present the same problem as males. Accessory nipples, warts on the skin, subcutaneous neurofibromas or dressings may also give spurious round shadows. A particularly good example of a spurious mediastinal mass appears in the lateral radiograph of a man who had had his arm amputated just below the shoulder (*Figure 3.151*).

Confusing shadows may also be produced by rib fractures, haematomas, and masses in or overlying the chest wall.

Other useful reviews of mediastinal tumours are by Doub (1950–51), Leigh and Weens (1959), Leigh (1963) and Hallgrimsson (1972).

4

Development of Tomography, Including Rotational Tomography

HISTORICAL REVIEW

Planigraphy and the Grossmann tomograph

Several workers (Bocage, 1922; Portes and Chausse, 1922; Pohl, 1927; Kieffer, 1929; Ziedses des Plantes, 1931; Bartelink, 1932) independently described techniques whereby a particular body section might be clearly reproduced while the layers above and below it were effaced. In these systems the x-ray tube and the film move during an exposure in parallel planes and in opposite directions, following a linear or a more complex (cruciform, circular or spiral) path. In each case the ratio of focus–object plane distance to object plane–film distance remained constant throughout although the focus–film distance varied. This system is illustrated in *Figure 4.1* and is the basis of many present-day tomographs.

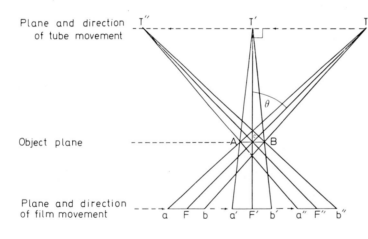

Figure 4.1. The Planigraph. Focus–object and object–film distancy vary continuously, but their ratio is constant $TO/OF = T'O/OF' = T''O/OF''$. The tube and film move on parallel paths. θ is the maximum angular displacement. It is not geometrically essential that the central ray be directed to the centre of the film throughout the exposure (Andrews, 1936; Twining, 1937), but it is highly desirable for the best results and is standard in all modern machines

A modified system which he termed 'tomography' was described by Grossmann (1935a, b). In this system the tube moves in an arc centred on the object plane, the film remaining parallel to the object plane although at varying distances from it (*Figure 4.2*).

The various forms of laminagraphy were extensively reviewed by Kieffer (1938).

Rotational tomography

The Grossmann system can be altered so that the x-ray tube is stationary and the central ray fixed, the object plane and the film rotating about parallel axes in line with the focus (*Figure 4.3*). This is the method described by Vallebona (1930), in which initially only the object plane rotated. Later it was elaborated by Bozzetti (1935), who called it stratigraphy.

Watson discovered the principle of rotational tomography in 1936 during experiments with a model using a stationary light source with the object and film or translucent screen rotating synchronously on separate parallel axes, such movement simulating the arcuate motion of the Grossmann tomograph. An x-ray tube and a fluorescent screen could be substituted for the light source and translucent screen. Watson built an apparatus, the Sectograph (British Patent Nos. 480,459, 1936, and 508,381, 1937).

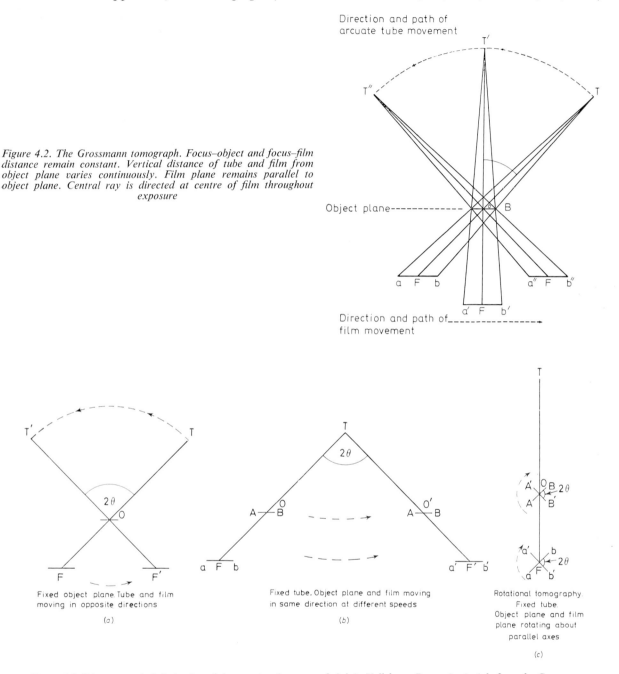

Figure 4.2. The Grossmann tomograph. Focus–object and focus–film distance remain constant. Vertical distance of tube and film from object plane varies continuously. Film plane remains parallel to object plane. Central ray is directed at centre of film throughout exposure

Figure 4.3. Diagrammatical derivation of the rotational tomograph (c) in Vallebona–Bozzetti principle from the Grossmann system (a) via a theoretical intermediary (b). It is of interest that for this intermediate system to form plane body section images, it is immaterial whether the object plane and the film move on parallel or curved paths. This illustrates the basic geometrical similarity between the Planigraph and the tomograph and their common relationship to the rotational system

This apparatus allowed a rotational movement of 360 degrees. Its motive power was 'a piece of string wrapped around the patient's turntable'. The operator had to pull the string and make the radiographic exposure. In 1939 and 1940, Watson reported the results of using this first apparatus and described his experiments. An improved model with motor drive was built, and Watson published in 1943 his results and illustrations of the use of this.

As Watson (1962) stated, 'The Sectograph was lent to hospitals in Birmingham, London and Bristol, but no useful work appears to have been done with it. It remained in Bristol for the duration of the war.' The usual British conservatism regarding new inventions, even British ones, had resulted in the apparatus not being used at all. It was returned to the Royal Cancer Hospital, London, following an extensive report on a large volume of work carried out by Vallebona and Amisano on the Zuder apparatus. The results of further work with the Sectograph were published by Stevenson (1950) (*see* Chapter 5). Stevenson's paper gives illustrations of Watson's two machines.

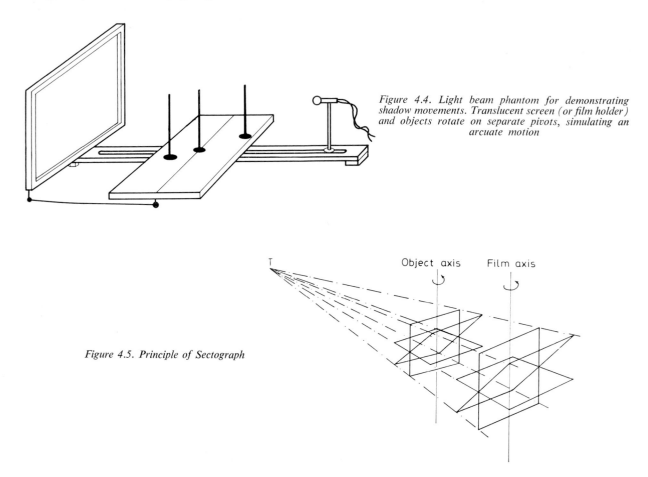

Figure 4.4. Light beam phantom for demonstrating shadow movements. Translucent screen (or film holder) and objects rotate on separate pivots, simulating an arcuate motion

Figure 4.5. Principle of Sectograph

Other workers, after experimenting with various systems, independently produced machines similar to the Sectograph. Amisano (1946) and Vallebona (1947a, b, 1948, 1949, 1950a, b, 1953) demonstrated the Zuder system (*see Figure 4.7*).

Gebauer (1949) produced an apparatus in which the patient's seat was attached to the column holding the film by a flexible drive. Hammer (1953) described a mechanism using magslip motors for connecting the film and patient turntables to give synchronous movement (the Hammer Transversotom). Frain and Lacroix (1947) employed a system in which the tube and film moved while the patient was stationary. In 1950 Frain *et al.* demonstrated the Radiotome (*see Figure 6.3*), in which the patient and the film rotate while the x-ray tube remains stationary.

Takahashi and Matsuda (1960), describing a prototype, and Takahashi (1969) developed a different type of transverse axial tomograph in which the patient lies horizontally instead of sitting or standing as with other types (*see Figure 4.8*). The tube and film rotate around the patient. A wedge filter evens out the radiographic exposure to give a clearer radiograph. With this apparatus it is possible to take tomograms from the top of the head to the soles of the feet. One major drawback of this machine, as commercially manufactured, is that it can be conveniently used only on small patients (the Japanese, for whom it was designed, are relatively small people).

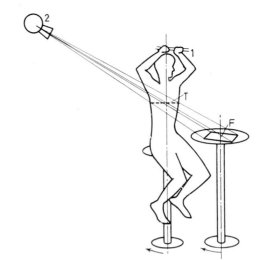

Figure 4.6. Principle of transverse axial tomography (Radiotome)

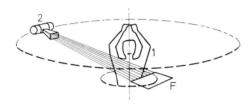

Figure 4.7. Principle of transverse axial tomography (Takahashi)

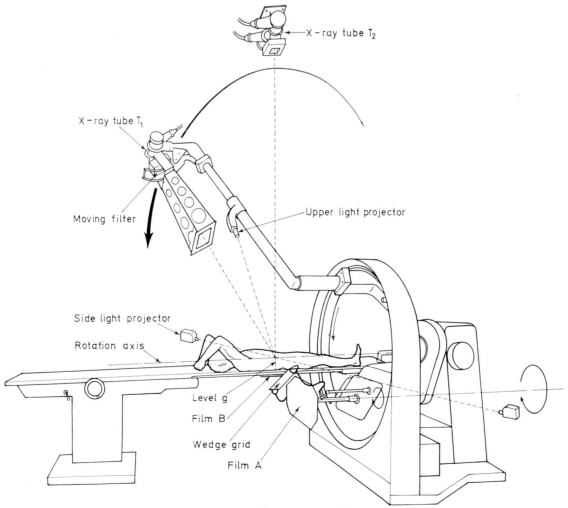

Figure 4.8. Schematic diagram of horizontal type of transverse axial tomograph

DEVELOPMENT OF THE TRANSVERSE AXIAL TOMOGRAPH
FOR INCLINED FRONTAL TOMOGRAPHY

Amisano, Piazza and Oliva (1950) showed that the Zuder apparatus for transverse axial stratigraphy, the Pantix-Strator, could also be used for rotational stratigraphy with the cassette placed vertically, the x-ray beam being horizontal. Frain *et al.* (1955) described tomography of the tracheo-bronchial tree with the Radiotome, using a film inclined parallel to the trachea and the main bronchi. This is

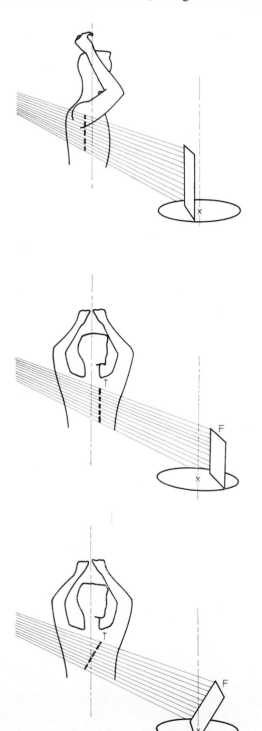

Figure 4.9. Principle of inclined frontal tomography. The cassette is inclined parallel to the plane to be examined, usually the tracheo-bronchial tree, but may also be inclined parallel to the spine or sternum. Placing the cassette behind or in front of the centre axis of the cassette turntable (X) gives a plane in front of or behind the centre of axis of rotation of the patient. The large object–film distance gives a magnification of 1·34:1 (see page 118)

the method which I have termed inclined frontal tomography. The principles of transverse axial and inclined frontal tomography are shown in *Figures 4.6–4.9.*

SOME PRINCIPLES OF ROTATIONAL TOMOGRAPHY

Ziedses des Plantes (1931) found that the thickness of the layer of which an acceptable image is formed diminishes as the angle through which the tube and the film move increases (angle θ in *Figures 4.1–4.3*), but that coincident with this, the contrast of the image and the sharpness of the outline are diminished. He also noted that for the same angular displacement the blurring effect was greater with a complex than with a linear movement. Grossmann (1935a, b) maintained that if the angle was sufficiently large, the blurring was adequate with a linear motion, which offers fewer constructional problems than a system using a complex movement. A small irreducible unsharpness of the image is produced by the non-point nature of the focal spot and the film screen combination employed.

Watson (1939) showed that the object and film axes must always be parallel and aligned with the focus. The object plane is always parallel with the film, and the film need not be coincident with the axis of rotation or parallel to it. The cassette may be flat or curved, and in the latter case a curved object plane is obtained; such a technique was elaborated by Paatero (1954), who called it Pantomography. Watson (1962) stressed that exact localization was important. He stated that postures which are not truly erect do not produce sections which are perpendicular to the vertical axis of the body, and that where there is an unavoidable tilt of the patient (or of the plane to be examined), the film can be tilted on its axis so that it is parallel to a transverse plane of the body.

The apparent thickness of a tomographic section, or 'selectivity', was discussed by Watson (1962) and also by Edholm (1960). For practical purposes a section is thinner or thicker according to the exposure angle, according to the ability of the recording medium to resolve detail, or arbitrarily according to the diameter of detail that it is desired to see. Watson showed the build-up of detail with a 60

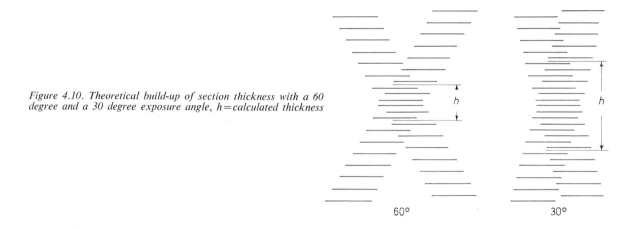

Figure 4.10. Theoretical build-up of section thickness with a 60 degree and a 30 degree exposure angle, h=calculated thickness

60°   30°

and a 30 degree exposure angle (*Figure 4.10*). The height of the diamond-shaped overlap can be calculated where the exposure angle and the diameter of the detail are known. However, for practical purposes, as the image in the region of the diamond apices would be completely indistinguishable, a section must be considered to be somewhat thinner than indicated by the height of the diamond. Willner (1956) calculated the thickness of the layer in rectilinear tomography as a mean value of half the amplitude. For transverse tomography the thickness would be less. Watson considered that owing to the non-point source, involuntary movement, slight mechanical imperfections and minute degrees of misalignment, it was difficult to resolve anatomical details less than 3 mm in diameter.

Greenwell and Wright (1965) found that to form a sharp image, the plane of a tomographic section must always be perpendicular to any flat surface and must follow the radius of a curved surface or pass through the widest diameter of a spherical or cylindrical structure (e.g. the trachea or larger bronchi). Only if such a valid section is obtained can any pathological significance be attached to apparent local destruction, narrowing or deviation from the normal position.

In inclined frontal tomography the films placed in front of or behind their axis of rotation will 'select' a plane in the object whose distance from the object axis is dependent on the magnification. This is essentially the same principle as that which underlies multisection radiography (Watson, 1953), a principle which can likewise be applied to transverse axial tomography. The films may also be placed obliquely or, as with transverse axial tomography, at right angles to the axis of rotation; the tube then has to be angled downwards to produce an image on the film, an angle of 20–30 degrees being commonly employed.

The relative merits of rotational tomography or stratigraphy (with patient and film rotating) and planigraphy (tomography with the x-ray tube and film moving) for the examination of the chest were discussed by Balestra and Oliva (1953). They concluded that the rotational method offered a larger angle with sharper detail and a shorter exposure time to set against the possibly disturbing effect of poor effacement of rib shadows.

5

Clinical Usage of Rotational Tomography—Historical Review

TRANSVERSE AXIAL TOMOGRAPHY

In English language publications there are few descriptions of the clinical uses of transverse axial tomography of the chest. Stevenson (1950), using Watson's second apparatus, showed examples of a right-sided aortic arch with azygos lobe, a double aortic arch, coarctation of the aorta, retrosternal goitre, bronchogenic carcinoma and pulmonary tuberculosis. In 1961, Hartley thought that 'transverse axial tomography can come to play an increasing and not diminishing part in the accurate assessment of the best method of treatment of malignant disease of the chest', and also wrote that transverse axial tomography demonstrated the region behind the bronchi and the carina, 'the retrocarinal space', with considerably more clarity than other methods. In 1965 he stated that 'the traditional tomograms (i.e. A.P. and lateral) will provide most of the information regarding the type of lesion, i.e. whether peripheral or central, intraluminal or peribronchial, early (localized) or advanced, whilst the transverse axial tomograms provide both corroborative evidence and information regarding mediastinal and particularly postcarinal spread'. A similar view was previously expressed by Hartley *et al.* in 1960.

As was discussed in Chapter 2, Drevvatne and Frimann–Dahl (1961) used transverse axial as well as A.P. and lateral tomograms to study the morphology of peripheral lung tumours and to demonstrate peribronchial infiltration spreading towards the hilum.

Books describing the technique and geometry of transverse axial tomography with some clinical illustrations have been written by Bonte, Brenot and Trinez (1955), by Gebauer and Schanen (1955) and by Farr *et al.* (1964). The last named volume contained a foreword by Blair Hartley and included an atlas of the normal anatomy of the thorax, using a double masking technique to give negative reproductions of the tomograms, which were accompanied by line drawings. Takahashi (1969) produced a well illustrated *Atlas of Transverse Axial Tomography and its Clinical Application*, using positive prints, artistic impressions and line drawings to depict the tomographic cuts. He outlined his method, with the patient lying horizontally as described in Chapter 4, and illustrated the normal anatomy from the head to the ankles, some pathological abnormalities, and the use of the technique in the planning of radiotherapy. Chest disease was represented by a tuberculous cavity, a metallic foreign body, enlarged mediastinal and hilar nodes, an interlobular effusion, an aneurysm of the descending aorta and a tuberculous abscess of the chest wall, but Takahashi did not fully discuss the clinical usefulness of the technique.

Other publications dealing with transverse axial tomography and with lung and mediastinal masses are listed below.

Balestra, Passeri and Macarini (1950)—lungs: examples of a pneumothorax situated anteriorly and extrapleurally, benign lung tumours and a fibrothorax.

Buzzi (1950)—mediastinum: two large mediastinal masses, the position of the oesophagus with barium sulphate in it, the position of the aortic arch, a right apical lung opacity, the air-filled trachea and the mediastinal glands.

Oliva (1950)—aorta.

de Maestri (1950) examined some children and showed an example of a large heart, pulmonary plethora and a retrosternal thymic mass.

Milani (1954) wrote: 'L'emploi de la stratigraphie transverse introduite et mise en valeur par le prof. Vallebona et par son école nous offre de nouvelles possibilitées d'apprecier l'état du médiastin, l'invasion des ganglions lymphatiques, le rapporte entre la tumour et l'espace du thorax etc.'

Schaudig and Kirst (1960)—mediastinum and bronchial carcinoma.
Pompili and Alè (1961)—thymus, thyroid and aorta.
Thomas and Stecken (1961, 1962)—lung and aorta.
Alè and Macchi (1953)—aorta.
Mattina, Curicale and Cricchio (1964)—mediastinum.

INCLINED FRONTAL TOMOGRAPHY

Inclined frontal tomography of the bronchi, using the Radiotome, was first described by Frain *et al.* (1954), working in Paris. Frain *et al.* (1955) showed five examples of the use of this technique—one normal case and four with bronchial narrowing or occlusion—and described their findings in 16 other abnormal cases. They used a tomographic angle of 180 degrees to give tomographic cuts approximately 1 mm thick. The discovery of this method of investigating the tracheo-bronchial tree apparently followed the attempted use of the technique to demonstrate tortuosity of the oesophagus and calcification in the aorta.

Three years later, Martin and Broussin (1958) from Bordeaux, using the C.G.R.* Pantomix, published five further examples of inclined frontal tomography to demonstrate hilar masses and stenoses of the larger bronchi. They used a tomographic angle of 100 degrees and inclined the film at an angle of 10–12 degrees to the vertical, taking tomographic cuts at 5 mm intervals and finding that the best cut was usually 12 cm from the posterior border of the chest, i.e. the cut which normally passed through the carina. In 1961 the same authors described two patients with gross mediastinal enlargement in the subcarinal region, which was not visible on plain radiography, and illustrated one of these.

Other papers describing experience with inclined frontal tomography are those by Rudler *et al.* (1955), Marlois (1956), Surmont, Markovits and Desprez-Curely (1961, 1962) and Markovits and Desprez-Curely (1962). All these authors worked in France. The last mentioned papers summarized the cumulative experience of 722 examinations on 498 patients and illustrated seven examples of the technique. Frain and Gaucher (1957) showed that the Radiotome might demonstrate the aortic arch, the descending aorta and the pulmonary vascular shadows. Frain and Duquesne (1962) used the Radiotome for oblique sagittal tomography.

Greenwell and Wright (1965) described results in patients examined at the Churchill Hospital. The technique has also been applied to studying the sternum (McKinlay and Wright, 1967) and the larynx (Ardran and Emrys-Roberts, 1965), using the same apparatus. Di Chiro (1964, 1965) applied the method to the tomography of the brain during air encephalography, and his supervisory radiographic research technologist devised a portable chair and rotating film platform for inclined frontal tomography of the brain and neck and the demonstration of calcification in heart valves (Morel, 1965). In the same year, Laubenberger (1965) from Germany described the use of the Siemens Transversal Planigraph for both inclined frontal and inclined right and left sagittal planes. This apparatus had previously been employed for inclined frontal tomography by Frey (1962).

The only papers in English describing the technique and reporting experience of it are by Markovits and Desprez-Curely (1962), Laubenberger (1965), Greenwell and Wright (1965) and Wright, MacLarnon and Morrison (1972). It has been largely ignored in Great Britain, although following the publication by Greenwell and Wright it has been adopted in some other centres, whilst others have tried to simulate the technique by inclining the patient after the manner of Kovats and Zsebök (1959) and Voigt (1964) or by inclining the lower cassette holder on the Polytome (Mayall, 1965).

A different method of rotational tomography has been employed for examining the teeth and jaws (Blackman, 1960).

* Compagnie Générale de Radiologie, Paris.

6

Tomographic Techniques the Author has Used and Some Practical Points

TOMOGRAPHIC TECHNIQUES

Linear (longitudinal) tomography using the Siemens Planigraph (Installed in 1952)

As was explained in Chapter 4, the Planigraph has focus–object and object–film distances which vary continuously during the radiographic exposure. The focus–object distance in the central position is 150 cm. The object–film distance in the same position measures 10 cm, assuming that the object is at the level of the table top; however, for most clinical procedures the object plane will lie above this level, usually at a distance in the range of 4–15 cm. An exposure angle of 20 degrees on either side of the midline (total 40 degrees) is used with an exposure time of 1·75 seconds for thin tomographic cuts, and an angle of 20 degrees with an exposure time of 0·9 seconds for thick layers.

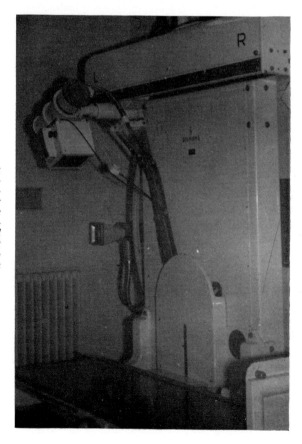

Figure 6.1. Siemens Planigraph (reproduced by courtesy of Sierex Ltd., London) with horizontally orientated tube for use with Radio-tome shown in background. The principle of this apparatus is diagrammatically shown in Figure 4.1. It can be used with the patient lying down or sitting up, i.e. in a horizontal or a vertical position. The vertical posture is preferred for lateral tomograms, since in this position there is no distortion of the mediastinum due to mediastinal movement towards the dependent side, as happens when a patient with a mobile mediastinum lies on his side. The vertical position also avoids the tendency for the dependent lung to be under-inflated. In addition, the sitting posture is more comfortable

Linear (longitudinal), oval or circular movement using the Siemens Multiplanigraph (Installed in 1967)

The Multiplanigraph has similarly varying focus–object and object–film distances, the distances in the central position for tomography being 108 and 8 cm respectively. Linear blurring can be carried out using an exposure angle of 10 degrees and an exposure time of 0·2 or 0·4 seconds to give a thick layer, or an angle of 30 degrees and an exposure time of 0·6 or 1·2 seconds to give a thin layer. The apparatus can also be used with a circular blurring motion of 40 degrees (360 degrees' rotation of the tube) and an exposure time of 2·5 or 5 seconds.

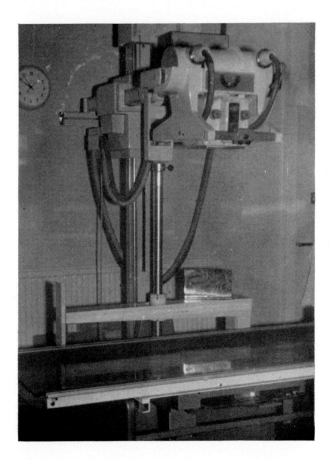

Figure 6.2. Siemens Multiplanigraph (reproduced by courtesy of Sierex Ltd., London). This apparatus has more 'tube wobble' than the Planigraph, largely because of the light-weight and detachable connections between the cassette tray and Bucky and the x-ray tube. It has a 'floating' table top, but can be used only in the horizontal position

Inclined frontal and transverse axial tomography using the Radiotome (Installed in 1962)

Transverse axial tomography

In performing transverse axial tomography, the alignment of the x-ray tube is of critical importance. The tube should be specifically assigned to working with the Radiotome, and once its central ray has been aligned correctly, lateral adjustment should be completely locked. I have used the tube inclined downwards at 26 degrees 30 minutes from the horizontal. The horizontal distance between the tube support and the centre of the patient's seat is 180 cm, and that between the centre of the patient's seat and the centre of the film turntable is 60 cm (*Figure 6.4*). This gives a magnification factor of 1·34 on the films. Single tomographic cuts are employed, using 15 × 12 in (380 × 305 mm), 14 × 14 in (355 × 355 mm) or 17 × 14 in (430 × 355 mm) films and cassettes as appropriate.

In order to simplify the adjustment of the x-ray tube between the downwardly inclined position for transverse axial tomography and the horizontally inclined position for inclined frontal tomography, I devised a clamp fixed on to the tube yoke to act as an end stop in downward rotation of the tube. If the tube is turned downwards as far as it will go, it will be adjusted to 26 degrees. For horizontal align-

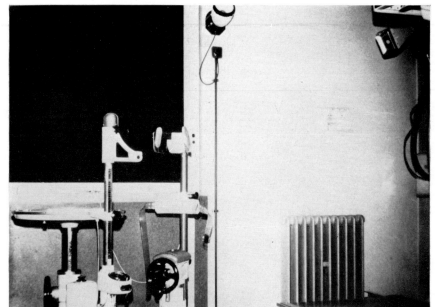

Figure 6.3 (a). Radiotome with x-ray tube aligned for transverse axial tomography

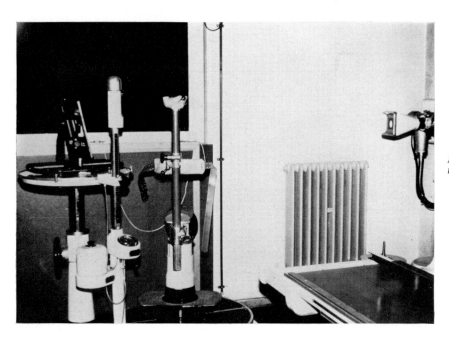

Figure 6.3 (b). Radiotome with x-ray tube aligned for inclined frontal tomography

Figure 6.4. Diagram showing horizontal distances employed in transverse axial tomography. In inclined frontal tomography the horizontal distances are the same as the focus–object and object–film distances

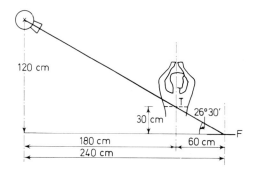

ment a spirit level has been fitted to the side of the tube. The tube can be moved vertically on its track by means of a cable hoist (*Figure 6.5*).

Inclined frontal tomography

For inclined frontal tomography the patient is positioned on the seat facing the upright column.

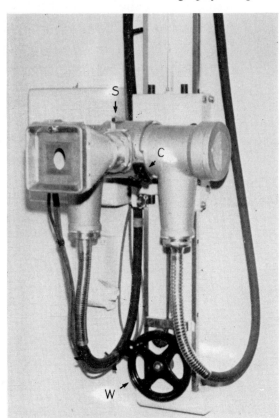

Figure 6.5. Photograph of x-ray tube used with the Radiotome, showing its height and inclination adjustment. S=spirit level; C=clamp; W=wheel of cable hoist

(Radiotome manufactured by Massiot-Philips, Paris. Illustrations by courtesy of Philips Medical Systems Ltd., London)

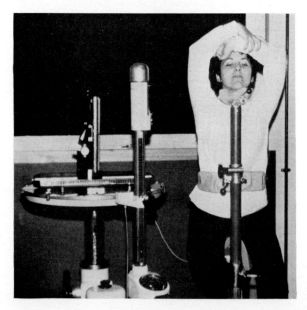

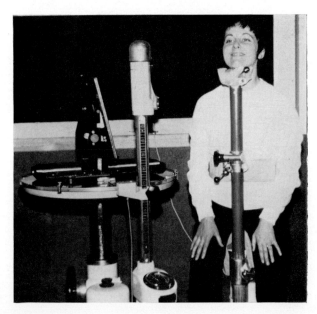

Figure 6.6 (left). Patient positioned for preliminary lateral radiograph with arms raised above the head

Figure 6.7 (right). Patient positioned for inclined frontal tomograms. Since the x-rays will form a useful image only when striking front of cassette (I use a 90 degree angle—45 degrees on either side of patient's spine), the patient's arms rest against his sides with the hands on the thighs. A strap is passed around the lower ribs

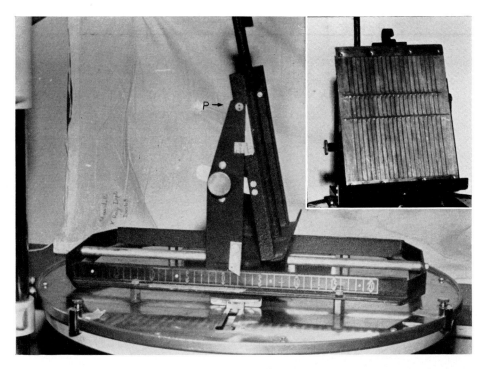

Figure 6.8. Accessory cassette holder used for inclined frontal tomography. P indicates pivot on which cassette is angled. Inset shows wire-lined grid for lateral view

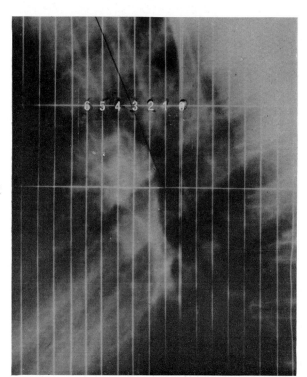

Figure 6.9. Preliminary lateral radiograph with grid superimposed. A line is drawn down centre of trachea. The figures represent tomographic cuts which may be taken

A strap is passed around his lower ribs to maintain his position while his chin rests on a pad on the top of this column (*Figures 6.6* and *6.7*). In order to determine the correct planes for tomography, a preliminary lateral radiograph is taken using an accessory cassette holder (*Figures 6.8* and *6.9*).

The preliminary lateral radiograph is rapidly processed, and during this time the patient is supervised to ensure that he does not move his chest out of position. On this radiograph is superimposed a grid (demonstrated earlier by Bret and Chollat, 1964) consisting of a rectangular plywood board on which are vertical wires spaced 1 cm apart, with a double wire in the centre to correspond with the axis of rotation of the film turntable. There are also two horizontal wires, one to mark the middle and one above this at the level of the horizontal axis, about which the cassette holder is angled forward (*P* in *Figure 6.8*). On this lateral radiograph, the angle the trachea makes with the vertical can be measured as well as the distance of the trachea in front of or behind the central axis of rotation at the level of the horizontal pivot (i.e. the upper horizontal wire).

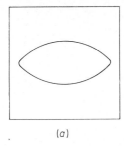
(*a*)

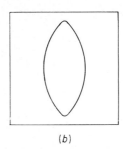
(*b*)

Figure 6.10. Diaphragm inserted in the tube cone. (a) Long axis horizontal as for transverse axial tomography; (b) long axis vertical as for inclined frontal tomography

The height of the patient is adjusted if necessary, and the cassette is tilted through the angle the trachea makes with the vertical. By rotating the film turntable through 90 degrees, patient and cassette are aligned so that the latter is parallel with a plane passing through the patient's shoulders, and also parallel to the trachea and the main bronchi. The movable part of the cassette holder is moved backwards or forwards on its longitudinal mounting bars an appropriate distance in front of or behind the axis of rotation as derived from the preliminary lateral film. In practice four, five or six films are exposed at intervals of 1 cm (as measured on the cassette holder), passing in front of, through and behind the trachea and the main bronchi. The film centimetres in fact represent intervals of 0·75 cm in the patient owing to the magnification of 1:1·34. An angle of 90 degrees and a speed of 4 seconds per revolution gives an exposure time of one second. The diaphragm inserted into the tube cone is the same as that used for transverse axial tomography, turned through 90 degrees so that its long axis is vertical.

SOME PRACTICAL POINTS ABOUT TOMOGRAPHY

(1) With all tomographic apparatus it is very important to ensure that the moving parts move in the desired lines, arcs, circles, etc., without any wobble and at the correct constant speed so as to produce radiographs of good sharpness and good diagnostic quality. Particular attention should be paid to the path of the tube, since this is usually one of the moving parts. In some machines the tube can be disconnected from the link with the Bucky and the cassette tray so that it can be used separately, and this may lead to some wobbling at this point. Similarly with tomographic attachments the lack of robustness due to flexibility of the linkage system may not be all that is desired.

(2) The radiographic exposure should start when the moving parts are already moving and should be terminated before they stop.

(3) The exposure time should be determined by the time set on the apparatus and not by the timer on the generator control unit, since if the latter prematurely terminates the exposure the fully desired time (or arc) will not be employed.

(4) The position of the radiographic exposure in the movement arc should always be known, since it is not always symmetrical on each side of the mid point of the movement. An asymmetrical radiographic exposure can be used to advantage—for example in renal work it may partly prevent the radiographic beam traversing the relatively dense liver—but it is best avoided in chest radiography.

(5) In the author's experience an erect posture seems preferable for lateral tomograms. A horizontal position is used for most A.P. pulmonary tomograms. Inclined frontal tomograms are used to show the hilar regions, larger air passages and mediastinum.

7

Rotational Tomography of the Chest Employing the Radiotome

GENERAL PRINCIPLES

The Radiotome apparatus was installed in 1962, and since that time approximately 300 transverse axial and 1,800 inclined frontal tomographic examinations of the chest have been made. Some preliminary experiments using a 'squirrel cage' phantom (*Figure 7.1*) showed that high quality tomograms were possible with this mechanism (*Figure 7.2*). The definition of the hollow tubes at the periphery

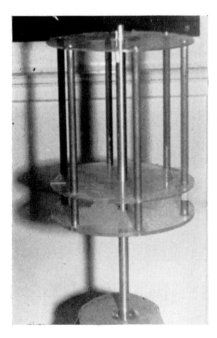

Figure 7.1. 'Squirrel cage' phantom positioned on the Radiotome. The centre rod is the 'centring rod' mentioned in Figure 7.3

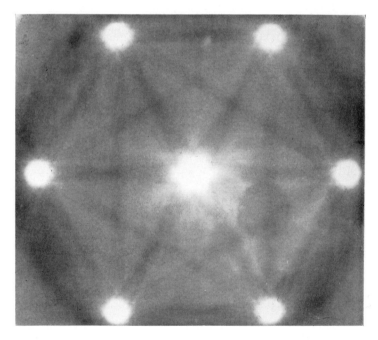

Figure 7.2. Transverse axial tomogram of 'squirrel cage' phantom showing good definition at both periphery and centre of radiograph

was as sharp as that of the metallic rod at the centre. The excellent apparent thinness of a tomographic cut and the fine vertical adjustment of the apparatus were demonstrated by the separating image of the obverse and reverse sides of an old penny (1d).

The method of ensuring that the tube, the patient and the cassette turntable are in correct alignment is shown in *Figure 7.3*.

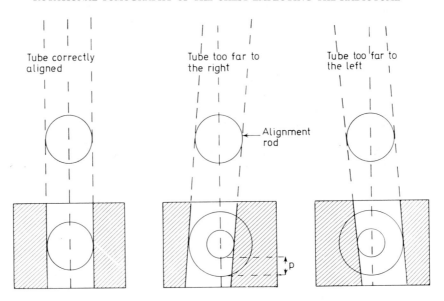

Figure 7.3. To check that the tube alignment is correct, i.e. that the central ray passes through the central axis of both turntables, two exposures are made of the alignment rod (the centre rod seen in the squirrel cage in Figure 7.2)—one with the turntable stationary and the other during a full 360 degrees rotation. From the width of any penumbra (p) which may be present, the tube alignment can be corrected

CLINICAL USE OF TRANSVERSE AXIAL TOMOGRAPHY

It is apparent from the greater number of patients who have been examined by transverse axial than by inclined frontal tomography that the former technique has been preferred for most diagnostic purposes. In this section I shall not only discuss my experience of the use of transverse axial tomography in assessing the spread of lung tumours, but shall consider its value in the diagnosis of mediastinal masses, since these must always be considered in the differential diagnosis of tumours which spread into the mediastinum. I shall also discuss the value of the technique in the elucidation of abnormalities of the aorta.

Lung tumours

With bronchogenic tumours, transverse axial tomography can give a good spatial orientation of the position of the tumour prior to radiotherapy (*Figure 7.4*). Contrary to the opinion of Blair Hartley (*see* Chapter 5, page 115), I have found that assessment of spread of tumour into the retrocarinal space—that is, the middle and lower parts of the posterior mediastinum—is very difficult. If the spread into this area of the mediastinum was massive (*Figure 7.5*), it was relatively easily seen on the transverse tomograms. However, where it was less marked, assessment was much harder.

It soon became apparent that false positive and false negative assessments occurred, and there appeared to be several reasons why this area of the mediastinum was difficult to assess by this method. In patients who were large or obese or who had cardiac enlargement, a pleural effusion or a large lung mass, the scattering effect from the greater amount of soft tissue rendered the mediastinal area between the heart and the spine less clear. A similar conclusion was reached by Lodin (1961) in his attempt to assess the descending aorta. In the case of tumours which were close to the mediastinum, it was often difficult to visualize any aerated lung tissue between the tumour and the mediastinum; hence the mass could appear to extend into the mediastinum when in fact, as found at thoracotomy, it did not. Radiographic contrast differences between different tissues on transverse axial tomograms are rather poor unless there is an abrupt change in density, for example that between aerated lung and the heart. Where there is a less abrupt transition, a less clear differentiation results.

With the Radiotome as installed at the Churchill Hospital, the rectified sine wave of the tube current supplied by a four-valve generator occasionally gives a stroboscopic effect. This is sometimes seen on radiographs containing shadows of very dense structures, particularly if metallic objects are present. It also tends to render transitional zones at the edges of particularly dense tissues less clear.

Because of the difficulty of assessing the posterior mediastinal and hilar regions by means of this technique, I have preferred to rely on other methods in studying lung tumours, using linear longitudinal tomography for peripheral lung tumours and inclined frontal tomography for the mediastinum, the hilar regions and the tracheo-bronchial tree.

Right

Left

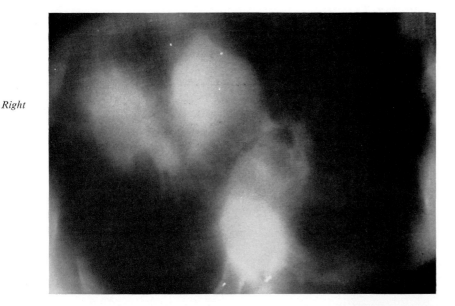

Figure 7.4 (above). Transverse axial tomogram showing position of an irregular tumour in right middle lobe. Note.—All the illustrations of transverse axial tomograms show left side of the patient on right side of the print, the figures being reversed right to left to give an orientation similar to that of the other radiographs. The reader should imagine that he is standing behind the patient looking at a horizontal section of him

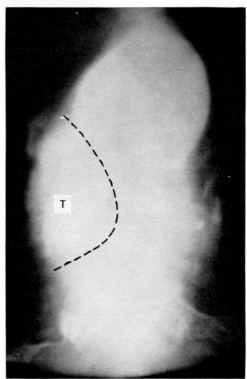

Figure 7.5 (right). Transverse axial tomogram showing involvement of retrocarinal space by a bronchial carcinoma. T=tumour

Masses in the oesophagus

For similar reasons, I found that assessment of the soft tissue masses associated with oesophageal tumours was almost impossible by this method.

Pericardial cysts

In the five patients who had pericardial cysts which were studied by transverse axial tomography, the position of the cysts in relation to the heart was readily shown in the pre-operative diagnostic assessment. They were most clearly seen when they lay anteriorly (*Figure 7.6*). In one patient, who was suffering from myasthenia gravis and in whom a possible thymoma was being sought, transverse axial tomography was the only method by which the cyst could be demonstrated at all. Plain radiographs failed to show any abnormality, and the demonstration of a mass low down in front of the heart was

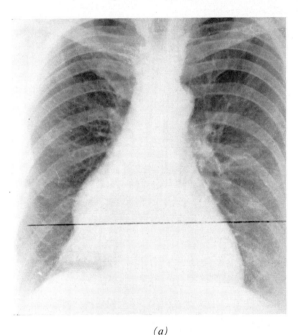
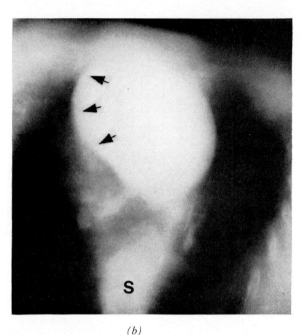

(a)   *(b)*

Figure 7.6. Pericardial cyst lying on right side of heart anteriorly, its shadow being continuous with that of the pericardium, in symptomless woman aged 59. S=spine

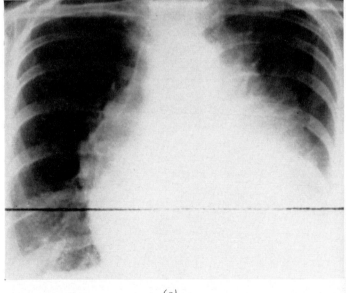

(a)

Figure 7.7. Anterior mediastinal haematoma; subsequently shown to be secondary to malignancy, but primary site of this was not identified. (a) P.A. chest. (b) Transverse axial tomogram through lower part of the heart and haematoma, which lies anterior to the heart and the pericardium

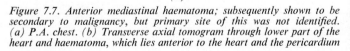

Horizontal lines on P.A. views indicate planes of tomographic sections   *(b)*

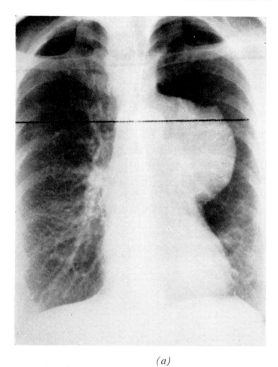

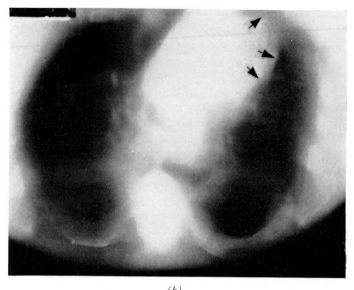

(b)

Figure 7.8. Thymic tumour in anterior mediastinum in a symptomless woman aged 59. Transverse axial tomogram (b) shows the mass lying anteriorly and to the left of the aortic arch. Aortogram (c and d) shows it to be a vascular tumour: a marked vascular 'blush' is seen and the blood supply is derived largely from the left internal mammary artery

(a)

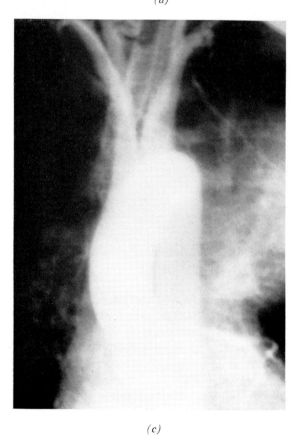

(c)

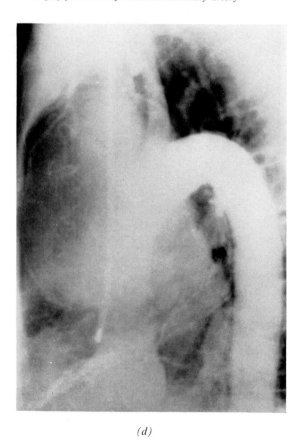

(d)

a rather surprising finding. Because of the relatively large size of the mass and its low position, a thymoma seemed unlikely and the possibility of a pericardial cyst was suggested. This was confirmed at exploration, when no evidence of a thymoma was seen.

dilatations of the descending aorta shown by transverse tomography are given in Figure *7.14*, while in *Figure 7.14c* this structure has been rendered invisible by increased adjacent soft tissue shadowing.

In the investigation of aneurysms one has to consider not only the lumen, which may be shown by aortography, but also the thickness of the wall, which means that the outer border must be defined. This border may not be readily seen on angiograms but may be visible on plain radiographs, especially if calcification is present. Tomograms can be of great value in the demonstration of this structure and of the soft tissue shadows of aneurysms, which are much wider than their lumina due to the deposition of layers of thrombus on their walls (*Figures 7.11b* and *7.15*).

False aneurysms pose a particularly difficult problem since the aneurysmal cavity may closely simulate a mediastinal tumour. Two examples appear in *Figures 7.12* and *7.15*. The first of these occurred in a symptomless patient aged 60 in whom a right superior mediastinal mass had been dis-

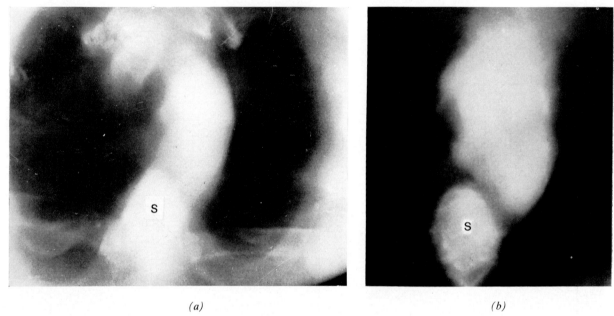

(a)   *(b)*

Figure 7.11. Transverse axial tomograms showing the aortic arch. (a) Dilated aortic arch in a patient with aortic valve disease. (b) Luetic aneurysm of the aortic arch. Calcification is shown in the wall of the aneurysm. S=spine

covered on routine chest radiography. Subsequent tomograms carried out just before thoracotomy showed that the mass was closely related to the ascending aorta. In the second case a woman aged 45 presented with a progressive stridor which had been increasing over a period of three months. The mass of the aneurysmal sac was demonstrated by inclined frontal tomograms as a very large, partly retrotracheal mass which markedly deviated and compressed the trachea. Subsequent aortography confirmed the aneurysmal cavity arising from the arch of the aorta. Serological tests for luetic disease were positive. In *Figure 7.16*, enlarged right paratracheal nodes give a similar appearance to the aneurysm shown in *Figure 7.15*.

It may also be difficult to distinguish without aortography between traumatic aneurysms of the aorta, especially the descending aorta, and masses alongside it. *Figure 7.17* shows a large bronchogenic cyst which lay alongside the aorta in a symptomless nurse aged 21. Congenital anomalies such as a 'double aortic knuckle (*see Figure 7.48*) or coarctation (*see Figure 7.46*) may occasionally be confused with other mass lesions, and the abnormality may be shown by tomography. Similarly, a horizontally passing descending aorta in a patient with a severe scoliosis may simulate a mass lesion (*see Figure 7.47*).

Masses alongside the aorta

The outer borders of these masses can be well demonstrated by transverse axial tomography

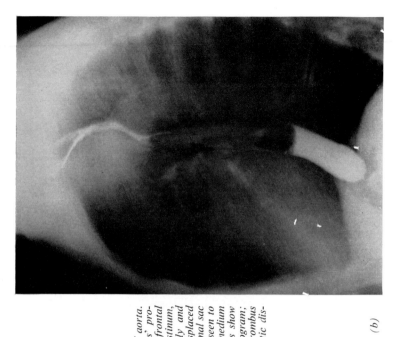

(b)

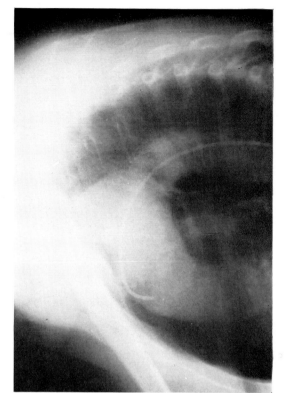

Figure 7.12. Aneurysmal sac arising from arch of aorta. The patient, a woman aged 45, had had 3 months' progressive stridor. Chest radiographs and inclined frontal tomogram (a) show large mass in superior mediastinum, displacing the trachea to the right and anteriorly and severely narrowing it. The oesophagus (b) is displaced posteriorly. Aortogram (c and d) shows an aneurysmal sac arising from superior aspect of aortic arch: this is seen to have a considerably thickened wall as the contrast medium does not reach as far as its outer border. (Arrows show outer border of aortic arch on tomogram and aortogram; the aortic wall is grossly thickened by mural thrombus formation). Serological tests were positive for luetic disease

(a)

(c) (d)

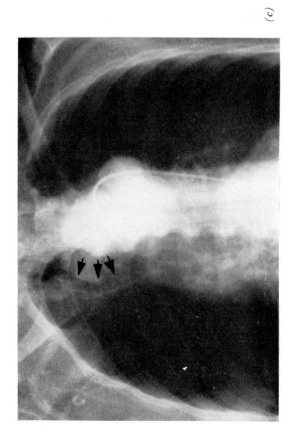

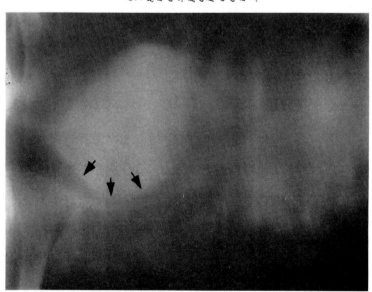

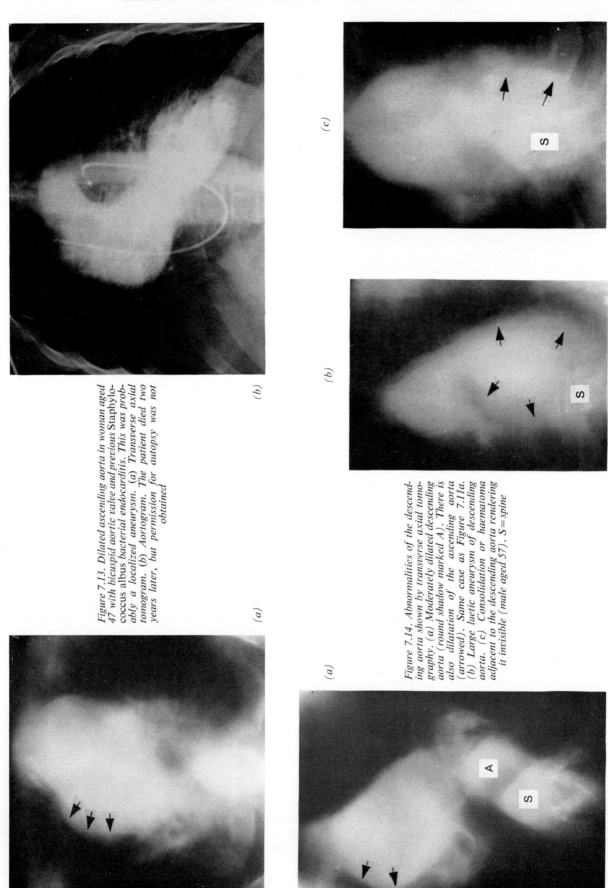

(b)

(a)

Figure 7.13. Dilated ascending aorta in woman aged 47 with bicuspid aortic valve and previous Staphylococcus albus bacterial endocarditis. This was probably a localized aneurysm. (a) Transverse axial tomogram. (b) Aortogram. The patient died two years later, but permission for autopsy was not obtained

(c)

(b)

(a)

Figure 7.14. Abnormalities of the descending aorta shown by transverse axial tomography. (a) Moderately dilated descending aorta (round shadow marked A). There is also dilatation of the ascending aorta (arrowed). Same case as Figure 7.11a. (b) Large luetic aneurysm of descending aorta. (c) Consolidation or haematoma adjacent to the descending aorta rendering it invisible (male aged 57). S=spine

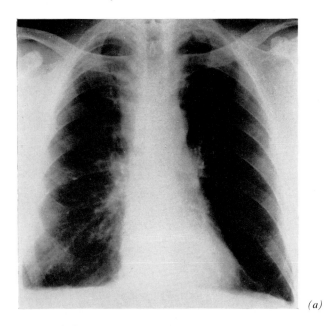
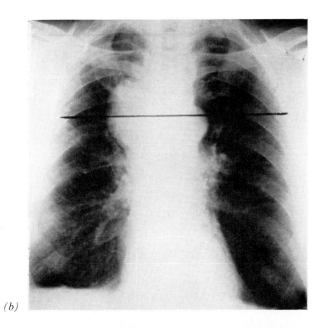

(a) *(b)*

(c) *(d)*

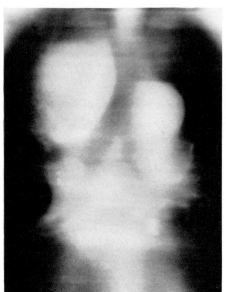

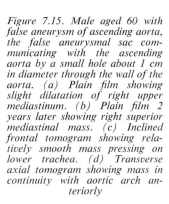

Figure 7.15. Male aged 60 with false aneurysm of ascending aorta, the false aneurysmal sac communicating with the ascending aorta by a small hole about 1 cm in diameter through the wall of the aorta. (a) Plain film showing slight dilatation of right upper mediastinum. (b) Plain film 2 years later showing right superior mediastinal mass. (c) Inclined frontal tomogram showing relatively smooth mass pressing on lower trachea. (d) Transverse axial tomogram showing mass in continuity with aortic arch anteriorly

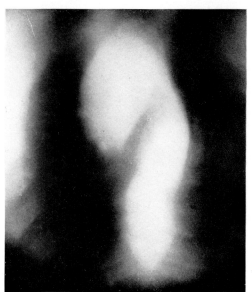

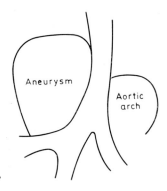

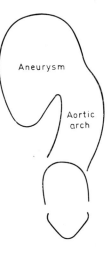

combined with inclined frontal tomography, but if there is any suspicion of an aneurysm the lumen of the aorta should be investigated by aortography, which may also demonstrate a vascular tumour blush.

Figure 7.18 shows a mass arising in the aortic wall which was a chance finding in a patient aged 63

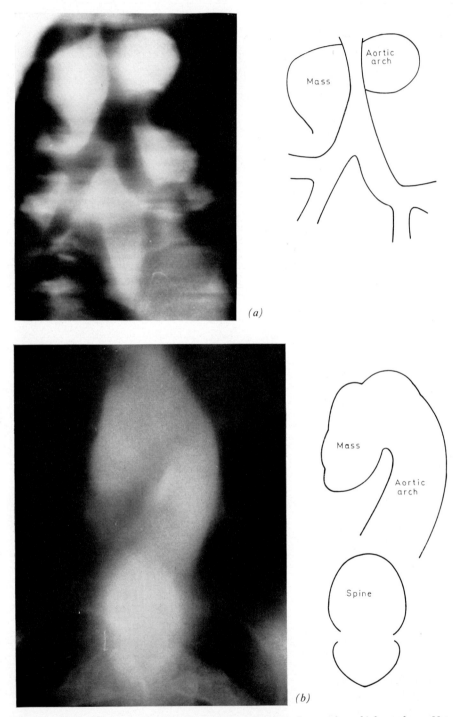

(a)

(b)

Figure 7.16. Enlargement of right paratracheal nodes secondary to bronchial neoplasm. Note similarity to false aneurysmal sac shown in Figure 7.15

years being treated for pernicious anaemia. The mass was indistinct from the aorta on transverse axial tomograms. An aortogram showed that it was not an aneurysm and that it had a faint tumour blush. Mediastinoscopy was carried out with no excessive bleeding, and on biopsy the mass proved to be a chemodectoma. This tumour probably arose from an aortic body within the aortic wall.

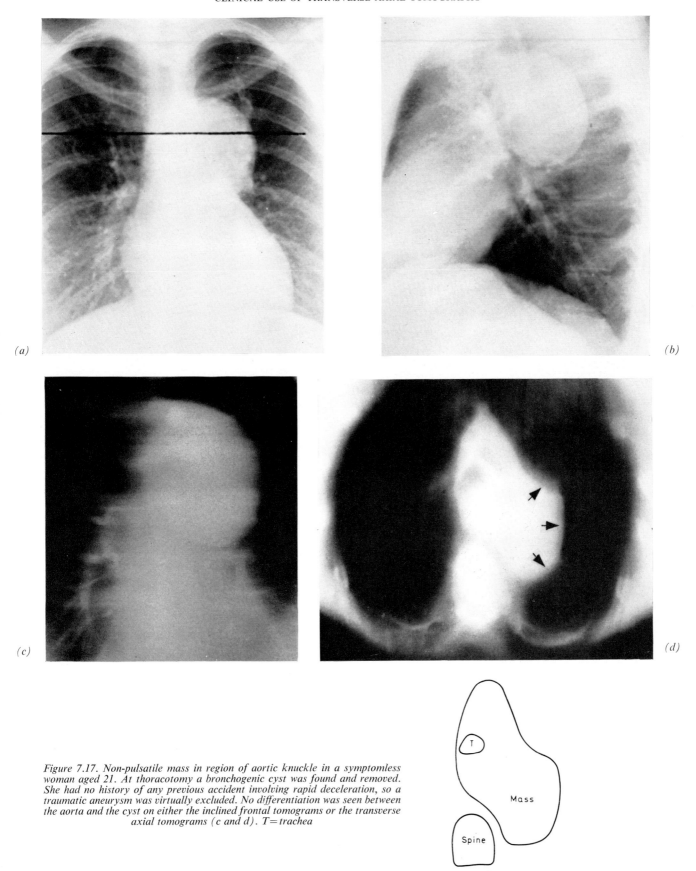

(a)

(b)

(c)

(d)

Figure 7.17. Non-pulsatile mass in region of aortic knuckle in a symptomless woman aged 21. At thoracotomy a bronchogenic cyst was found and removed. She had no history of any previous accident involving rapid deceleration, so a traumatic aneurysm was virtually excluded. No differentiation was seen between the aorta and the cyst on either the inclined frontal tomograms or the transverse axial tomograms (c and d). T = trachea

135

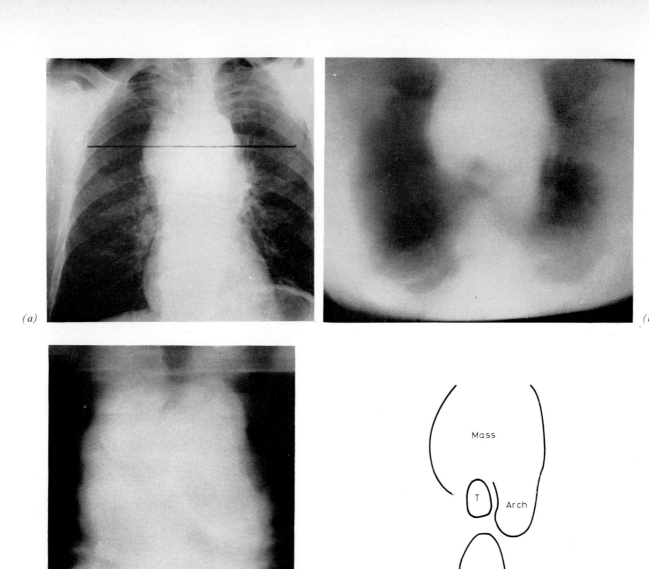

(a)

(b)

(c)

Mass

T

Arch

Figure 7.18. Chemodectoma of aortic wall in a patient aged 63. (a) Plain film. (b) Transverse axial tomogram showing mass on both sides of anterior part of aortic arch. (c) Inclined frontal tomogram showing mass on both sides of mediastinum. (d) Aortogram: normal aortic lumen, faint vascular blush in the tumour. T = trachea

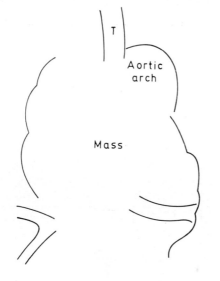

T

Aortic arch

Mass

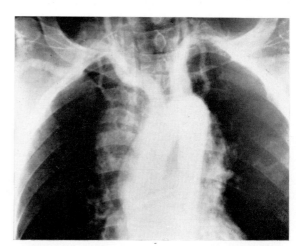

(d)

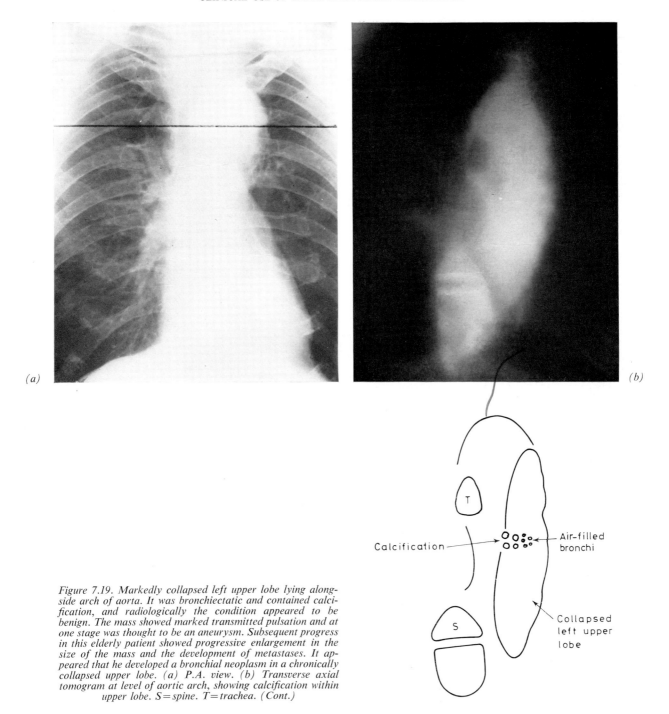

Figure 7.19. Markedly collapsed left upper lobe lying alongside arch of aorta. It was bronchiectatic and contained calcification, and radiologically the condition appeared to be benign. The mass showed marked transmitted pulsation and at one stage was thought to be an aneurysm. Subsequent progress in this elderly patient showed progressive enlargement in the size of the mass and the development of metastases. It appeared that he developed a bronchial neoplasm in a chronically collapsed upper lobe. (a) P.A. view. (b) Transverse axial tomogram at level of aortic arch, showing calcification within upper lobe. S = spine. T = trachea. (Cont.)

In another case (not illustrated) a similar mass was found in a symptomless man aged 21. This was a smooth right upper mediastinal mass, closely related to the ascending aorta and not separated from it on the tomograms. Aortography revealed no abnormality. At thoracotomy a thoracic seminoma was found in the right antero-superior mediastinum alongside the ascending aorta. In this case the tumour possibly arose from a dermoid cyst. The patient's testes were clinically normal and a lymphangiogram showed normal para-aortic nodes. An older patient with a thoracic seminoma, normal testes and a normal lymphangiogram had marked enlargement of lymph nodes on both sides of the mediastinum.

The difficulty of differentiating nodal masses alongside the arch of the aorta from an aneurysm is further illustrated in *Figure 7.19*. This patient, an elderly fairground owner, had a collapsed left upper

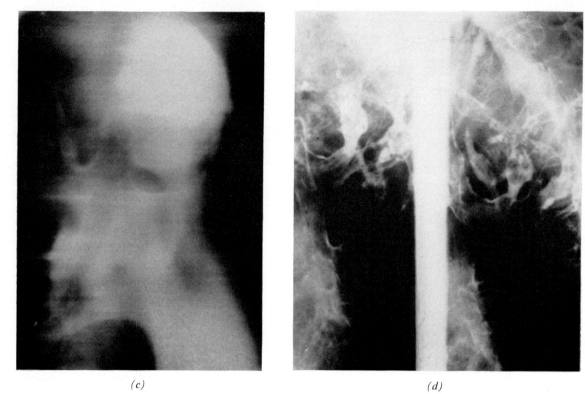

(c)   *(d)*

Figure 7.19. (c) Inclined frontal tomogram. The left main bronchus is elevated and distorted. (d) Bronchiectatic changes within what appeared to be a chronically collapsed upper lobe

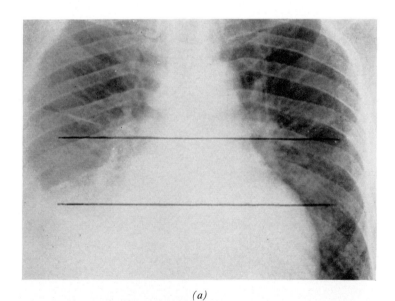

(a)

Figure 7.20a–d. Young adult immigrant from Indian subcontinent with right pleural effusion and gross enlargement of subcarinal and lower mediastinal lymph nodes due to tuberculosis. (a) P.A. view; horizontal lines indicate plane of section of the transverse axial tomograms (b and c). (d) Inclined frontal tomogram. RMB and LMB=right and left bronchi. A=descending aorta.

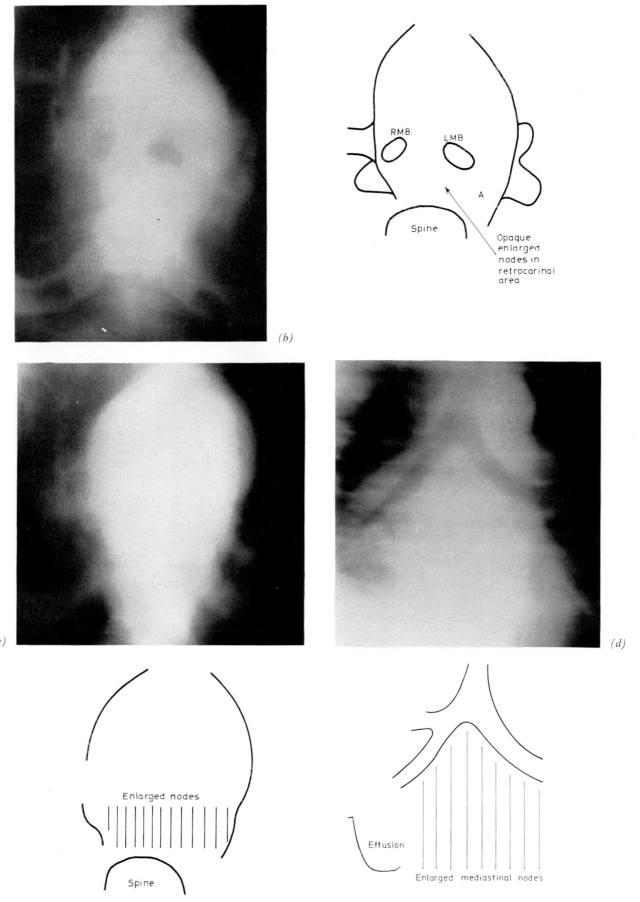

Figure 7.20 (cont.)

lobe lying against the mediastinum. Calcified left upper hilar nodes were present, and the bronchogram revealed bronchiectatic change in what appeared to be a chronically collapsed left upper lobe. Fluoroscopy erroneously gave the impression of expansile pulsation suggestive of an aortic aneurysm. As the serology proved negative, an aortogram was carried out which showed a normal lumen. Subsequently the shadow alongside the aorta slowly and progressively enlarged. The patient developed pulmonary metastases and a pleural effusion. It appeared that he had had a bronchial neoplasm developing peripherally in a left upper lobe which was chronically collapsed, probably as a result of a tuberculous infection in childhood.

An early paper describing the use of a bronchogram to help in the differentiation between an aneurysm of the aorta and a bronchial carcinoma is that of Lian, Huguerin and Brawermann (1933).

VALUE IN DEMONSTRATING ENLARGED NODES NOT CAUSED BY NEOPLASM

Transverse axial tomograms are sometimes very helpful in demonstrating enlarged mediastinal nodes in patients with lymphadenopathy due to infection or reticulosis. *Figure 7.20* shows the tomograms of a young male patient from the Indian subcontinent who had a small right pleural effusion and a mild pyrexia of uncertain origin. The tomograms demonstrated a gross lower mediastinal lymphadenopathy which, in this instance, is perhaps better seen in the transverse axial than in the inclined frontal views. A pleural biopsy confirmed the presence of tuberculosis.

VALUE IN PLANNING RADIOTHERAPY OF LUNG AND MEDIASTINAL TUMOURS

Transverse axial tomograms may help in treatment planning in the following ways.

(1) By showing the extent of the tumour. This may be particularly important in those relatively small tumours whose site renders them inoperable, but where there is a good chance of palliation or even a possibility of cure with radical (high dosage) irradiation.

(2) By aiding in the field arrangement:

(*a*) To avoid over-irradiation of the spinal cord.

(*b*) To prevent the irradiation of too much lung in the pathway of the treatment beam to the tumour and so help to avoid the production of excessive radiation fibrosis and the reduction of pulmonary vascularity.

(*c*) To assess the position of the heart fairly accurately, thus allowing it to be used as an entry portal for radiotherapy. Although minor ECG changes may be produced by the therapy, the heart is usually less affected than other tissues such as the lung and the spinal cord.

(3) By assisting in the calculation of radiation dosimetry in an attempt to compensate for tissue inhomogeneity (*see* Ellis, Feldman and Oliver, 1964).

CLINICAL USE OF INCLINED FRONTAL TOMOGRAPHY

I have used inclined frontal tomograms in the study of various types of disease processes in the lungs and mediastinum for the demonstration of disease, for its differential diagnosis, and for showing the extension of the disease process into the hilar regions or the mediastinum.

Many of the patients attending the various departments of the Churchill Hospital, including the Chest Clinic and the Thoracic Surgery and Radiotherapy Departments, who had suspected or confirmed lung tumours have been investigated by this method since 1963. Initially for 15 months, virtually all patients admitted to the Thoracic Surgical Unit with suspected or known bronchial neoplasm were examined in order to assess the value of the technique. It was hoped that during this time the appearances seen on the tomograms would not influence the surgical decision as to whether an exploratory thoracotomy was to be carried out, so that operative correlation might be obtained in most cases. However, some of the grosser deformities demonstrated by the method, together with other findings at bronchoscopy or the anaplastic nature of the neoplasm as discovered on biopsy, undoubtedly influenced selection for surgery as the series continued. A detailed analysis of the first 206 cases is given in Tables 7.1–7.3, and of 688 patients seen over a four-year period in Table 7.4.

RADIOLOGICAL APPEARANCES OF TRACHEO-BRONCHIAL TREE

Normal appearances

An inclined frontal tomogram of a normal case is reproduced in *Figure 7.21* together with an explanatory drawing. All the larger air passages including the trachea, the carina, the main bronchi and the main upper and lower lobe branches (including the right intermediate bronchus between the origins of the upper and middle lobes) are well shown. The proximal portions of the upper lobe segmental bronchi are easily distinguished. However, neither the right middle lobe nor the apical segmental

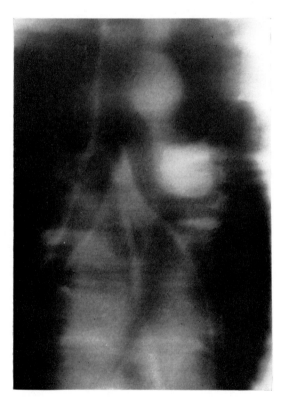
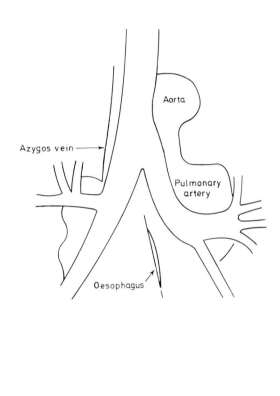

Figure 7.21. Normal anatomy as shown by inclined frontal tomography

bronchi of the lower lobes are demonstrated by this technique, since they run almost at right angles to the plane of section. In order to demonstrate these, lateral tomography is required. This may be carried out on the Radiotome with the film either vertical or inclined parallel to the trachea and the lower lobe bronchus (*see Figure 7.25*).

The thickness of the bronchial walls is well seen, as are mediastinal structures such as the aorta, the pulmonary artery and the hilar vessels. The oesophagus usually appears as a partially air-filled structure below the carina, and the medial border of the right pleural cavity is often well demonstrated. In the lower part of the hilar regions, on each series of tomograms the pulmonary veins can usually be distinguished from arteries by their course into the left atrium. The azygos vein is not as a rule fully distended with the patient in the sitting position. The ghost shadows of the spine and ribs run horizontally across the tomograms.

Abnormal appearances

The following are some of the many types of anatomical abnormality which may be recognized on inclined frontal tomograms.

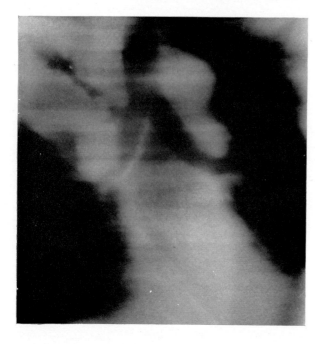

Figure 7.22. Bronchial carcinoma; rounded tumour in right upper lobe bronchus. The bronchi distal to this are dilated. Right upper lobe collapsed, and enlarged nodes in right hilum

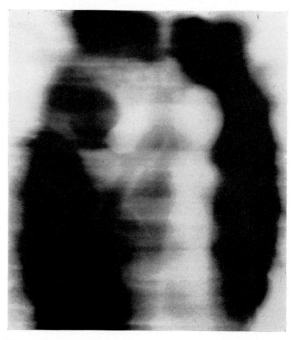

Figure 7.23. Bronchial carcinoma. Very narrowed right upper lobe bronchus leading into large air-filled cavity in collapsed upper lobe

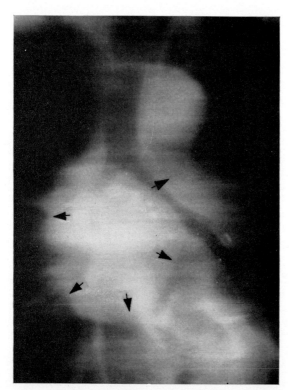

Figure 7.24. Bronchial carcinoma. Very large mass of enlarged nodes in right hilum and subcarinal region, with gross narrowing of both main bronchi. These findings were almost invisible on plain radiographs. The patient had had an increasing 'wheeze' with exercise for 6 weeks

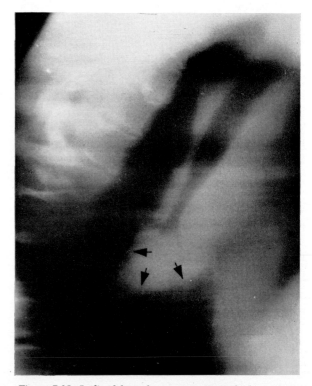

Figure 7.25. Inclined lateral tomogram. Bronchial carcinoma; blocked right lower lobe bronchus just distal to origins of middle lobe and lower lobe apical bronchi. The soft tissue mass of the tumour is also demonstrated (arrowed)

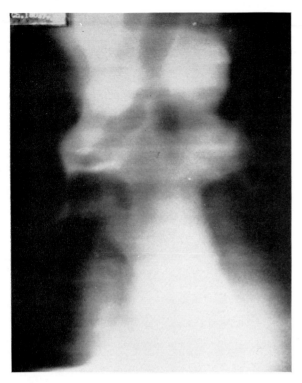

Figure 7.26. Bronchial adenoma. Smooth mass projecting from right upper lobe orifice into right main bronchus. The right upper lobe is collapsed

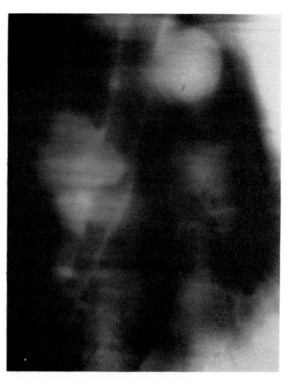

Figure 7.27. Fairly large endobronchial mass in intermediate bronchus, causing an audible wheeze. There is a very much larger extrabronchial tumour, lobulated in appearance

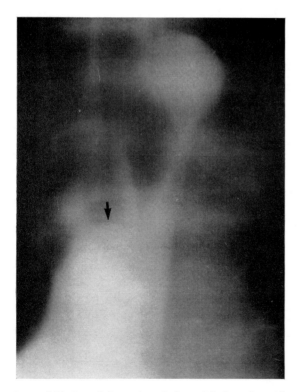

Figure 7.28. Rounded mass in right lower lobe bronchus with collapse of the right lower lobe

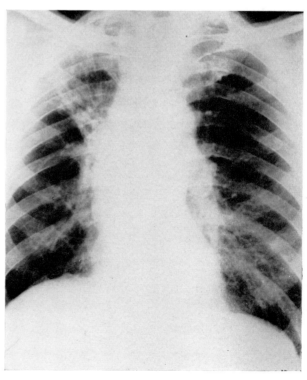

Figure 7.29 (a). P.A. view. Partial collapse of right upper lobe. Note mediastinal deviation, crowding of right upper ribs and decreased volume of right lung

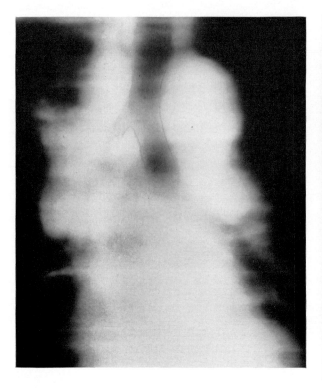

Figure 7.29 (b). Inclined frontal tomogram. Concentric stenosis and shortening of right main bronchus with right hilar and right paratracheal node enlargement

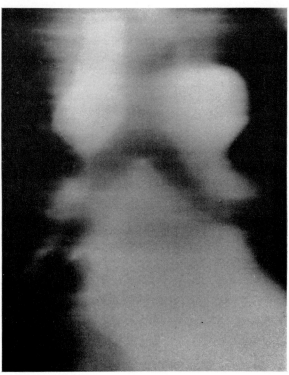

Figure 7.30. Bronchial carcinoma; enlarged nodes in right upper mediastinum

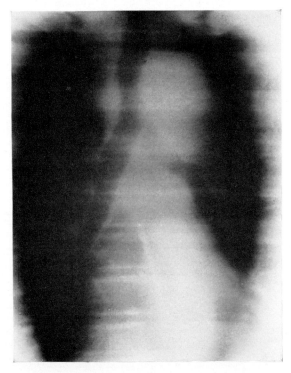

Figure 7.31. Bronchial carcinoma; enlarged nodes around aortic arch and pulmonary artery

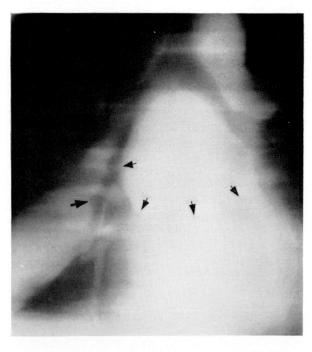

Figure 7.32. Inclined frontal tomogram showing collapse of the lateral basic segment of right lower lobe, with its bronchus occluded (large arrow), and enormous subcarinal nodal enlargement (small arrows)

(1) Displacement of mediastinal structures, particularly the main air passages.

(2) Alterations in the contour of the air passages resulting from external compression, intrinsic narrowing or stenosis, or bronchial block.

(3) Filling defects within the air passages.

(4) Enlargement of broncho-pulmonary, hilar or mediastinal nodes.

(5) Enlargement of mediastinal structures such as the aorta, the pulmonary artery and the oesophagus.

(6) Mediastinal tumours.

(7) Collapse or masses within the adjacent lung.

An important point to realize is that when the air passages do not lie entirely within the plane of

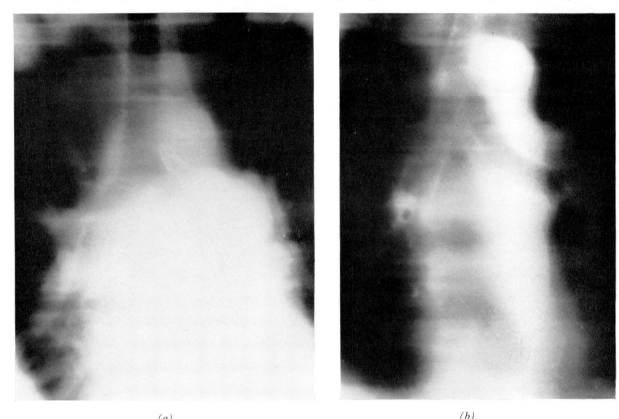

(a)   *(b)*

Figure 7.33. (a) Extensive left hilar, left mediastinal and subcarinal spread of tumour from left lower lobe. (b) Four weeks later, following tumour chemotherapy, the appearances have virtually returned to normal

section on any single tomograph, a composite image can be constructed from two or three adjacent cuts. This is most likely in cases of collapse or fibrosis.

Examples of abnormalities demonstrated by inclined frontal tomography and by inclined lateral tomograms are given throughout this volume and especially in *Figures 7.22–7.50*. In these tomograms, hilar and mediastinal abnormalities are usually well demonstrated, as are the larger air passages. The tomograms are particularly valuable in that they show not only strictures, blocks or filling defects within the air passages, but also the surrounding soft tissue masses. In this respect they are far superior to bronchograms, which demonstrate only the endobronchial abnormalities. In addition, the tomograms may show the characteristics of an endobronchial abnormality more clearly because the relatively viscous bronchographic medium may not be able to pass through a strictured area which will still allow a little air to pass through. In patients with severe narrowing of the main bronchi (*Figure 7.24*), bronchography or bronchoscopy may be a hazardous undertaking, whilst little inconvenience is experienced by a patient undergoing tomography. In many cases with almost invisible masses on plain films or with symptoms suggestive of mediastinal masses, inclined frontal tomograms may show surprisingly large tumours. It is these cases which prompt a reassessment of the 'normal' low kV chest

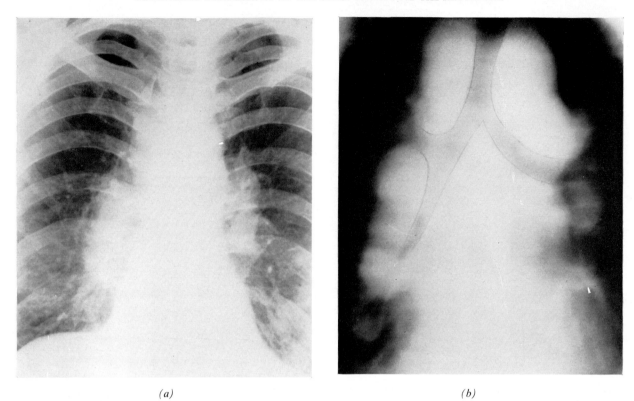

(a)   *(b)*

Figure 7.34. A patient with sarcoidosis. Plain radiograph (a) had been interpreted as showing a right hilar mass, but inclined frontal tomogram (b) clearly demonstrates diffusely enlarged nodes in both hilar regions and throughout the mediastinum

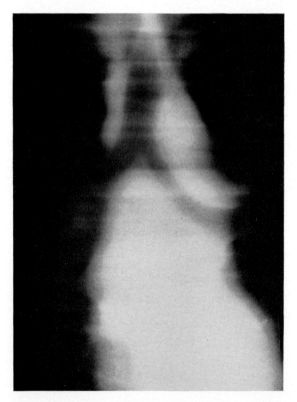

Figure 7.35. Predominantly unilateral left hilar, left upper mediastinal and subcarinal nodal enlargement caused by sarcoidosis

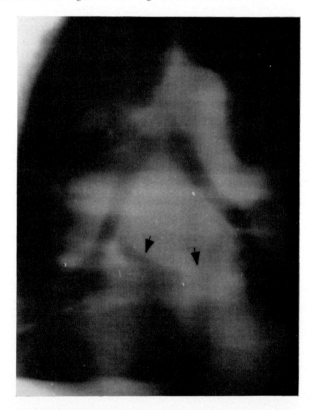

Figure 7.36. Bilateral hilar and subcarinal nodal enlargement due to sarcoidosis. Arrows show subcarinal node enlargement

radiographic techniques commonly used, because if the techniques are so inadequate that such lesions are not recognized, there is much less chance of smaller and surgically treatable lesions being found. Even the demonstration of large masses of nodes is important in the planning of radiotherapy and the consideration of anti-tumour chemotherapy and in studying the response of these masses in the patients so treated (*Figure 7.33*).

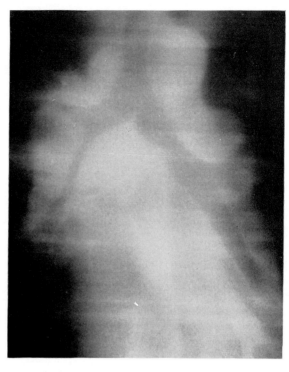

Figure 7.37. Mediastinal and hilar node enlargement may also be caused by rheumatoid granulomas. Biopsy was obtained by media-stinoscopy

Figure 7.38 (below). Bacterial pneumonia in anterior segment of right upper lobe and apex of right lower lobe. Enlarged nodes (arrowed) are well demonstrated in inclined frontal tomogram (b). The nodal enlargement cleared in 6 weeks

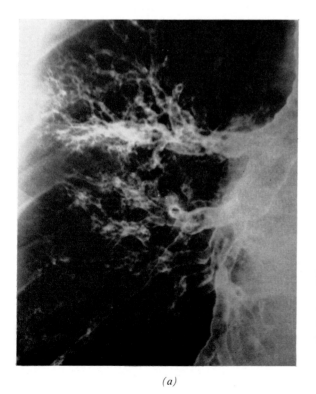

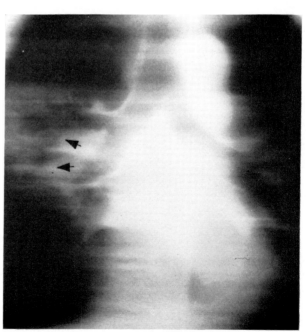

(a)

(b)

Nodal enlargement

Nodes may be enlarged not only due to tumour metastasis but also in reticulosis (*Figure 7.43*), in sarcoidosis (*Figures 7.34–7.37*), or in infections such as pneumonia (*Figures 7.38* and *7.39*) or tuberculous mediastinitis. Such nodal enlargement has to be distinguished from enlargement of pulmonary vascular structures, of the great veins or of the aortic arch. As was discussed in the section on transverse axial tomograms, superior mediastinal tumours are sometimes very difficult to differentiate from dilated vascular structures on tomograms alone. Such differentiation may require an aortogram to show the lumen of the aorta and also tumour circulation if present. However, tomograms do help in defining the shape and position of the mass. When investigating lung tumours, one needs to be constantly aware of the possibility of

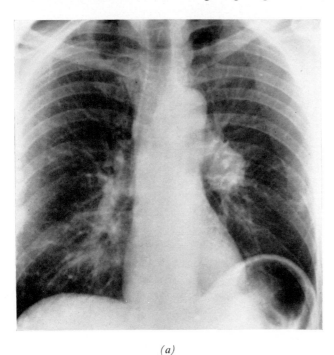

Figure 7.39. (a and b) Adult male with massive left hilar, superior mediastinal and subcarinal node enlargement due to pneumonia; small focus in left lower lobe. (c) Eight weeks later the nodal enlargement had completely resolved

(a)

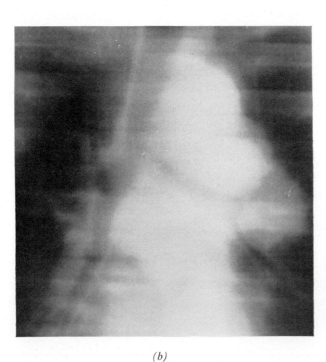

(b)

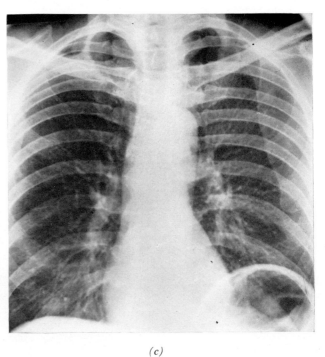

(c)

148

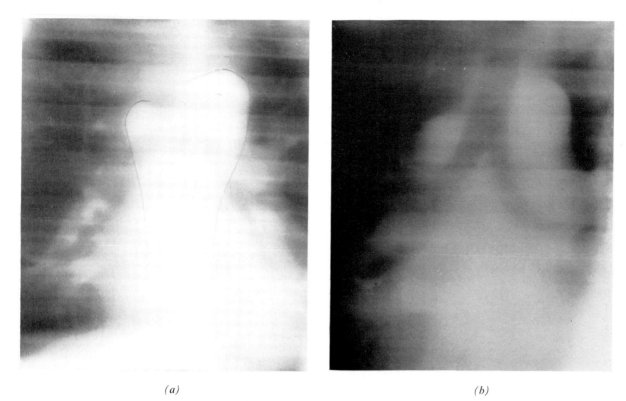

(a) *(b)*

Figure 7.40. Double aortic knuckle in a symptomless patient. Inclined frontal tomograms showing (a) descending aorta and (b) right side of arch mimicking a dilated azygos vein or enlarged nodes in the azygos region

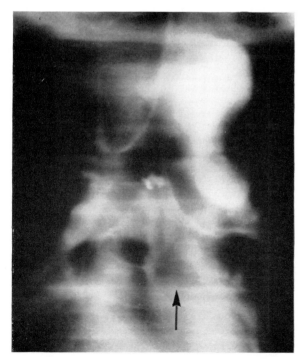

Figure 7.41. Coarctation of the aorta. There is a double aortic knuckle, which is high in position. Note also calcification in subcarinal nodes and gas in hiatus hernia (arrowed)

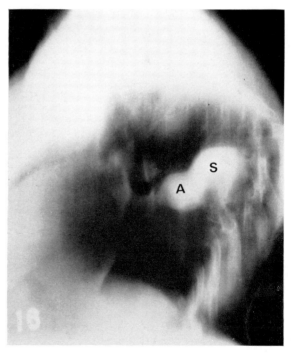

Figure 7.42. Lateral tomogram: transversely passing descending aorta in a patient with severe scoliosis. The aorta (A) mimics a lung tumour. S = spine

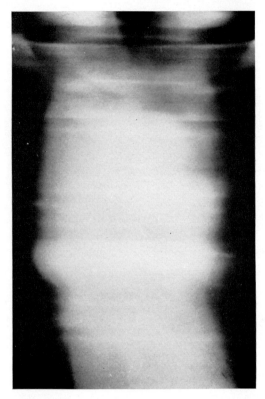

Figure 7.43. Inclined frontal tomogram showing large mass of enlarged nodes in anterior mediastinum in the region of the thymus in a patient with reticulosis

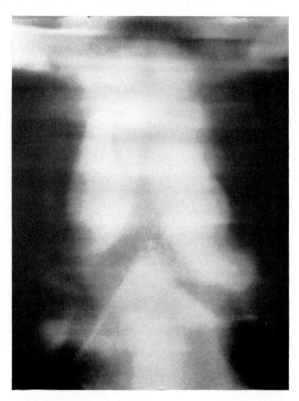

Figure 7.44. Inclined frontal tomogram of a symptomless young man with neurofibromatosis of the vagi. The tumours extended down through the mediastinum into the mesentery

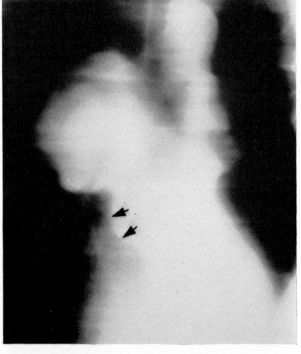

(a)

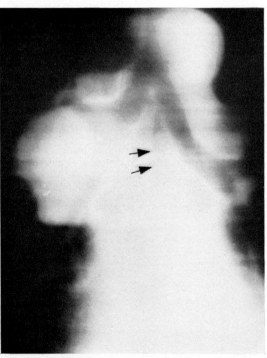

(b)

Figure 7.45. Chemodectoma of right hilum. The mass has spread around the larger bronchi, but no evidence of enlarged nodes is seen and none were found at operation. Tomographic cut (b) is taken 1·5 cm posterior to tomographic cut (a). Arrows in (a) indicate right border of left atrium, and in (b) the air-filled oesophagus

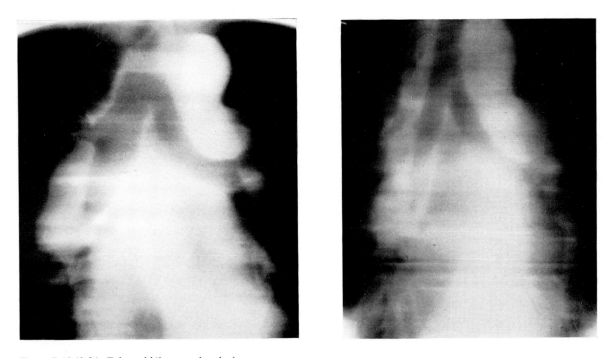

Figure 7.46 (left). Enlarged hilar vascular shadows

Figure 7.47 (right). Conical narrowing of right intermediate and lower lobe bronchi with surrounding soft tissue mass; bronchial carcinoma

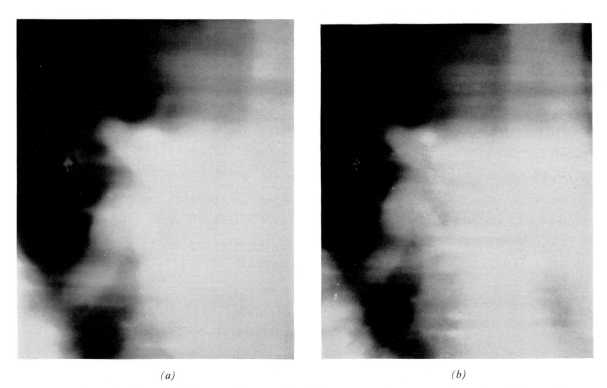

(a)   *(b)*

Figure 7.48. Effects of Müller and Valsalva experiments on size of pulmonary vascular structures in a patient with large pulmonary vessels, particularly the pulmonary veins. (a) Müller experiment (negative pressure). (b) Valsalva experiment (increased pressure); diameter of vascular shadow (lower lobe vein) is reduced from 1·9 to 1·5 cm

other anomalies such as the double shadow of the aortic arch in a patient with a double aortic knuckle (*Figure 7.40*) and in another with a mild coarctation (*Figure 7.41*). Similarly, the horizontally passing aorta in a patient with a severe scoliosis may be confused with a lung tumour (*Figure 7.42*). Other mediastinal masses such as thymic masses (*Figure 7.43—see also Figure 3.129*) or, rarely, neurofibromatosis of the vagi (*Figure 7.44*) must also be differentiated. A hilar mass produced by a pulmonary chemodectoma is shown in *Figure 7.45*.

As can be seen from the illustrations, nodal enlargement in the superior mediastinum or the hilar regions is usually obvious, but minor degrees of enlargement may not always be visible. Vascular enlargement is usually differentiated (*Figure 7.46*—compare with *Figure 7.47*), and as the patient sits up for inclined frontal tomograms, a distended azygos vein will rarely be seen. Pneumonia may give rise to nodal enlargement, usually lasting only a few days or weeks (*see Figures 7.38* and *7.39*). In the retrocarinal and retrocardiac areas, particular caution is necessary in interpreting the tomograms. A mass of nodes will usually give rise to an irregular opacity situated posteriorly to the normal opacity of the left atrium. Normally, the pleural stripe on the medial border of the right lung and the shadow of the oesophagus are seen in this plane. Failure to see them usually suggests the presence of enlarged nodes, tumour or an inflammatory process in this situation.

Another means of distinguishing between enlarged nodes and vascular hilar structures, or between enlarged right-sided paratracheal nodes and the azygos vein, is by taking tomograms while the patient performs the Müller and Valsalva manoeuvres. In this way it is possible to obtain changes in intrathoracic pressure of the order of 80–100 cm of water. Two tomograms (or two series of tomograms) are taken while the patient attempts (1) to breathe out against a closed glottis after a maximum inspiration and (2) to breathe in with a closed glottis after a maximum expiration. Precautions are taken to minimize any change in the patient's position and to make the tomograms otherwise comparable. During these experiments, vascular structures change in size while no effect is produced on enlarged nodes (*Figure 7.48*).

Such a method was used by Lindgren (1946) to diagnose arterio-venous aneurysms in the lungs and by Westermark (1944) and Amundsen (1953) to distinguish between pulmonary vessels and enlarged hilar nodes. Amundsen employed simple longitudinal tomography and gave seven examples of the use of the technique. He also employed a water manometer to standardize the pressure differences, but this is impracticable when using rotational tomography.

SCOPE AND ACCURACY OF THE TECHNIQUE—FIRST 206 CASES

The scope of inclined frontal tomography and its accuracy in demonstrating bronchial tumours and their hilar and mediastinal metastases have been assessed in detail in 136 of the first 206 patients examined

TABLE 7.1

Conditions Investigated by Inclined Frontal Tomography

	Number of cases
Bronchial neoplasm	134
Bronchial adenoma	2
Sarcoid and reticulosis	7
Incompletely resolved pneumonia	19
Aortic abnormalities	6
Large pulmonary artery shadows	4
Thymic masses	3
Thyroid	2
Post-operative or post-irradiation	3
Oesophageal lesions	2
Tuberculosis	4
Bronchiectasis and chronic infections	5
Pneumoconiosis	1
Normal	10
Other	4
Total	206

by this method. Table 7.1 shows the range covered by these first 206 cases, which have been analysed in detail to give an idea of the value of the technique.

Two of the patients with inflammatory lesions had enlarged nodes. In one case the nodes quickly returned to normal. The other patient was explored since cells which were suspicious of neoplasm had been found in the sputum, and a pneumonectomy was performed. The specimen showed a largely destroyed upper lobe with granulation tissue, abscess formation and fibrosis, but no evidence of neoplasm. Fifteen of the 24 patients with incompletely resolved pneumonia, bronchiectasis or chronic infection also had bronchograms; these showed the bronchiectasis rather better, since the bronchial dilatations were often too peripheral for adequate assessment by inclined frontal tomography. In cases of incompletely resolved pneumonia the tomograms frequently showed the distorted bronchi almost as well as the bronchograms. In later cases, bronchiectasis and lung base honeycombing were often well demonstrated on inclined frontal tomograms, as were fluid-filled bronchi distal to a bronchial block.

In the two cases of adenoma there were endobronchial masses. In one of these patients there was an associated hilar mass, while the other had no evidence of this or of enlarged lymph nodes. Careful correlation of all the radiological investigations with the operative findings was undertaken in the 129 cases of bronchial neoplasm in this series.

Comparison with other investigations

Plain chest x-rays (P.A., penetrated P.A. and lateral)

In 109 cases the inclined frontal tomograms gave further information about the air passages and about mediastinal or hilar enlargements. In 5 cases the information gained may have been misleading (*see page* 154).

Other tomograms

Other tomograms, taken to show the presence or shape of a peripheral lung lesion, which included the hilar region did not demonstrate the enlarged mediastinal nodes as well as did the inclined frontal tomograms. Lateral tomograms were taken on the Radiotome in six cases when it appeared that the lesion and the hilum were not well shown with a lesion in a segment of the lung at right angles to the section of the inclined frontal cut, i.e. in the anterior segment of an upper lobe or the apex of a lower lobe (*see Figure 7.25*). Fifteen patients had transverse axial tomograms taken to study possible nodal enlargements behind the heart, around the aortic arch or in the thoracic inlet, but assessment of mediastinal nodal enlargement or direct extension of a tumour into the mediastinum was found to be very difficult by this method unless it was very marked (*see Figure 7.5*).

Bronchography

Nine patients had bronchograms, which showed segmental blocks a little more clearly than the inclined frontal tomograms (*see Figure 8.14*). For visualization of the larger bronchi, the two methods gave comparable results (*see Figure 8.13*). The tomograms in addition provided information about hilar and mediastinal enlargements which was not obtainable from the bronchograms except indirectly if the bronchi were displaced or narrowed.

Bronchoscopy

The purpose of bronchoscopy is not only to inspect the main air passages but also to take a biopsy of any lesion or suspicious area which may be seen. Tomograms would appear to be complementary to bronchoscopy because they show the surrounding soft tissue structures as well as the air passages. Nodal enlargement may also be inferred from bronchoscopy if the trachea or the larger bronchi show defects produced by pressure from without, or if the carina is flattened or widened. Ideally, tomograms should be taken first so as to direct particular attention to suspicious areas of the tracheo-bronchial tree.

Table 7.2 correlates the tomographic with the bronchoscopic findings. In these cases the degree of correlation was good. The differences indicate weaknesses in one or other method of examining the air passages. In an upper lobe, if the endobronchial lesion is distal to a segmental orifice, the lesions

of the bronchial tree. These authors suggested the following five projections to show each part of the lung.

(1) *Right upper lobe*—right posterior projection with the left side of the chest elevated 22 degrees from the table top.

(2) *Right middle lobe*—right posterior projection with the left side of the chest elevated 72 degrees.

(3) *Right lower lobe*—right lateral projection with the pelvis elevated from the table so that the body makes an angle with the table top of about 25 degrees.

(4) *Left upper lobe*—45 degrees posterior projection.

(5) *Left lower lobe*—left lateral projection with the pelvis elevated to angulate the body about 25 degrees from the table top.

Such a technique seems too complicated for routine clinical use.

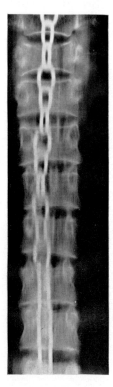

Figure 7.51. Tomograms of a brass chain and dried dorsal spine. (a) Longitudinal movement with the spine in the plane of tomographic focus gives poor blurring of the chain. (b) Transverse movement has a good blurring effect

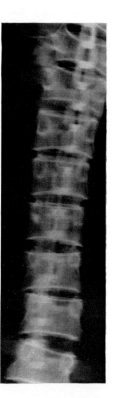

(a)   *(b)*

Another method of demonstrating the larger air passages and the tracheo-bronchial tree, zonography, employs circular tomography using a narrow angle (Westra, 1966).

In tomography the direction of movement blur should be that best suited to the removal of confusing shadows. This point, often poorly understood, is further illustrated by the following experiment. Tomograms were taken of a part of the dorsal spine from a dried skeleton with a superimposed metal chain, using blurring movements in longitudinal and transverse directions (*Fig. 7.51a* and *b*). In *Figure 7.51a*, taken with longitudinal movement, some of the cross-linked portions of the chain have been blurred out, while the larger longitudinally orientated parts are barely blurred. In *Figure 7.51b*, with the crosswise movement, much more blurring has taken place, though the shadows of the cross-linked part of the chain largely remain.

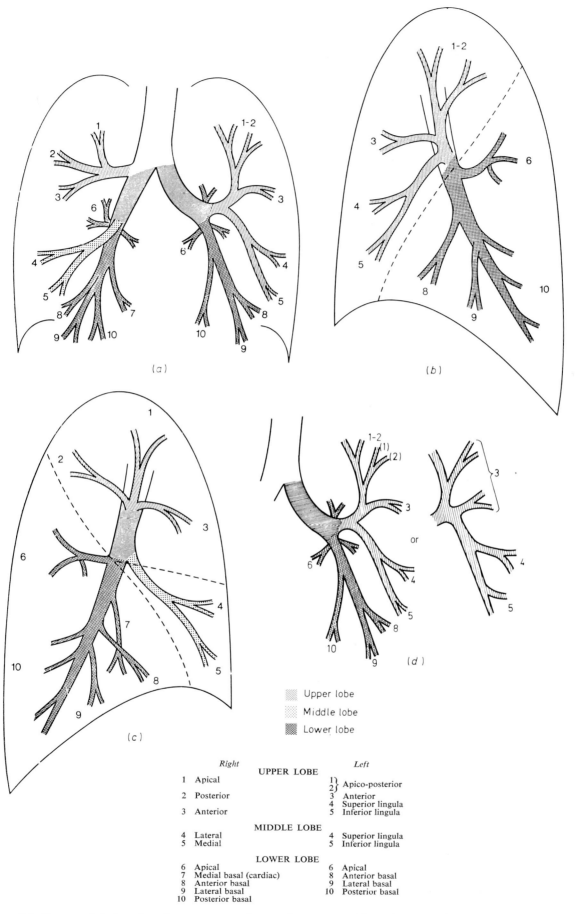

Right		Left
	UPPER LOBE	
1 Apical		1⎫ Apico-posterior
		2⎭
2 Posterior		3 Anterior
		4 Superior lingula
3 Anterior		5 Inferior lingula
	MIDDLE LOBE	
4 Lateral		4 Superior lingula
5 Medial		5 Inferior lingula
	LOWER LOBE	
6 Apical		6 Apical
7 Medial basal (cardiac)		8 Anterior basal
8 Anterior basal		9 Lateral basal
9 Lateral basal		10 Posterior basal
10 Posterior basal		

Figure 8.3. Diagram of the broncho-pulmonary segmental nomenclature approved by an International Committee (1949) and by the Thoracic Society. (a) Anterior view. (b–d) Lateral and left oblique views. (After Pallardy and Remy)

his side and is then tipped head downwards for 20 minutes. He is asked not to cough strongly, as the inspiratory effort preceding such coughing will result in contrast medium being re-aspirated peripherally into the lung. He should gently expectorate the medium which has drained into the larger bronchi. In this way about 75 per cent of it will be recovered, a little usually passing into the alveoli and some being swallowed. The patient is warned of the possible development of surgical emphysema and is instructed to press over the puncture site before performing any strenuous coughing manoeuvres.

When carrying out bronchography for the possible diagnosis of tumour, attention to detail, both in the bronchial filling and in radiography, is very important. Should poor filling of the bronchi occur because the patient coughs (he may be apprehensive or may have had a recent cold), a poor bronchogram may result. One should always endeavour to gain the patient's confidence, and if this is achieved very little trouble will ensue. Slight coughing during the introduction of a contrast agent suspended in water,

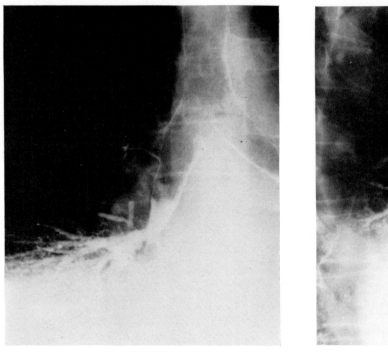
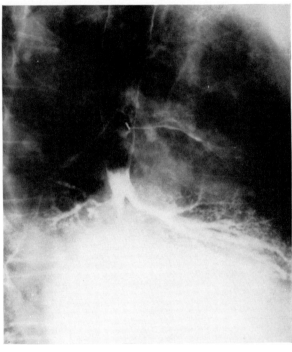

(a)   (b)

Figure 8.4. Patient aged 74 with right basal pleural effusion. On inclined frontal tomograms it was not possible to see the right lower lobe bronchus. The bronchogram shows conical narrowing of this bronchus

such as Hytrast, may be beneficial since the watery medium will tend to adhere more readily to the bronchi and a sharp cough will not of itself cause as much clearing as with an oily medium.

It is important to possess a detailed knowledge of *bronchial anatomy* (*Figure 8.3*). From this it will at once be apparent that the bronchi of the right middle lobe, the apex of each lower lobe and the posterior segment of the upper lobe are best seen in lateral views. Indeed, the middle lobe bronchi are often well seen only in a lateral view, and if the left side has also been filled, good visualization of this part of the bronchial tree may be well-nigh impossible. A bilateral bronchogram taken with full-sized films only is, in my view, almost useless except for the detection of grosser abnormalities. For this reason, in cases of possible tumour where it is necessary to examine both sides, I examine one side at a time. With the technique used, only one side of the bronchial tree becomes opacified. When both sides have to be examined on the same occasion, the right side should always be done first so as to enable its bronchi to be radiographed adequately, the lingula bronchi being readily demonstrable on an oblique view (with the patient rotated to the left—the left oblique view shown in *Figure 8.3d*).

In sick or elderly patients a simplified technique, using less contrast medium to fill only a single lobe, may suffice (*see Figures 8.4* and *8.25*).

I prefer examination under local anaesthesia since (1) it allows a little more time for the subsequent radiography, (2) the examination can be carried out expeditiously, and (3) it can be preceded by tomography, which in my view is complementary to bronchography. I do not agree with Le Roux and Duncan (1964), who advocated doing all bronchograms under general anaesthesia, that the technique described above carries an 'element of mystique' or lends 'an air of profundity to the experienced bronchographer'.

Alternative ways of performing bronchography under local anaesthesia have been discussed by various authors including Vickers (1949). Vickers discussed the many techniques then available, including the simple 'passive deglutition method' in which the pharynx is first anaesthetized with 10 per cent cocaine. When the anaesthesia is at its height, the patient is given 15–30 ml of contrast medium to swallow, but because of the anaesthesia he inhales it. Other methods have involved tipping the contrast medium over the back of the tongue, or the pernasal or peroral catheterization of the trachea (for example, using Rosenthal's cannula or Métras' sounds—*see* Appendix 7). The first descriptions of the use of a catheter to catheterize a part of the bronchial tree were by Huguenin (1928) and Huguenin and Delarue (1933).

Modifications of the crico-thyroid technique have been suggested by Craven (1965); by Rossi, Shahinfor and Ruzcika (1965), who inserted a short catheter into the trachea by means of the Seldinger technique; and by Willson (1961), who passed a short polyethylene catheter through the needle. The advantage of these modifications is that they prevent the accidental injection of contrast medium into the neck. However, they do make a larger puncture hole in the crico-thyroid membrane, and they are more liable to be followed by surgical emphysema of the neck which can be distressing to the patient. For this reason I prefer to use a simple needle and feel that if a basic rule is observed, namely that *the needle tip must at all times lie within the trachea while the contrast medium is being injected*, there is no real danger of injection into the soft tissues of the neck. The air aspiration test is simple to perform. The needle must lock on to the syringe and, provided that air can easily be aspirated into and out of the syringe, *the needle must be in the trachea*. This test should be repeated after every 1–2 ml of contrast medium have been injected and after every swallowing movement or change in the patient's position.

General anaesthesia

I have not used general anaesthesia in the detection of bronchial deformities due to lung tumours, but have reserved this method for examining the bronchial tree in young children. It has, however, been employed by others, and one or two points must be discussed.

The anaesthesia is best achieved with barbiturates (such as thiopentone), nitrous oxide and oxygen. Fat-solvent gases such as ether and halothane should be avoided as these may increase absorption of the contrast medium. The latter is inserted into a main or lobar bronchus via a catheter which passes down into the trachea through either an endotracheal tube or a bronchoscope. Following injection of the medium, the patient is turned on to one or other side as appropriate and three maximal inflations of the lungs are performed. Relaxant drugs facilitate the contrast injection, and the maximal inspirations are performed by squeezing the anaesthetic bag. The cessation of spontaneous respiration should persist during the subsequent radiography. After a brief fluoroscopy, spot and/or overcouch films are taken as described for examinations under local anaesthesia.

VALUE OF BRONCHOGRAPHY IN DETECTING LUNG AND BRONCHIAL TUMOURS

HISTORICAL SURVEY

Following the work of Sicard and Forestier, bronchography became popular for the demonstration of bronchiectasis, deformities of the bronchial tree secondary to abscess or tuberculosis, and cavities or fistulae complicating these conditions. It was even held that Lipiodol might have a therapeutic antibacterial or antiseptic effect, but this view was soon dispelled (*see* Huizinga and Smelt, 1950).

Chandler (1932) noted that the differentiation of a lung abscess from a new growth was rendered more difficult by the tendency of the latter to produce a secondary bronchiectasis. He also found that a bronchial block due to a tumour was often conical in outline.

In the same year, Davidson (1932) stated: 'Often the introduction of 15–20 cc of Lipiodol would demonstrate bronchial obstruction and the typical picture of a "blocked bronchus" seen in the x-ray department of a chest hospital was, to all intents and purposes, diagnostic of a primary carcinoma.'

Farinas (1933, 1934) employed a technique in which Lipiodol was injected through a urethral sound into the appropriate main or lobar bronchus. He found that the bronchial deformity seen in cancer varied with the type of tumour. With polypoid tumours a filling defect might be demonstrated in the bronchi, whereas with infiltrating types of growth a stenosis would be present. This, if not complete, appeared as an incomplete concentric stenosis with irregular borders and was seen especially in the larger bronchi. With a more advanced stenosis the block would be complete. Farinas observed that at the point of an obstruction the walls of a bronchus were irregular due to the malignant infiltration which might extend to the surrounding parenchyma. Irregular cavitating lesions might also be filled. A bronchial carcinoma situated distal to the larger bronchi can give two different appearances: if it is relatively near the hilum a compression of the main, second and third order bronchi may be seen, while if it is distant from the large bronchi the displacement of the bronchial tree may be gross, with small bronchioles and alveoli distorted around the tumour mass.

Westermark (1938) studied the factors producing bronchostenosis. He mentioned neoplasm only briefly, being mainly concerned with inflammatory conditions. He wrote: 'Bronchial cancer does not generally appear on the radiogram* until at a very late stage. Since, however, bronchial cancer already at an early stage produces bronchostenosis, we are able also at this stage to diagnose the condition. For the diagnosis in question it is necessary to carry out bronchography. This examination must be carried out in all cases of chronic atelectasis to exclude or confirm the presence of cancer. The growth appears here as a confluent defect with torn and stiff edges.'

Poppe (1948), discussing the role of bronchography in the diagnosis of bronchiectasis and early carcinoma, referred to the pitifully low rate of operability due to late diagnosis of bronchogenic carcinoma as providing ample evidence that improved diagnostic measures were needed, of which bronchography should be one.

Schinz et al. (1953) pointed out that a bronchogram could demonstrate a tumour growing in a bronchial wall by revealing that the lumen of the bronchus had become stenosed or irregular. With more extensive stenosis, the contrast medium might pass through the irregular narrow portion or be stopped proximally to it.

Dijkstra (1958) discussed the value of bronchography in the detection of bronchial neoplasm and illustrated several cases of irregular stenosis and segmental or lobar occlusion. He pointed out that peripheral lesions might not show any bronchial abnormality.

Wilt et al. (1959) from Columbus, Ohio, analysed the usefulness and accuracy of bronchography in the differential diagnosis of bronchogenic carcinoma. They reviewed bronchograms of 1,408 patients, including 236 with proven bronchogenic carcinoma, taken between 1952 and 1955. They used both spot and large films and found that the abnormality suggestive of a bronchogenic carcinoma consisted simply of a blocked bronchus. The cut-off was usually abrupt, especially in the smaller bronchi; in the main bronchi or the intermediate bronchus, a tapered block might occur. The *persistent bronchial block* of a carcinoma was compared with the distorted but still patent bronchial pattern of an infective process. A bronchial block considered diagnostic of bronchogenic carcinoma was demonstrated in 213 cases, though 3 of these were later shown to be due to actinomycosis, cholesterol pneumonia or chronic interstitial pneumonitis. Twenty-six patients with tumours had normal bronchograms, the lesions in these cases being described as parenchymal masses or nodules, hilar or mediastinal masses, infiltrations or abscesses. The authors felt that while it was easy to see why a peripheral lesion might not produce a visible bronchial block on account of the involvement of the distal portion of the bronchial tree, it was difficult to understand why masses near the hilum did not give rise to a characteristic block in a higher percentage of cases.

Molnar and Riebel (1963) continued the review of the experience of bronchography in Columbus, Ohio, in patients with peripheral lung lesions. They reviewed 667 bronchograms in patients who had had peripheral pulmonary lesions examined between 1952 and 1962 and reported the following findings.

(1) Sizeable, chronic, peripheral inflammatory processes affected the bronchial tree more readily than did their malignant counterparts.

* This is the correct term for an exposed and processed x-ray film. Strictly speaking, 'radiograph' should refer to the x-ray machine, just as 'photograph' should really refer to a photographic camera, though common usage has reversed the terminology.

(2) The accuracy of bronchography was higher in the diagnosis of inflammatory lesions than in that of malignancy.

(3) Lesions, whether inflammatory or neoplastic, commonly failed to affect the bronchial segments if they were located close to the pleura or the lung apex.

Molnar and Riebel illustrated their findings with regard to peripheral masses, segmental infiltration, cavitation, superior mediastinal masses and multiple or bilateral consolidations.

Rinker *et al.* (1968) reviewed the bronchograms of 104 patients with bronchial carcinoma, 97 of these being histologically proven cases. They noted six signs of malignancy found on bronchograms.

(1) *Amputation* of a bronchus usually occurred near its origin. The involved bronchus often showed a meniscus pointing away from the hilum at the site of occlusion. The authors considered such a meniscus to be different from that produced by benign intrabronchial processes such as adenomas, which tended to widen the bronchus proximally to the point of occlusion and showed a meniscus pointing towards the hilum.

(2) *Sharp cut-off* of a bronchus was generally seen at a bronchial origin. There was usually little or no narrowing proximal to the occlusion.

(3) A *stretched or bent* bronchus was mostly produced by a tumour mass which displaced a segment of the bronchus, leaving the proximal and terminal portions in their normal positions. This could be a sign of primary carcinoma but could also occur with metastic tumours.

(4) *Symmetrical narrowing* of a bronchus, with irregular encroachment of the lumen, was due to invasion of the bronchus by tumour prior to its complete occlusion.

(5) '*Rat-tail*' *narrowing* was seen as a narrowing of the bronchus with a lack of the normal arborization as it extends peripherally.

(6) *Thumb-print indentation* of the involved bronchus was a reflection of direct invasion of a bronchus by a tumour mass. It was usually seen in the trachea and the main bronchi, and often denoted secondary mediastinal involvement by the tumour.

Other papers evaluating bronchography in cancer of the lung have been published by Di Rienzo (1949), Therkelsen and Sorensen (1953), Anaker (1955), Stuts and Vieten (1955), Nissenbaum (1964) and Mason and Templeton (1966).

THE AUTHOR'S VIEWS

Before one can make any proper assessment of the bronchi by means of bronchography, a detailed knowledge of bronchial anatomy and its common variations is essential. The first good description was given by Professor Aeby in 1880. He noted that the right main bronchus was wider than the left and descended more vertically from the trachea. He also attached considerable importance to the so-called eparterial bronchus. Brock (1946) published a well illustrated monograph on the anatomy of the bronchial tree in particular relation to his theory that 'bronchial emboli' are the cause of many lung abscesses. At an international meeting in London on 21 July, 1949, a nomenclature for the bronchial tree was agreed, and this should always be used to avoid confusion.

Common anatomical variations include (1) the anterior segmental bronchus of the left upper lobe arising with the apico-posterior segment instead of with the lingula; (2) segmental bronchi or groups of segmental bronchi of an upper lobe arising from the trachea or from a main bronchus; (3) a sub-apical bronchus in either or both lower lobes. Occasionally the bronchial anatomy in the two lungs is reversed, as in situs inversus.

When studying a bronchogram, it is always important to remember that this examination should really be complementary to bronchoscopy, tomography or both. One should consider how much of the bronchial tree can normally be seen at bronchoscopy and how much of it may be examined by bronchography. A diagrammatic representation of this is given in *Figure 8.5*.

With increasing experience of interpreting tomograms and comparing them with the complementary bronchograms, the number of bronchograms carried out has considerably decreased.

Bronchial deformities

Bronchial deformities can be grouped as follows by their positions in the lung.

(1) Central (larger bronchi).

(2) Middle (segmental and sub-segmental bronchi).

(3) Peripheral.

Central area

In the central bronchi, the trachea and the main, intermediate and lobar bronchi, tumours may be demonstrated by the following signs.

(1) Filling defects, which may be rounded or irregular and may have a narrow or a wide base.

(2) Distal bronchiectasis or mucocoeles caused by such filling defects.

(3) Concentric narrowings, which are often irregular in shape, or may extend along the bronchus for a distance of a few centimetres to give an appearance similar to a linitis plastica of the stomach or colon.

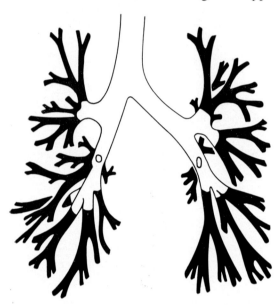

Figure 8.5. Drawing of the bronchial tree comparing the part which may be examined by bronchoscopy (white) with the extra portion which may be examined by bronchography (black). Note.—For an extremely well illustrated description of the method of bronchoscopy and the possible findings, each with colour prints and line drawings, see Stradling, 1968

(4) Complete occlusions, which are irregular in shape. Whether the meniscus of the contrast medium points distally into the blocked bronchus or the reverse seems to depend on how much tumour tissue lies within the lumen of the bronchus.

(5) Shortening of the bronchus due to the tumour.

(6) Irregularities of the wall of a patent bronchus.

(7) Bronchial compression or displacement from an adjacent tumour mass or enlarged nodes. This is usually better appreciated by means of tomography, which will also demonstrate the soft tissue shadow of the mass on the nodes.

Examples of such deformities are shown in *Figures 8.6–8.13.*

Middle area

The segmental and sub-segmental bronchi are much smaller in diameter, and finer details of changes within their lumens are less likely to be seen.

(1) Filling defects are less common than in the larger bronchi.

(2) Irregularities in the contour of the bronchial walls may be present.

(3) The bronchi may be blocked with an irregular cut-off.

(4) The bronchus may be displaced by a tumour mass.

These conditions are illustrated in *Figures 8.14–8.28.*

Peripheral parts of the bronchial tree

In the outer third of the lung, the diameter of the bronchi is even smaller and characteristic deformities within the bronchi are even less likely to be visible. However, there are three main groups of changes that may be present.

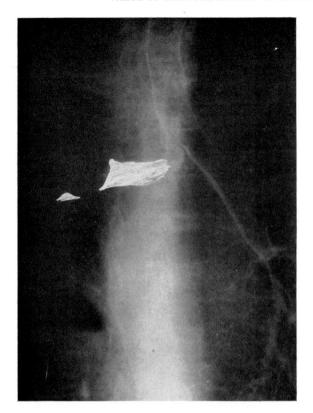

Figure 8.6. Large adenoma in right main bronchus
(retouched print)

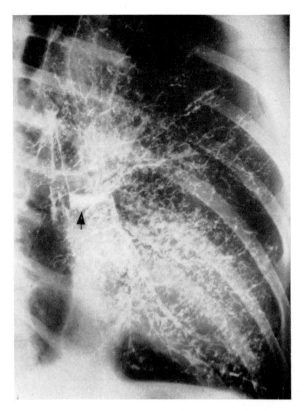

Figure 8.7. Adenoma occluding left lower lobe bronchus

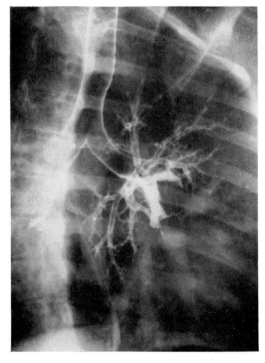

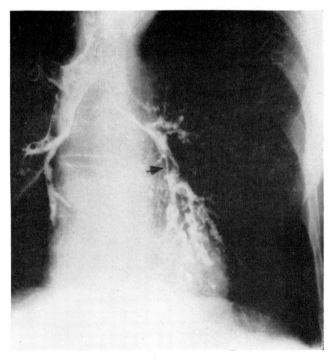

Figure 8.8 (left). Stricture of left upper lobe bronchus and basic bronchi of left lower lobe due to bronchiectasis follicularis secondary to fungus infection. Distal to the strictures the bronchi are visible as dilated soft tissue shadows (mucocoeles). Only the apical bronchi of the left lower lobe have filled normally

Figure 8.9 (right). Small rounded tumour in left lower lobe bronchus with bronchiectasis distal to it. Bronchial carcinoma

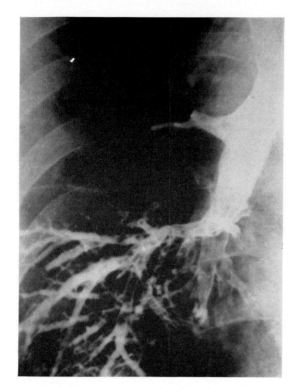

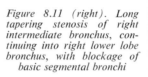

Figure 8.10 (left). Concentric narrowing and shortening of right upper lobe bronchus due to neoplasm

Figure 8.11 (right). Long tapering stenosis of right intermediate bronchus, continuing into right lower lobe bronchus, with blockage of basic segmental bronchi

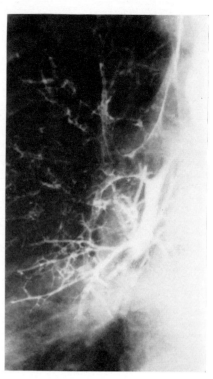

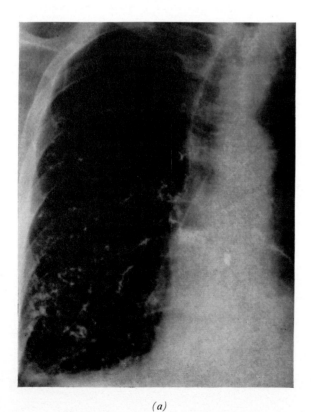

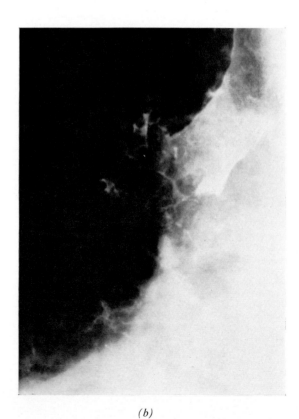

(a)   (b)

Figure 8.12. Bronchial neoplasms causing complete obstruction of right intermediate bronchus. (a) Rounded tumour. (b) Irregular tumour

(1) Deformities of several smaller branches due to their involvement by the peripheral tumour.

(2) Displacement of the bronchi by the tumour.

(3) A normal or near normal appearance, with the bronchi going through the tumour. This is especially encountered with sarcomas and reticuloses (*see Figures 8.31* and *10.32*). A 'leafless tree' appearance is occasionally seen with alveolar or bronchiolar cell carcinomas (*see Figure 10.7*).

A peripheral rounded tumour may give rise to no bronchial deformity.

Only rarely have I seen contrast medium enter a malignant cavity, the characteristics of which are better studied by tomography.

There may be bronchiectasis and/or mucocoeles distal to a stricture or to an endobronchial filling defect.

Illustrations of the above signs appear in *Figures 8.29–8.31.*

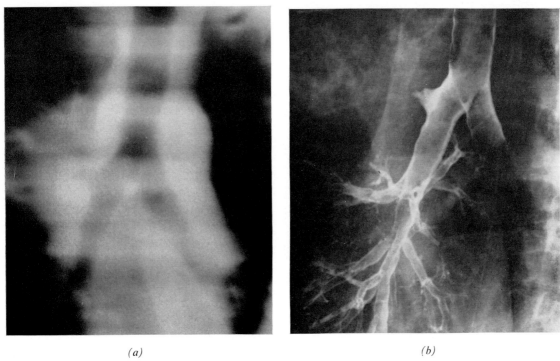

(a)　　　　　　　　　　　　　　　　　　　　*(b)*

Figure 8.13. Concentric narrowing of right upper lobe bronchus due to bronchial neoplasm. The inclined frontal tomogram shows the soft tissue shadow better than the bronchogram. Both examinations show the bronchial deformity equally well

Note.—As is pointed out in Chapter 9, a peripheral lung tumour may give rise to a more central bronchial deformity caused by (1) enlarged nodes or (2) bronchial wall metastasis.

Figure 8.32 shows peripheral shadowing in the right upper lobe when there was a normal bronchogram. Twelve months later a repeat bronchogram revealed concentric narrowing of the right upper lobe bronchus with deformity extending along the adjacent main and intermediate bronchi. At the time of the first bronchogram the patient had had a normal bronchoscopy. One wonders whether the tumour originated in the right upper lobe bronchus or whether it was peripheral in origin with later secondary spread to the central bronchi.

In addition, metastases occasionally arise in the walls of bronchi from tumours developing at distant sites. Schoenbaum and Viamonte (1971) have reported patients with endobronchial metastases from tumours of the breast and thyroid and also from cutaneous melanomas.

Differential diagnosis

Appearances produced by bronchial tumours must be distinguished from those of benign lesions. Filling defects may sometimes be caused by mucous plugs*, a broncholith or an inhaled foreign body. Strictures may be caused by past tuberculosis, by injury or rarely by syphilis (Ingram, 1950). If present

* As in asthma or pulmonary eosinophilia.

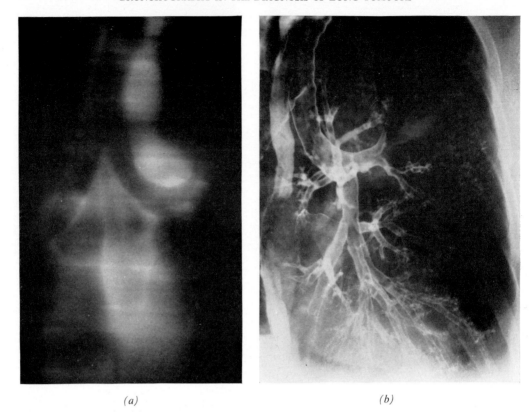

(a)   *(b)*

Figure 8.14. Carcinoma arising in anterior segmental bronchus of left upper lobe with gross left hilar involvement. The bronchial stenosis was seen on both the inclined frontal tomogram (a) and the bronchogram (b), but the tomogram also showed soft tissue shadow of enlarged hilar nodes and displacement of left main bronchus downwards and medially

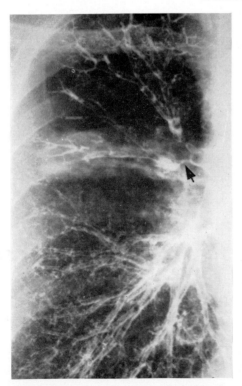

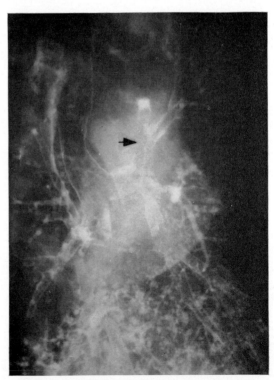

Figure 8.15. Complete blockage of posterior segmental bronchus of right upper lobe with stenosis of origins of apical and anterior segmental bronchi

Figure 8.16. Long filling defect on medial side of apico-posterior segmental bronchus of left upper lobe. The apical branch is dilated above the intraluminal mass

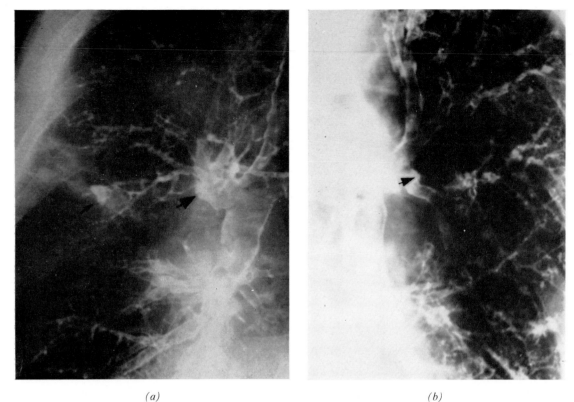

(a)   *(b)*

Figure 8.17. (a) Sharp 'cut-off' of anterior segmental bronchus of right upper lobe (large arrow). The lobe remains partly aerated, and contrast has passed into a bullous cavity within this segment from a small branch within the posterior segment. (b) Sharp 'cut-off' of anterior segmental bronchus in left upper lobe due to neoplasm

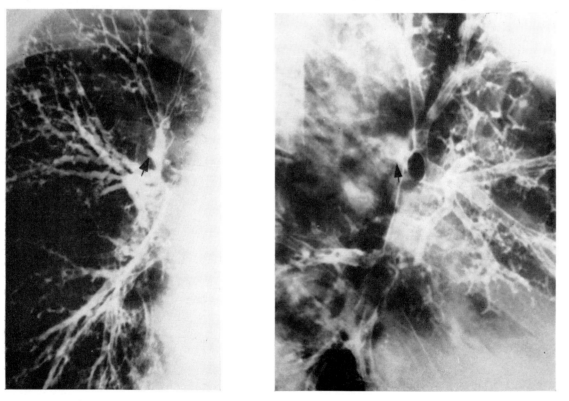

Figure 8.18 (left). Sub-segmental stenosis of apical segmental bronchus of right upper lobe due to carcinoma
Figure 8.19 (right). 'Pigtail' deformity of posterior segmental bronchus of right upper lobe due to bronchiectasis follicularis, a benign condition. Retained secretions are present in the bronchi distal to the obstruction

173

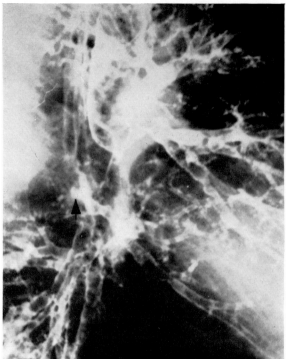

Figure 8.20. Irregular deformity of a small bronchus produced by a bronchial neoplasm

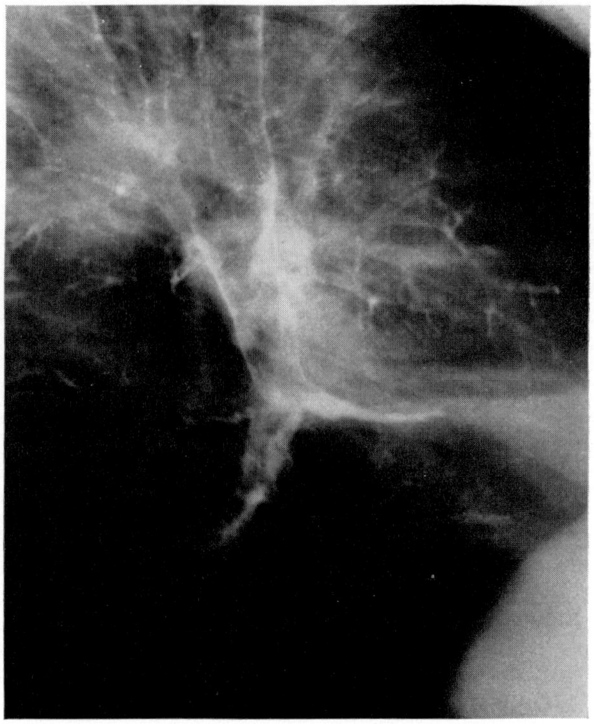

Figure 8.21. Typical 'rat-tail' narrowing of right middle lobe bronchus due to carcinoma

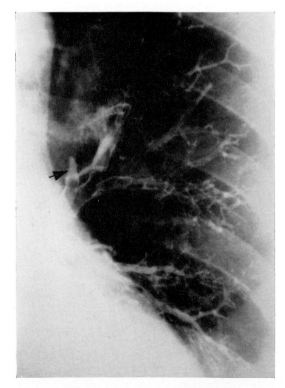

Figure 8.22. Short tapering and stenosis of apico-posterior segmental bronchus of left upper lobe due to carcinoma

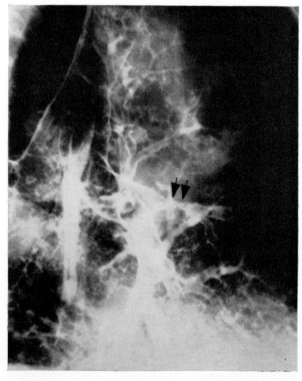

Figure 8.23. Irregular stenosis of left upper lobe bronchus due to carcinoma (magnified view)

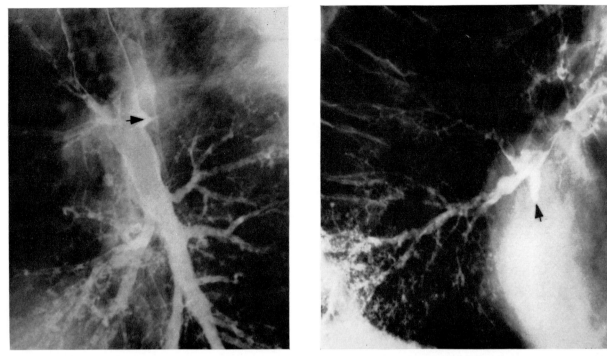

Figure 8.24 (left). Rapidly tapering block of posterior segmental bronchus of right upper lobe. This was almost invisible in the A.P. and oblique views, but is well demonstrated in this lateral view taken under fluoroscopic control. It was due to a bronchial carcinoma

Figure 8.25 (right). Modified bronchogram using only 5 ml Dionosil Oily to demonstrate stenosis of right middle lobe bronchus. The patient, a man aged 80, had had a right lower lobe pneumonia. As this cleared, a biconvex shadow at the lower end of the oblique fissure enlarged. The bronchogram clearly demonstrated that this was not an encysted effusion

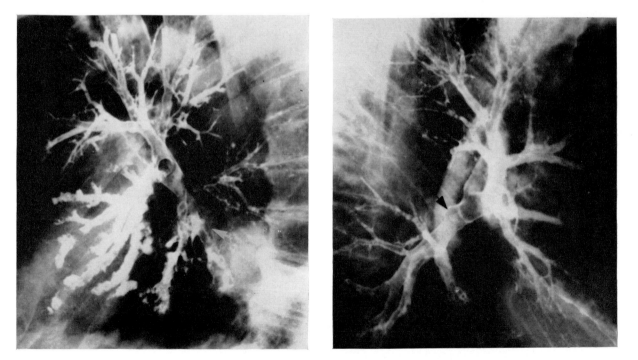

Figure 8.26 (left). Bronchial neoplasm with bronchial block arising in a patient with pre-existing bronchiectasis

Figure 8.27 (right). Stenosis of apical segmental bronchus of left lower lobe. The patient had had three episodes of pneumonia in this segment over a period of 3 years; he was actually referred for a barium swallow examination to exclude an oesophageal lesion causing inhalation, but a bronchogram was carried out first. At operation the tumour was still endobronchial. This case illustrates a flat meniscus at the site of the block (arrowed)

in the larger bronchi, usually they are smooth and do not extend for any distance along the wall of the bronchus, and the lung distal to them may show considerable scarring or tuberculous bronchiectasis. Progressive strictures are also seen in some patients with endobronchial sarcoidosis. Scarring following pulmonary infarction may give rise to multiple smooth bronchial strictures (Walker and Wilson, 1967). The case shown in *Figure 8.33* was complicated by old tuberculous hilar glands, and although the pathological diagnosis as well as the patient's recent history was consistent with infarction, it is possible that the old tuberculosis contributed to the deformity in this case. Infarction may also produce a chronic peripheral lung lesion.

Other strictures mimicking a neoplasm may be produced by fungus infections or by keratinized plaques in a bronchus leading to bronchiectasis follicularis (*Figures 8.8, 8.19*). Blind bronchial buds are

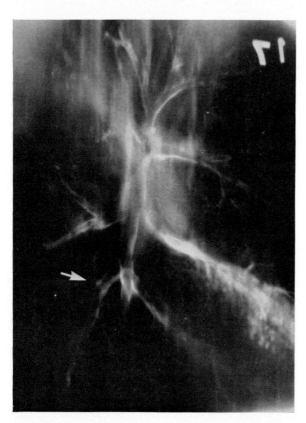

Figure 8.28. Tomo-bronchogram showing sub-segmental bronchial block in posterior basic segment of right lower lobe due to neoplasm. The right lower lobe was resected. Eight years later the patient developed a second tumour in the left upper lobe

sometimes caused by failure of a bronchus to develop properly, but the smooth 'cup' of the diverticulum usually prevents confusion (*Figure 8.34*). Similarly, a post-operative deformity (*Figure 8.35*) rarely causes any difficulty in diagnosis. Occasionally a bronchogram will help in differentiating the abnormal vascular shadows which may be associated with a congenital bronchial deformity.

The main problem in the differential diagnosis of a bronchial neoplasm by bronchography lies in the differentiation from inflammatory disease. Typically a pneumonia will show patent bronchi running through an area of consolidation (*Figure 8.36*), but such an appearance is rarely seen in malignant consolidation, particularly that due to a reticulosis (*see Figures 8.31* and *10.32*). More commonly, partial collapse associated with an incompletely resolved infection will give rise to crowding of the bronchial branches in a segment or lobe (*Figure 8.37*). Such branches may well be distorted or deformed, especially in the more virulent infections such as staphylococcal pneumonia. Incomplete filling of the individual branches may be seen if the patient has residual secretions in the bronchi or has received insufficient physiotherapy before the examination. Rarely a lung abscess or an emphysematous cyst will fill with the bronchographic contrast medium (*see Figure 8.17a*).

More difficulty is experienced when a bronchial carcinoma complicates a long-standing pulmonary disease process such as tuberculosis, bronchiectasis, sarcoidosis or post-operative scarring (*see* Chapter

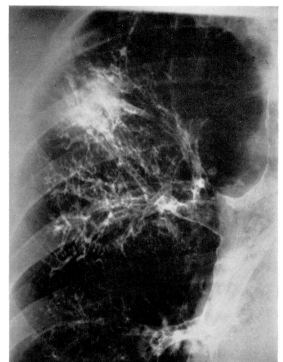

Figure 8.29. Irregular tumour in outer third of right lung. Several smaller bronchi are distorted by the tumour, which is well demonstrated by conventional tomography. (a) Magnified bronchogram. (b) Conventional tomogram (two tomographic cuts)

(a)

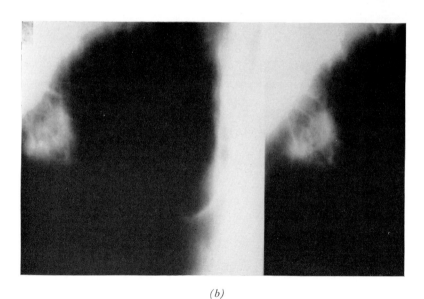

(b)

3). The bronchial deformity may be remote from the area of the pre-existing disease (*see Figure 8.26*) or may lie close to it and not be easily recognized (*Figure 8.37*).

Another difficult differential diagnosis occurs with peripheral solid or cavitating lesions (*Figure 8.37*), which may show little or no bronchial deformity. Most often a pleural shadow (*Figure 8.38*) associated with only inflammatory changes in the underlying lung will be due to a loculated collection of fluid or an empyema. However, this appearance can be mimicked by a pleural tumour or by a very peripheral lung tumour which is extending into the chest wall, and an irregular 'frayed' edge to the apparent pleural shadow may then suggest its true nature (*see Figure 9.4a*). Bronchial tumours may involve the bronchi more centrally than the primary peripheral lesion due to spread of tumour through the lung or to intra-

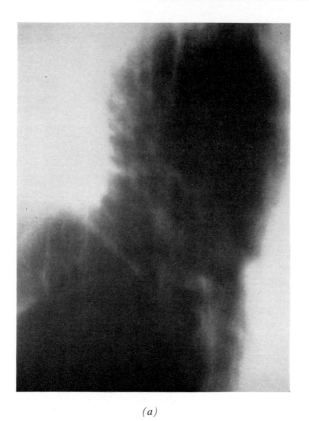

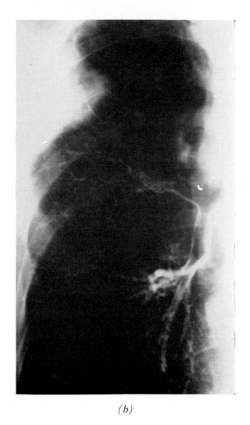

(a)   *(b)*

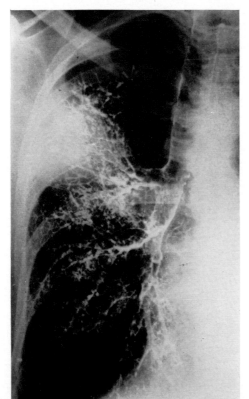

Figure 8.30 (above). Irregularly bordered peripheral mass in right upper lobe. (a) Conventional tomogram. (b) Bronchogram: the tumour is too peripheral to show any bronchial deformity

Figure 8.31. Consolidation of right upper lobe due to lymphosarcoma, with patent bronchi. The patient has remained well for 15 years following right upper lobe resection. Another example of reticulosis with patent bronchi passing through a mass is shown in Figure 10.32

pulmonary or hilar lymph nodes, with secondary invasion of the bronchus. Such involvement is indicated by the appearance seen in *Figure 9.4b*.

Comparison with tomography

As already stated, I consider that tomograms are complementary to bronchograms in that on the former, soft tissue shadows outside the bronchi are readily seen as well as the air-filled bronchi. In

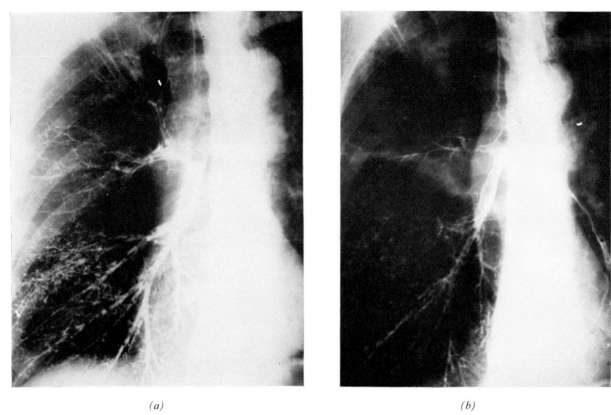

(a)   *(b)*

Figure 8.32. (a) Small peripheral shadows in right upper lobe; normal bronchogram. (b) Twelve months later: enlarged right hilum and concentric narrowing of right upper lobe bronchus with deformity extending along adjacent main and intermediate bronchi

peripheral lesions of the lung, tomograms often give much more information than bronchograms about the anatomy of disease processes (*see Figures 8.13* and *8.30*).

With more proximal tumours the deformities resulting from the pressure of hilar and juxta-hilar masses on the larger bronchi may not be appreciated on the bronchograms, although they will be clearly seen on tomograms and especially on inclined frontal tomograms. The presence of dense consolidation or fluid renders rather indistinct the detail which might otherwise have been shown by tomography. Air-filled bronchi are readily demonstrable in an area of consolidation, but if the lung is collapsed it may not be possible to visualize the bronchi in this way. Bronchography then has the advantage of enabling a study of the position, number and morphology of the bronchi in the diseased area. The presence of a bronchial block, of peripheral bronchi displaced by a loculated effusion or by empyema, or of underlying bronchiectasis may reveal the cause of the disease process.

Figure 8.39 shows in diagrammatic form the various types of bronchial deformity which may be produced by bronchogenic tumours.

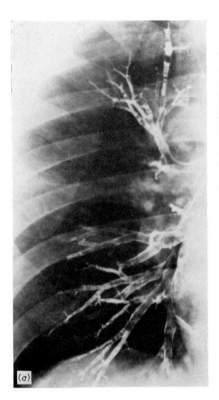

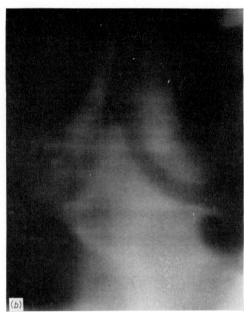

Figure 8.33. Scarring following pulmonary infarction giving rise to a prominent right hilum and stenosis of the anterior and posterior segmental bronchi of the right upper lobe

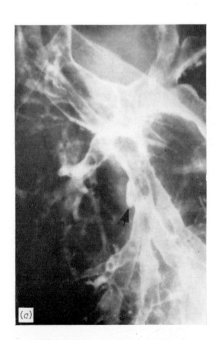

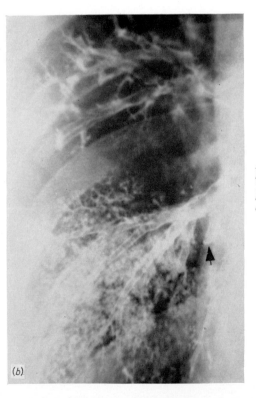

Figure 8.34. (a) Blind 'bronchial bud'. (b) Blind 'bronchial bud'. The patient, who also had minor bronchiectasis, had blind bronchial buds on both sides of the chest

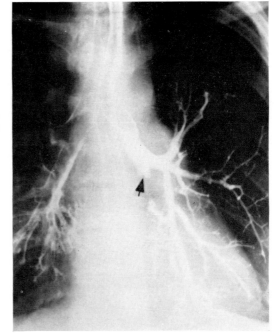

Figure 8.35. Bronchial stump following resection of left lower lobe for bronchiectasis. This stump has an elevated centre due to the surgical closure

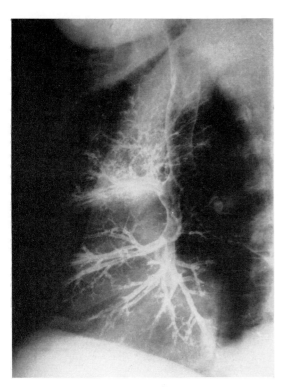

(a)

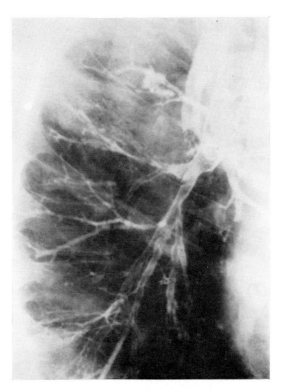

(b)

Figure 8.36. (a) Bacterial pneumonia with consolidation of right upper lobe which was slow to clear. The bronchi throughout the upper lobe are patent. (b) Slowly resolving inflammatory change in apical segment of left lower lobe with some crowding of sub-segmental branches in upper and middle parts of apical segment (which normally has three sub-segments). Lateral tomogram also showed slight residual collapse

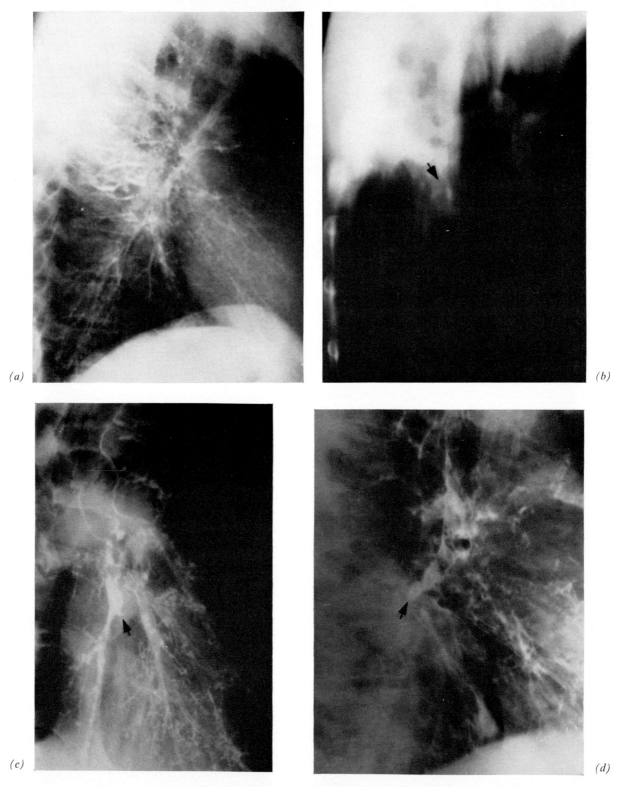

Figure 8.37. This case shows the difficulty of making a diagnosis of bronchial neoplasm when there is already pre-existing disease in the same or a neighbouring portion of lung. (a) Bronchogram showing bronchiectasis in apical segment of left lower lobe. This male patient had a resection of this segment because of repeated infections in it. (b) Eleven years later, plain radiographs showed a possible small shadow adjacent to the left hilum. A.P. tomograms did not show the lesion well, but again suggested a small round shadow below the left hilum and behind the heart. Lateral tomograms showed marked scarring in the area of the previous resection, with a small nodule below it (arrowed). (c) A bronchogram at this time showed a sub-segmental block in the left lower lobe with dilated fluid-filled bronchi distal to it, but this was unrecognized at the time. (d) A further bronchogram almost two years later showed a completely blocked left lower lobe bronchus

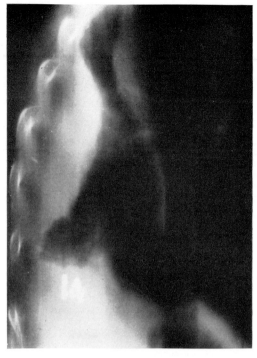

(a)

Figure 8.38. Pleural thickening at right base posteriorly due to a loculated empyema. (a) Lateral tomogram. (b) Bronchogram

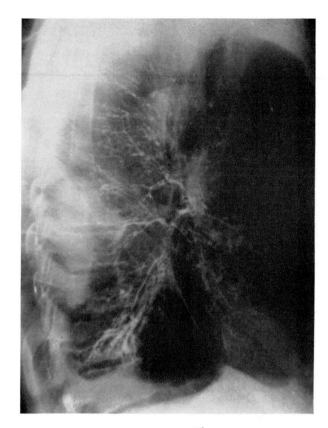

(b)

(*a*) Endobronchial mass

(*b*) Asymmetrical or irregular bronchial narrowing

(*c*) Mucocoeles or bronchiectasis

(*d*) Tumours below or at axil of side branch

Shouldering

(*e*) Rat-tail narrowing

(*f*) Conical narrowing

(*g*) Pigtail deformity

(*h*) Rounded cut-off with meniscus due to endobronchial tumour

(*i*) Sharp cut-off of side branch

(*j*) Deformities caused by extrabronchial masses

(*k*) Shortening of a bronchus caused by a tumour in the bronchial wall

(*l*) Rudimentary bronchial bud

(*m*) Benign strictures

Figure 8.39. (a–k) Some types of bronchial deformity which may be produced by bronchogenic tumours and demonstrated by bronchography. For comparison, (l) and (m) show bronchial blocks due to benign conditions; a 'stump' or sharp cut-off may also be present following surgical resection (see Figure 8.35)

9

Lymphatic Drainage of the Lungs and Thorax

Because of their size and function, lymphatic vessels were not observed until 1563, when Eustachius discovered the thoracic duct in the horse and termed it the *vena alba thoracis*. Thomas Bartholinus wrote his *Vasa Lymphatica* in 1653. William Cruickshank (1786) distinguished 'superficial absorbents' from those which were 'deeper seated', both sets of vessels draining into the glands at the root of the lungs. A

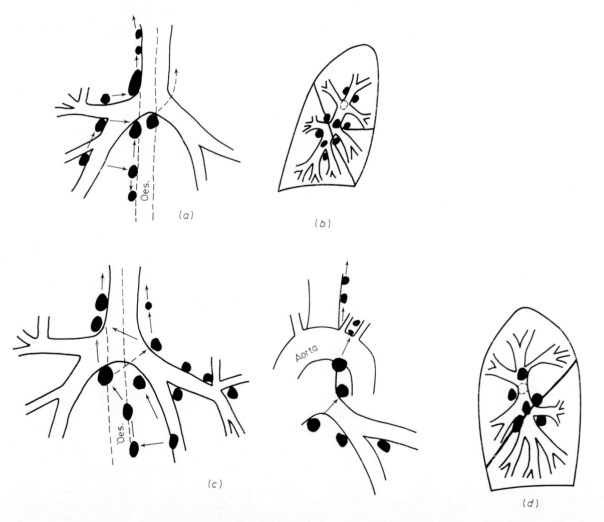

Figure 9.1. Diagrams of the lymph nodes draining the lungs (after McCort and Robbins, 1951, and Nohl, 1962). Right lung: (a) A.P. and (b) lateral views. Left lung: (c) A.P. and (d) lateral views

year later Mascagni (1787), in a book dealing with the lymphatics of the whole body, showed up the sub-pleural and deeper lymphatics by injection of mercury and noted the position of the major lymph nodes in the angles of the bifurcations of the major arteries and bronchi. He also observed that crossed drainage into the left or right side of the superior mediastinum could occur from the contralateral lung or hilar nodes. A reproduction of his drawing of the lymphatics and lymph nodes of the thorax appears in the frontispiece. The lymph nodes draining the lungs are also shown in diagrammatic form in *Figure 9.1*.

Following Mascagni's work, Becker (1826) classified the lymph nodes of the thorax into parietal and visceral, distinguishing three groups: (1) those lying on the trachea, (2) those at the bifurcation of the trachea, and (3) those situated in the hila of the lungs. Just over 50 years later, Parrot (1876) wrote, 'les ganglions bronchiques sont comme le miroir du poumon'. Kuss (1898) elaborated on this concept with reference to pulmonary tuberculosis in childhood, giving the first description of the primary focus ('le foyer pulmonaire primitif') later also studied by Ghon (1912).

At the end of the nineteenth century, many publications appeared dealing with the anatomy of the lymph nodes of the chest in relation to pulmonary tuberculosis. Leaf (1898) noted the relationship of the left sub-aortic nodes to the left recurrent laryngeal nerve. Sukiennikow (1903) studied the topographic anatomy of the bronchial and tracheal lymph nodes, described spaces alongside the trachea and

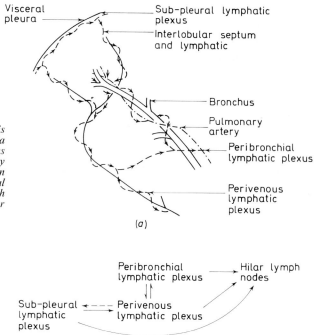

Figure 9.2. Lymphatic drainage of the lung. According to this schematic diagram, the spread of a tumour may take place via the sub-pleural, peribronchial and perivenous lymphatic plexuses and their interconnections. Such spread is most commonly proximal, to the hilar nodes and peribronchial lymphatics (often with secondary involvement of the central or more proximal bronchi), but may also occur to the pleura with reversed lymph flow. The arrows indicate the normal direction of flow (After Trapnell, 1970)

nodes below the carina, and observed the gradual lateral deviation of the node chains as they pass upwards towards the thoracic inlet. He thought that nodes were mainly of two types: (1) nodes lying at the bifurcations of the trachea or bronchi, and (2) interconnecting nodes. On the other hand, Engel (1926) considered that nodes were usually associated with the pulmonary artery and its branches. Steinert (1928) believed that the hilar nodes were related to both vessels and bronchi, and also noted anastomotic vessels linking the paratracheal chains. Rouvière (1932) published a detailed study of the lymphatic system, including a chapter on that of the mediastinum and the lung. This subject was later studied in more detail by Rouvière's pupils, Cordier, Papamiltiades and Cedard (1958).

McCort and Robbins (1951), discussing the roentgen diagnosis of intrathoracic lymph node metastases in carcinoma of the lung, reported a study of the sites of metastases in 103 patients who had undergone thoracotomy for bronchial carcinoma. They found that there was a tendency for right upper lobe tumours to spread to the paratracheal nodes earlier than those arising in the left upper lobe. They also

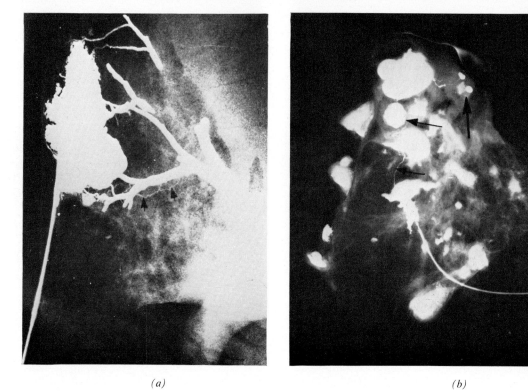

(a)   *(b)*

Figure 9.3. (a) Injection of contrast medium into a sub-pleural lymphatic and bronchi, showing contrast medium passing through the lung into the peribronchial lymphatic system. Note that the peribronchial lymphatics may deviate away from a bronchus and later in their course return towards it. (b) In this specimen, a lower lobe obtained from a patient with tuberculosis, the Lipiodol passed through a cannulated sub-pleural lymphatic (small arrows) to the hilum (large arrow)

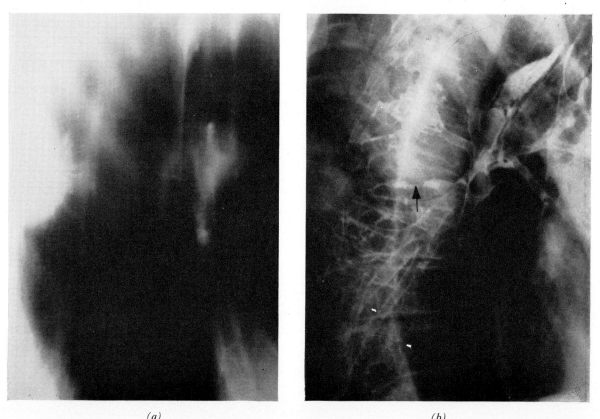

(a)   *(b)*

Figure 9.4. Irregular peripheral mass with 'frayed' edge in apex of right lower lobe. (a) Lateral tomogram. (b) Bronchogram showing stenosis of apical segmental bronchus, almost certainly due to more proximal spread of tumour through the peribronchial lymphatics

186

found that several tumours showed contralateral mediastinal nodal involvement, and postulated that when a node becomes filled with tumour and can no longer function as a filtering organ, the lymph flow is forced into other channels. They further stated: 'Since it is unlikely that the valve system of the lymphatics can remain competent in the presence of blockage and dilatation, adjacent anastomotic channels take up the load. For this reason, the lymph nodes which will become involved by carcinoma arising in any given anatomic unit cannot be predicted with certainty, no matter how thoroughly normal lymphatic pathways are understood.' The nodal enlargements were seen on plain radiographs, through deviation of the barium-filled oesophagus, or through pressure on bronchi as shown on bronchograms.

Nohl (1962) studied both the lymphatic and the haematogenous spread of lung tumours. He particularly pointed out the drainage of the left lower lobe through the subcarinal nodes and thence to the right paratracheal nodes. (*See also* Nohl-Oser, 1972.)

The peripheral lymphatics of the lung have been studied by several workers, including Miller (1937, 1947) and Trapnell (1963, 1967, 1970). These workers have confirmed the view that there are two groups of lymphatics in the lungs, one in the sub-pleural space (or in the pleura according to Trapnell),* and the other deep in the lungs in relation to the bronchi and the blood vessels. Willis (1679) first showed the presence of valves in the sub-pleural lymphatics. Councilman (1900) reported that valves were present in the interlobular vessels and that they pointed towards the pleura, though Trapnell (1963, 1970) considers on good evidence that they mainly point in the opposite direction. A diagram of the intrapulmonary lymphatics is given in *Figure 9.2*.

As shown in *Figure 9.2* and in the pulmonary lymphangiograms carried out on freshly excised lungs (*Figure 9.3*), a lung tumour may spread through the lymphatic system to the pleura, to the hilar nodes, to vessels alongside the bronchi and the pulmonary artery (the peribronchial vessels), or to vessels around the pulmonary veins (the perivenous lymphatics). Spread of tumour to these sites, and into the peribronchial vessels in particular, may give rise to secondary involvement of a bronchus at a more proximal site in the lung. The bronchus then becomes fixed or rigid as determined by bronchoscopy or narrowed with a peribronchial mass as seen on radiography, particularly on bronchograms or tomograms (*Figures 8.32* and *9.4*). Such secondary proximal bronchial involvement may be mistaken for the primary tumour at bronchoscopy, by the pathologist examining a surgical specimen or at autopsy (a point noted by Spencer, 1968). Spencer also postulated that metastases to the adrenals and kidneys and to the abdominal nodes may be caused by retrograde lymph flow in a caudal direction from the hilar nodes.

Peribronchial infiltration may be suggested on radiographs by peribronchial or perivascular 'streaky' shadows (*see Figures 3.22* and *3.25*) as well as by more proximal bronchial deformities.

Trapnell (1972) also points out that lymphatics in the inferior pulmonary ligament may pass to the abdomen without necessarily passing through any intrathoracic lymph nodes. They may be filled with tumour cells in patients with lymphangitis carcinomatosa. Occasionally these vessels are demonstrated at lymphangiography. Not only may bronchial tumours spread to the abdomen in this way, but these vessels may explain why a renal tumour sometimes gives rise to a hilar lymph node metastasis (*see* Wright and Bishop, 1973). They may also explain the uncommon (when other than hepatic) abdominal presentations of bronchogenic carcinoma. Sinclair and Gravelle (1967) reported various abdominal presentations of bronchogenic carcinoma, finding metastases not only in the para-aortic nodes, the liver, the retroperitoneal tissues, the tail of the pancreas, the kidneys and the adrenals, but also in the wall of the colon simulating a primary bowel tumour.

In addition, there are submucosal lymphatics in the bronchi through which either extension of the primary tumour or development of secondaries in the peribronchial vessels may take place. Nohl (1962) pointed out that a tumour may extend proximally through these vessels for several centimetres from its main bulk, thus allowing a positive biopsy at a more proximal site and also giving rise to stump recurrences after lung resection, similar findings being previously noted by Cotton (1959) and by Griess, McDonald and Clagett (1945).

---

* However, in the technique which I have employed for demonstrating the pulmonary lymphatics—namely the injection of 0·1 ml patent blue sub-pleurally as soon as the chest is opened at thoracotomy, thus allowing about 30 minutes of natural lung perfusion before the resection is completed, and the subsequent cannulation of a lymphatic on the surface of the lung as for other lymph-angiograms, the pleura first being penetrated and then the lymphatic cannulated—these lymphatics seem to me to be very mobile below the visceral pleura. Trapnell used autopsy specimens inflated with formalin vapour, which may have caused some fixation.

10

Special Radiographic and Isotope Procedures in the Assessment of Lung and Mediastinal Tumours

ANGIOCARDIOGRAPHY

In 1950 Dotter, Steinberg and Holman advocated venous angiography, performed by the rapid injection of contrast medium into the veins of both arms, in the pre-operative assessment of bronchial carcinoma. They used this technique to demonstrate possible mediastinal involvement as shown by complete or partial occlusion of the left pulmonary artery close to its origin, by complete or partial occlusion of the great mediastinal veins (sometimes with polypoid-looking defects in the superior vena cava), by mediastinal vessels displaced or deformed by metastases, and by pericardial thickening.

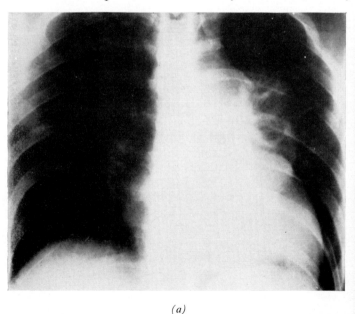

(a)

Figure 10.1. Large tumour abutting on to upper left border of pericardium. Lateral view shows that the tumour was situated anteriorly. Angiocardiogram fails to show any deformity of pulmonary trunk or pulmonary arteries

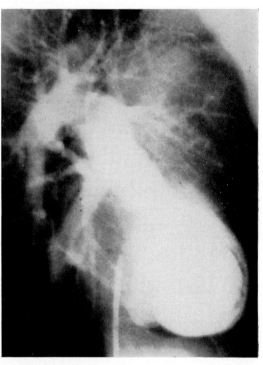

(b)

These workers studied 53 proved cases of lung carcinoma and found that of 25 patients who had been considered inoperable, 3 were able to have resections at exploratory thoracotomy, while out of the 22 patients who had been thought to have no angiocardiographic evidence of inoperability, 10 proved inoperable at exploratory surgery. They emphasized that non-neoplastic conditions, either on their own or complicating a neoplasm, could cause or simulate any of the changes ascribable to neoplasm, and stated: 'No patient should be denied exploratory surgery on the basis of angiocardiographic changes alone'.

Amundsen and Sörensen (1956) injected contrast medium into the superior vena cava in order to give better opacification of the heart and great vessels. They studied 41 patients, 37 of whom had proven lung or mediastinal tumours. Seventeen of the latter were judged by angiocardiography to be inoperable and this opinion was verified in 12 cases by thoracotomy, the remaining 5 having no operation.

Steinberg and Finby (1959) found, in 250 proven cases of lung cancer examined by angiocardiography, that 30 per cent of the tumours involved the great vessels (the superior vena cava and the major pulmonary arterial branches). In over 50 per cent, lobar and segmental pulmonary arterial involvement was demonstrated, thus permitting pre-operative evaluation of the pulmonary circulation. When a vascular anomaly was confined to a lobe or a segment, a lobectomy could be planned, and where there was bilateral pulmonary disease, by evaluating the pulmonary circulation they could avoid carrying out a pneumonectomy in a potential respiratory cripple. They agreed with Lyons and Vertova (1958) that irregularities and occlusions of the pulmonary arterial tree could be regarded as early signs of pulmonary cancer, but pointed out that since lung diseases, notably tuberculosis, distort the pulmonary vascular system, caution in attributing such changes to cancer is advisable.

Sanders, Delarue and Lau (1962) and Sanders, Delarue and Silverberg (1970) have also used angiocardiography alone or combined with mediastinoscopy. In the combined series they claimed a correct assessment in 95 per cent of the patients.

These are some of the apparently few workers who still use angiocardiography routinely to assess operability. Others employ it occasionally to prove or disprove an associated pericardial effusion or pericardial involvement (*Figure 10.1—see also* discussion in Chapter 3).

HEART SCINTISCAN

If the patient's blood is labelled with a suitable isotope (for example, ^{113m}In bound to transferrin), it is often possible to demonstrate the presence of pericardial effusions provided that these are larger than 300 ml (*Figure 10.2*). This is done either by showing on a radiograph that the size of the cardiac chambers is less than that of the cardiac silhouette or by demonstrating a 'clear zone' around the cardiac chambers when the blood and the lungs are labelled at the same time. The method is essentially similar to that used to determine the placental site (*see* Wright, 1970c).

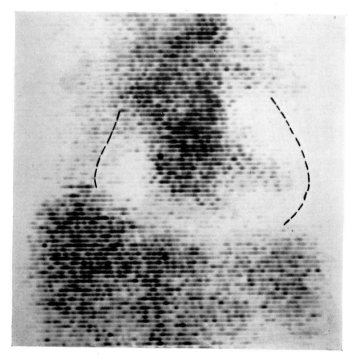

Figure 10.2. Scintiscan of patient with a large pericardial effusion. The pericardial border, as determined radiographically, is indicated by the broken lines. The liver is displaced from the lower heart border by the fluid. The blood has been labelled with ^{113m}In bound to transferrin

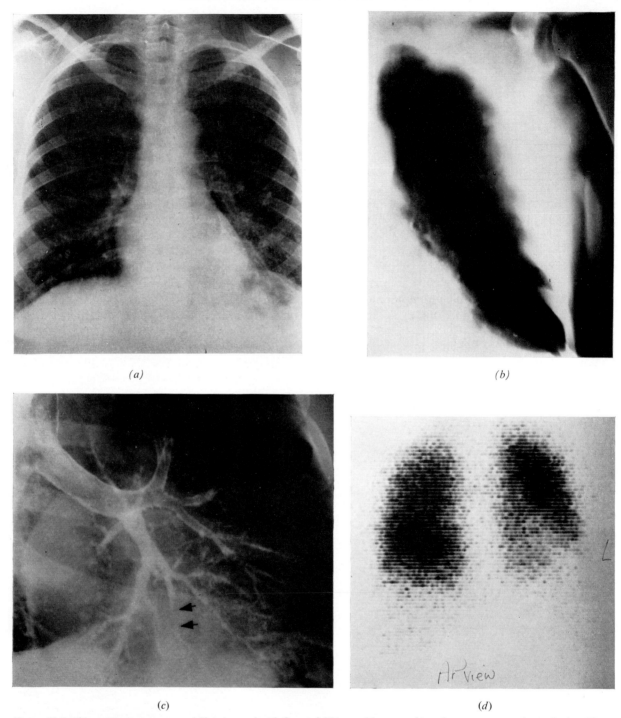

(a) *(b)*

(c) *(d)*

Figure 10.7. This patient, a woman aged 50, presented with finger clubbing and hypertrophic pulmonary osteo-arthropathy (see Figure 3.101). (a) Plain radiograph showed multiple small calcified foci throughout both lungs due to previous chickenpox pneumonia. (b) Tomograms showed these shadows more clearly and also revealed an area of collapse in left lower lobe. (c) Bronchogram showed relatively long stenosis and compression deformity of anterior basic segmental bronchus of left lower lobe, with loss of smaller bronchial branches. (d) Scintiscan showed well marked perfusion defect at left base (bronchiolar carcinoma)

In pulmonary scintiscanning, particulate aggregates of the order of 20–100 μ in diameter, labelled with a suitable radioactive isotope such as ^{131}I or ^{113m}In, are injected intravenously to lodge in the pulmonary capillaries. Their detection is either with a rectilinear scanner or with a stationary detector such as a gamma camera. The technique has been widely employed to detect perfusion defects in the lungs secondary to pulmonary emboli. It will also demonstrate other perfusion deficits, including those secondary to lung cancer, which may be gross or less marked. Secker Walker and Goodwin (1971) suggested that pulmonary scintiscanning might be more accurate in determining inoperability of lung tumours than plain chest radiographs, and pointed out that as the tumour approached the main bronchus as judged by bronchoscopy or the hilum as judged by radiography, the relative perfusion of the affected lung diminished.

My own experience has indicated that pulmonary vascularity may be more impaired than initially appears from plain radiographs. It has also shown that peripheral defects in the pattern of pulmonary vascularity may be present with less advanced tumours (*Figures 10.5–10.7*), and has tended to confirm the impression of Oeser, Ernst and Gerstenberg (1969) (*see* Chapter 3) that relatively early in the progress of a tumour there may be an alveolar–vascular reflex which reduces the calibre of the pulmonary vessels on the side of the tumour (*see Figures 3.83–3.86*). My experience has been limited to about 100 cases, and the technique has not been used for the general assessment of lung tumours but only in order to answer specific diagnostic questions. I have employed ^{113m}In particulate aggregates for lung scanning because of the ease of preparation of the particles, which includes autoclaving, a procedure which is not applicable to macro-aggregated albumin preparations.

My method of preparing the ^{113m}In particles has been based on the original method described by Stern *et al.* (1966), but has differed from this in the use of a much higher pH to avoid the formation of smaller particles (*see* Appendix 9). My scans have been made with a dual 5 inch detector system (SELO scanner) or a Nuclear Enterprise Mark IV gamma camera. One advantage of the latter apparatus is that as the record is taken much more quickly, usually in under one minute as opposed to 20–30 minutes with the scanner, less movement of the patient and particularly of the diaphragm will occur during the taking of the record. Another advantage is that the patient can sit up.

Secker Walker and Provan (1969) and Secker Walker *et al.* (1971) found that when perfusion of the affected lung was less than one-third of the total, the tumour was likely to be unresectable. They were also able to detect perfusion defects due to other diseases, such as localized emphysematous cysts, in the contralateral lung (*Figure 10.6*). Reduced perfusion is also caused by collapse (*see Figure 10.25b*).

Maynard *et al.* (1969) likewise noted that the vascular impairment of a lung was often of greater magnitude than plain chest radiographs had suggested. They found that hilar lesions produced greater changes than peripheral lesions on the scan and thought that except in isolated cases, lung scans were likely to be of little value in the early diagnosis of carcinoma. They did not think that scans could determine resectability, but suggested that they might be of some use as an indication of response to radiotherapy. (Scans following radiotherapy often reveal a reduced pulmonary vascularity, secondary to the radiation fibrosis, which may at times be so gross as to indicate an almost functionless lung.) Garnett, Machell and Macleod (1969) reported that the good correlation of scintiscanning with differential bronchospirometry had allowed them to abandon the latter in favour of lung scanning.

PULMONARY INHALATION AND TRANSMISSION SCANNING

Following inhalation of a radioactive isotope such as ^{133}Xe, the isotope may be found trapped in a lung or in part of a lung if there is air trapping such as occurs behind a bronchial block or in an emphysematous cyst or bulla. By this means air trapping can be demonstrated in up to 80 per cent of central bronchial tumours and may also be detected in some that are peripherally situated (Ackery, 1971). Such findings emphasize the importance of obstructive emphysema.

By using an isotope in a large flat container, it is possible to utilize the transmission of the gamma rays as an index of pulmonary vascularity and to determine whether this is unilaterally reduced (that is, with increased transmission of the radioactivity). For this purpose it is necessary to employ an isotope with fairly low energy in its γ emission, for example, ^{99m}Tc, 140 keV.

PULMONARY FLUORODENSITOMETRY

This is an extension of the technique of electrokymography which has been used mainly to study cardiac pulsation (Henny and Boone, 1945; Bartley, 1960; Lissner, 1962). It has also been utilized in the

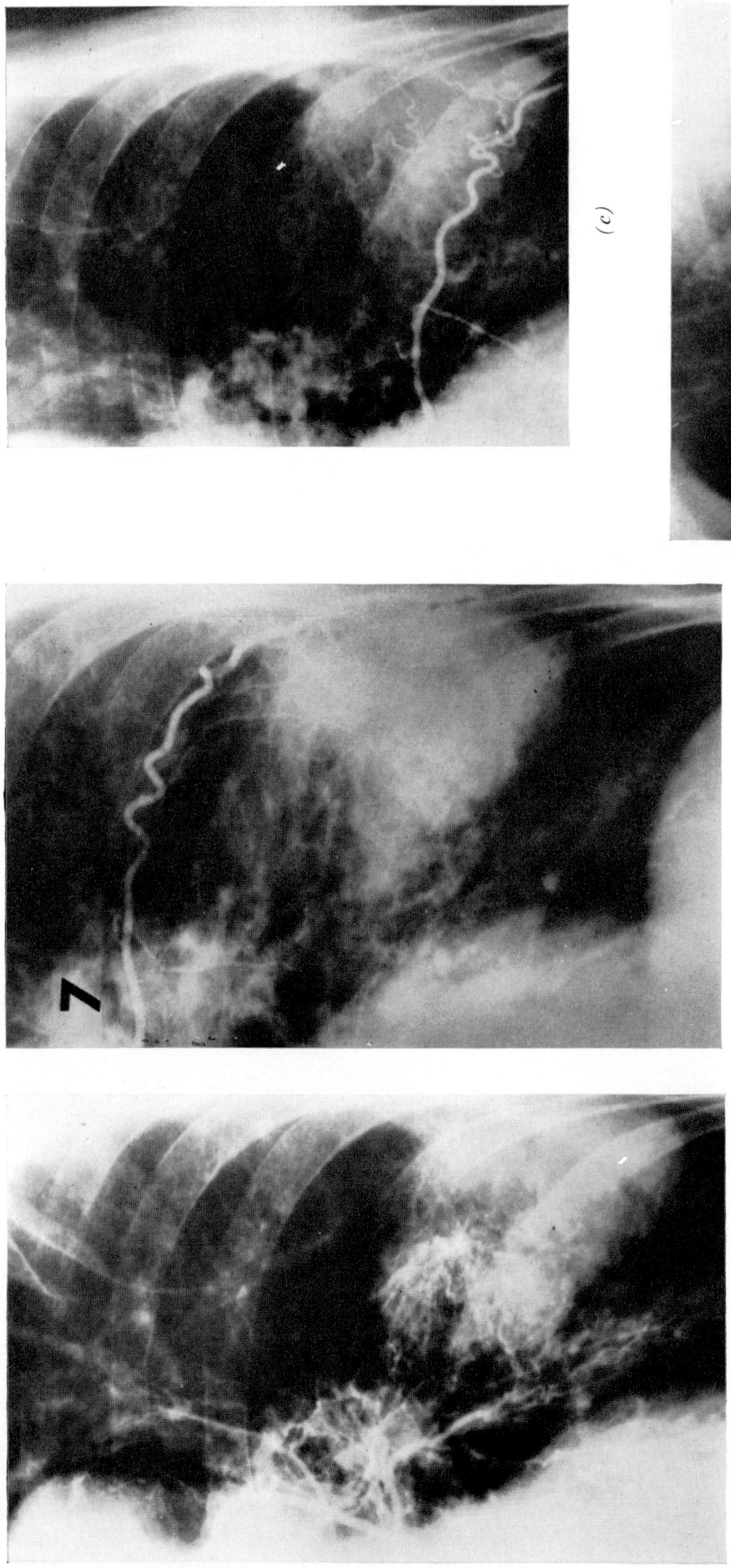

Figure 10.8

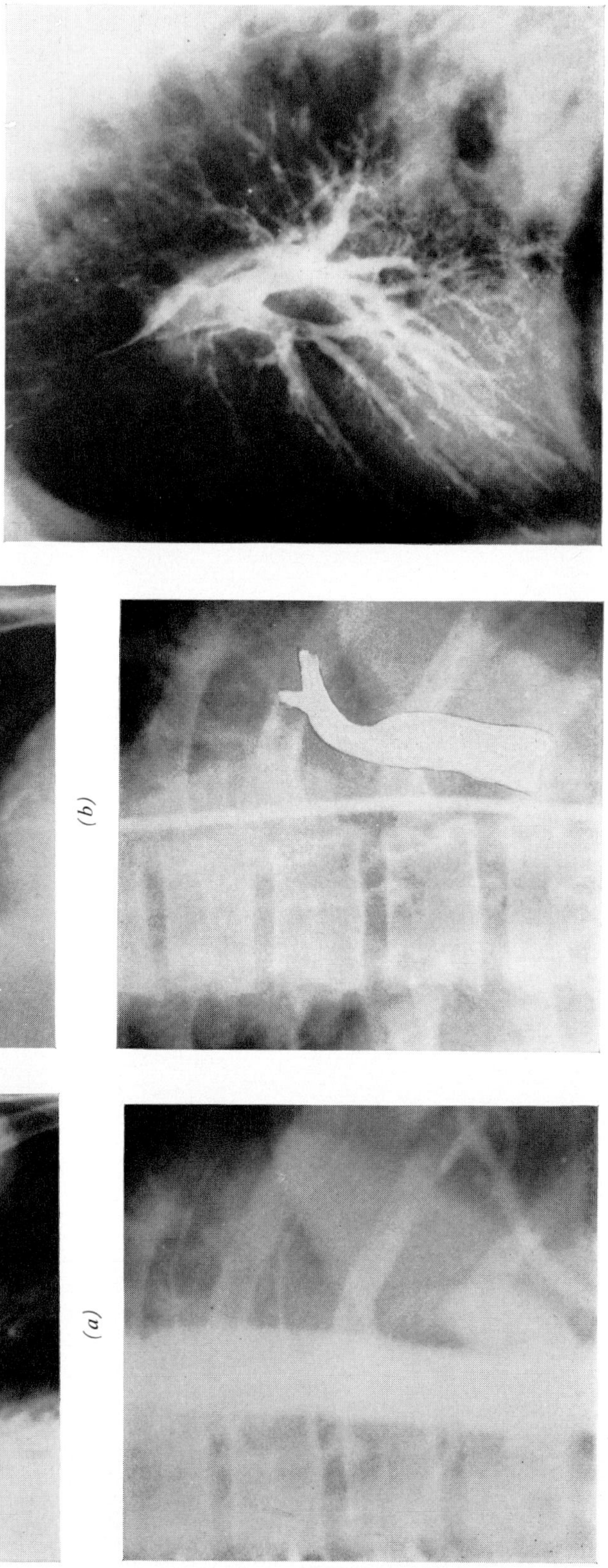

Figure 10.9

(c)

(c)

(b)

(b)

(a)

(a)

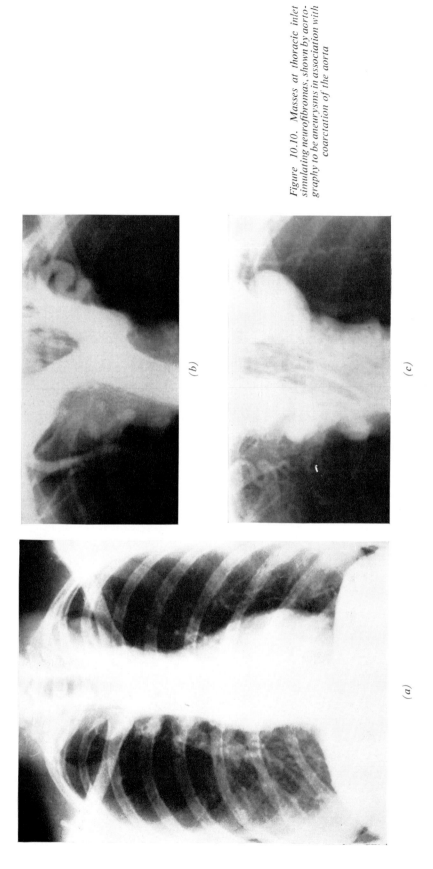

Figure 10.8. (a) A vascular bronchogenic tumour is demonstrated by bronchial arteriography. (b and c) Extension of tumour into chest wall is shown by intercostal arteriograms. The figures 7 and 9 refer to arteries lying below seventh and ninth ribs

Figure 10.9. Very large 'bronchial artery' arising from aorta below the diaphragm in patient with a sequestrated segment in left lower lobe. (a) Relatively early arterial phase of aortogram. (b) Eight seconds later the large artery is well demonstrated. (A very slow circulation time in these lesions is not uncommon.) (c) Lateral view of left bronchogram, showing absence of any bronchi going to the sequestrated segment

Figure 10.10. Masses at thoracic inlet simulating neurofibromas, shown by aortography to be aneurysms in association with coarctation of the aorta

study of pulmonary vascular pulsations, particularly in patients with bronchial carcinoma, and in the assessment of pulmonary ventilation. Marchal and Marchal (1963) found that in over 80 per cent of bronchial neoplasms the pulmonary vascular pattern was reduced or absent, whereas this did not happen with pulmonary metastases. Sutherland, Leask and Samuel (1968) studied 20 patients with bronchial carcinomas and found a reduction not only in the vascularity but also in the ventilation of the affected lung. As with isotope scintiscanning, it is possible to examine the contralateral lung as well.

BRONCHIAL AND INTERCOSTAL ANGIOGRAPHY AND AORTOGRAPHY

The value of bronchial and intercostal arteriography has been studied and reviewed by Nordenström (1967c, 1969b), Darke and Lewtas (1968), Düx et al. (1969) (who also reviewed other angiographic and venographic techniques), Botenga (1970) and Grainger (1970).

Bronchial angiography may be performed either by the injection of contrast medium into the thoracic aorta or by selective bronchial angiography, a technique pioneered by Viamonte (1964, 1965), Newton and Preyer (1965) and Boijsen and Zsigmond (1965). Wood and Miller (1938) and Cudkowicz and Armstrong (1953) considered that bronchogenic tumours might receive their main blood supply from the bronchial arteries while metastases might obtain most of their blood supply from the pulmonary arteries, a view supported by Darke and Lewtas. It has also been suggested by Cudkowicz and Armstrong that haemoptysis may be related to the higher pressure in the systemic bronchial circulation supplying the primary bronchial tumours than in the pulmonary arterial supply to metastatic deposits. My own view is that haemoptysis seems much more likely to be related to the bronchial ulceration and infection which are frequently present in cases with endobronchial extension, or to the initial endobronchial location of lung tumours. However, metastases from distant sites do sometimes have an endobronchial position (Schoenbaum and Viamonte, 1971). In a few cases, secondary deposits derive a demonstrable blood supply from the bronchial arteries as shown by Turner-Warwick (1963), Noonan, Margulis and Wright (1965) and Boijsen and Zsigmond (1965).

In about two-thirds of the bronchial neoplasms investigated by bronchial angiography, abnormal angiographic appearances have been noted. These can be summarized as follows.

(1) The bronchial arteries may be abnormally dilated and tortuous. However, such dilatation is usually less than that seen in chronic inflammatory lung conditions, especially in bronchiectasis, in which arterio-venous shunts are often present.

(2) There may, as with tumours elsewhere in the body, be abnormal ('pathological') vessels with a coarse calibre variation along their course and a rapid circulation through them.

(3) There may be a systemic–pulmonary anastomosis with direct shunting of contrast material through the tumour into the pulmonary circulation around and distal to the tumour.

Spread of tumour to the hilum or mediastinum may be demonstrated by the finding of an abnormal circulation in these areas as well. If it is suspected that the tumour has spread to the chest wall, selective intercostal arteriography may show an abnormal circulation in the chest wall and thus confirm the presence of tumour there. *Figure 10.8* illustrates the value of combined bronchial and intercostal angiography.

The techniques of bronchial and intercostal arteriography have not been used in many centres for the following reasons.

(1) They are difficult and rather time-consuming.

(2) About one-third of bronchial tumours do not exhibit any angiographic abnormality, whilst many inflammatory conditions show hypervascularity, making the differentiation of a benign from a malignant condition difficult unless typical signs are present.

(3) The bronchial arteries are variable in number and in their site of origin, and failure to catheterize the bronchial artery supplying the tumour may give a 'false negative' result.

Aortography is occasionally of great value in demonstrating a large aberrant 'bronchial' artery if a sequestrated segment of lung is present (*Figure 10.9*), or in confirming the presence of a coarctation of the aorta giving rise to multiple aneurysms within the chest wall, which may be confused with neurofibromatosis (*Figure 10.10*—compare with *Figures 3.136* and *7.44*).

SUBCLAVIAN AND INTERNAL MAMMARY ARTERIOGRAPHY AND AORTOGRAPHY

The use of aortography and internal mammary arteriography in the differential diagnosis of anterior mediastinal masses is exemplified in *Figures 7.8* and *7.12*, which show a thymoma and an intrathoracic aneurysm simulating a thyroid mass.

Subclavian and internal mammary arteriography has also been used by Boijsen and Reuter (1966) to help in differentiating anterior mediastinal masses. They reported 17 cases including thymomas, metastases from bronchogenic carcinoma, goitre, dermoid cyst and sarcoidosis.

VENOGRAPHY

Venography may be performed to show thrombosis in the superior vena cava or caval compression or displacement by a tumour or by enlarged lymph nodes. It is most conveniently carried out from the arms, as is done by other authors including Guozdanovic and Oberhofer (1953); however, it can also be carried out via an intra-osseous route, such as the vertebral spinous process or a rib, to show the vertebral venous system and the azygos and hemiazygos systems (Viamonte, 1965; Wolfel, Linberg and Light, 1966; Janover, Dreyfuss and Skinner, 1966).

Rinker *et al.* (1967) used the combined techniques of superior vena cavography and azygography to study 63 patients with suspected bronchial carcinoma. They found six signs of neoplastic involvement of these veins: (1) complete obstruction of either venous system; (2) a partial or segmental block; (3) reflux of contrast material from the azygos system up the superior vena cava or into the inferior vena cava; (4) displacement of part of the azygos or caval system; (5) delayed emptying of the arch of the azygos vein; and (6) involvement of the superior vena cava or the innominate veins with a normal azygos system. Wolfel, Linberg and Light (1966) commented after reviewing 86 examinations: 'In general the azygogram adds little of any informative nature as to the status of the mediastinum than what is already known by plain roentgen means. In ascertaining resectability, a normal azygogram is of no value, while an abnormal azygogram is a strong indication of inoperability.'

When carrying out superior vena cavography, I prefer to have the patient standing erect with his arms elevated above the horizontal plane and held gently by assistants, who simultaneously inject contrast medium into veins in both antecubital fossae. Usually 50 ml are injected into each arm within 5–10 seconds while the patient performs the Valsalva manoeuvre. The flow of contrast medium into the great veins and towards the heart is observed by television fluoroscopy and recorded on videotape, and large (14 × 14 in) spot films are taken when maximum opacification of the great veins has occurred. Examples of a normal examination, a displacement of the superior vena cava and a thrombosis secondary to tumour are shown in *Figures 10.11–10.13*. It is usually impossible to distinguish between filling defects in the veins due to thrombi and those due to tumour, but the latter are much less common. Inflammatory conditions may also cause displacement of or secondary thrombosis in veins (*see* Steinberg, 1966).

Patients who are too ill to stand may be examined lying down (preferably tipped head up) or in the sitting position.

Spot films taken with the explorator are preferred to the serial changer (1) because fluoroscopic monitoring allows spot films to be taken at the correct time and avoids the necessity of taking numerous films, most of which will provide little information, and (2) because it permits the use of a Bucky diaphragm, thus giving much clearer radiographs.

LYMPHANGIOGRAPHY

Lymphangiography is rarely used in the assessment of metastases from lung tumours. *Figure 10.24* shows a block to the passage of the contrast medium through the abdomen due to metastases in the para-aortic region, with no demonstrable bone destruction. In *Figure 10.13b*, blockage of the lymphatic drainage from the right arm was present secondary to superior mediastinal enlargement.

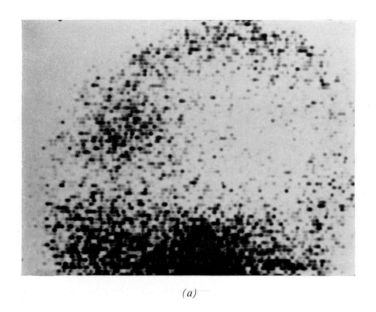

(a)

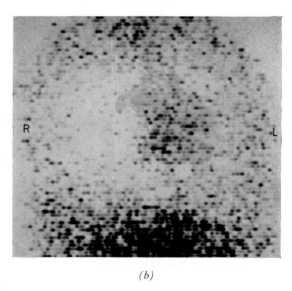

(b)

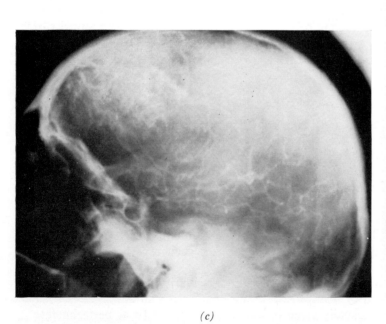

(c)

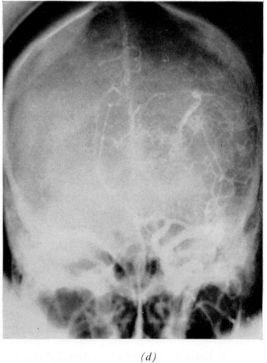

(d)

Figure 10.14. (a and b) Lateral and A.P. views of large secondary deposit from a bronchial carcinoma as demonstrated by brain scan using
¹¹³ᵐIn chelate. (c and d) Lateral and A.P. views of the same secondary tumour as shown by carotid angiography. There is marked abnormal
vascularity in the tumour and considerable displacement of the anterior cerebral vessels to the right. The plain chest radiograph and inclined
frontal tomogram of this patient are shown in Figure 3.10

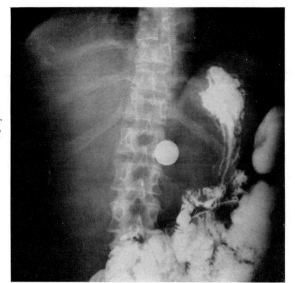

Figure 10.15. (a) Marked enlargement of soft tissue shadow of liver. Right side of diaphragm is elevated. The barium-filled stomach and colon are also displaced

(a)

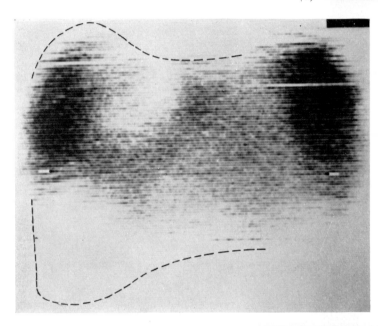

(b) Liver scan using ¹¹³ᵐIn colloid. Multiple large 'cold' defects are present in the liver. (With this colloid the spleen is also usually well demonstrated.)

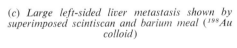

(b)

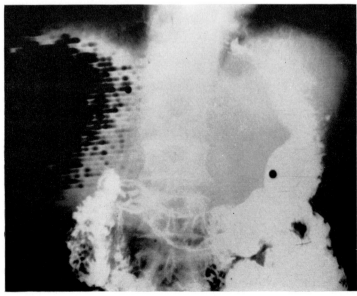

(c) Large left-sided liver metastasis shown by superimposed scintiscan and barium meal (¹⁹⁸Au colloid)

(c)

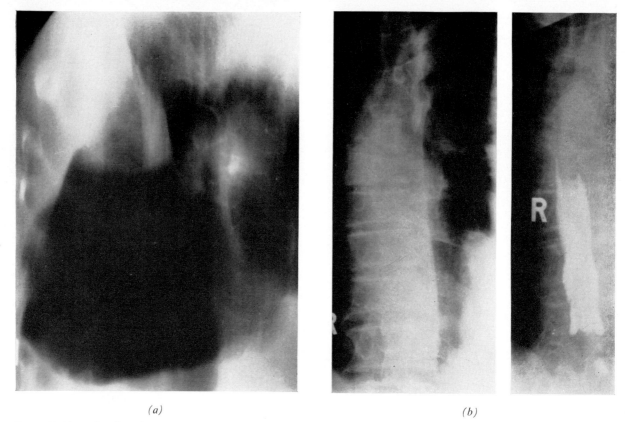

(a)   *(b)*

Figure 10.16. Wedge-shaped tumour in apex of left lower lobe with extension into pleura and also into the spine producing paraplegia. Spinal block was shown by myelography. The patient had a spinal cord decompression and radiotherapy and recovered for a period of 8 months. (a) Lateral tomogram. (b) A.P. dorsal spine and myelogram

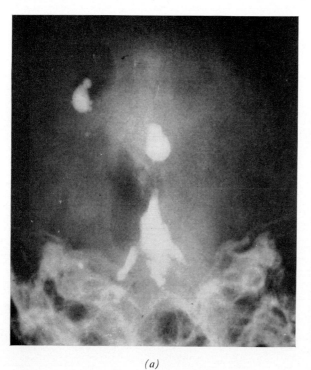

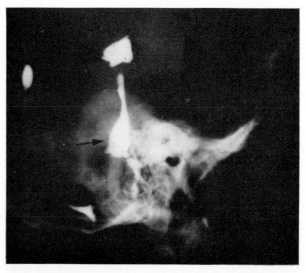

Figure 10.17. Positive contrast ventriculogram showing deformity of fourth ventricle and also its marked forward displacement, indicating bilateral cerebellar masses (secondary deposits from a bronchogenic tumour). (a) A.P. view. (b) Lateral view

(a)   *(b)*

202

biliary tract, to some extent even during the procedure, this does have the disadvantage that an accumulation of isotope in the biliary tree may result in a confusing record when one is searching for metastases. Most workers therefore prefer an isotope-labelled colloid (I use a ^{113m}In colloid) which will be taken up by the reticulo-endothelial cells of the liver and spleen. Ludin and Künzli (1969) compared selective angiography with venography and isotope scanning in tumours of the liver and found that whilst angiography and venography—especially trans-umbilical venography via the usually still patent adult umbilical vein—might show smaller tumours, the isotope studies were more convenient to carry out.

A major problem in liver scanning is movement of the organ during the scanning procedure. Since the latter takes 15–20 minutes per view when using a rectilinear scanner, considerable movement of the liver must take place even during shallow respiration. For this reason, and also in order that multiple views may be taken over a similar period of time, a stationary detector such as a gamma or Anger camera may demonstrate more lesions, even though its standard of resolution may be lower than that of the scanner.

Some brain and liver scans are shown in *Figures 10.14, 10.15* and *3.132.*

NEURO-RADIOLOGICAL PROCEDURES

These procedures will not be considered here in detail, only a few points being stressed.

In the spine, many metastases extend outside the normal confines of the vertebral body so as to produce extradural compression on the spinal cord or nerve roots. This compression will generally be demonstrated by myelography (*Figure 10.16*), and multiple levels of deformity of the theca are frequently found even, at times, when the plain radiographs of the areas appear normal.

Within the cranium, metastases may occur in the cerebral hemispheres, the mid-brain or the cerebellum. Scintiscans, angiography (*see Figure 10.14*) or air studies may be used to demonstrate these lesions or deformities secondary to their presence. In the posterior fossa, positive contrast ventriculography may supply clearer pictures of deformities of the fourth ventricle secondary to cerebellar masses

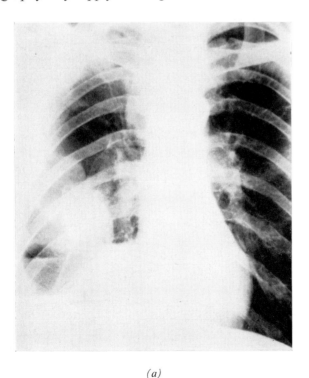
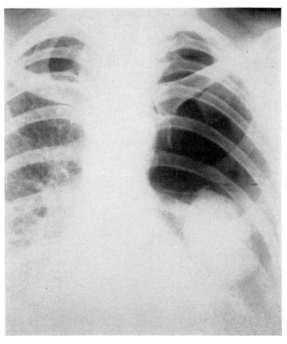

(a)   *(b)*

Figure 10.18. (a) Right-sided artificial pneumothorax showing multiple pleural masses due to mesothelioma. (b) Artificial pneumothorax demonstrating that an anteriorly situated mass in left side of chest arises in the chest wall and from a rib. It was a chondroma. The plain radiograph is shown in Figure 3.149

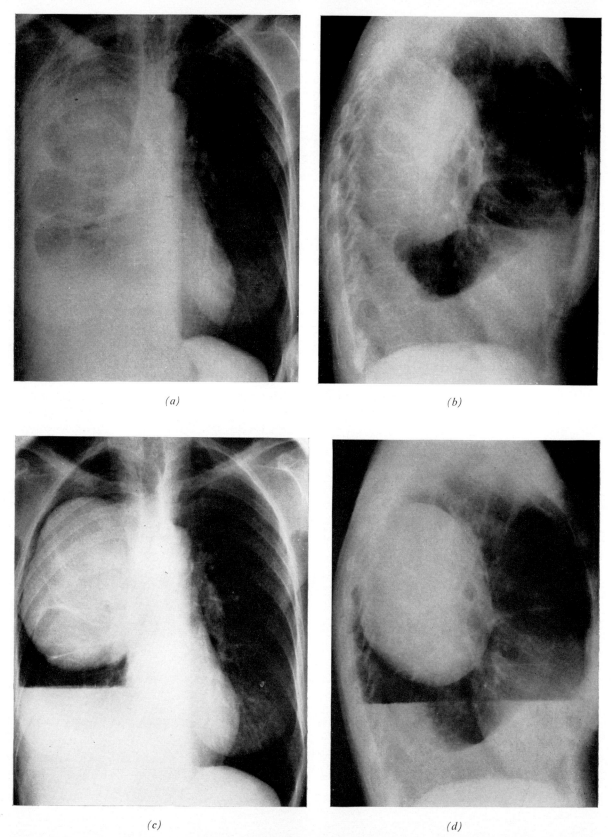

(a)   *(b)*

(c)   *(d)*

Figure 10.19. Accidentally induced pneumothorax at pleural paracentesis, showing that the supposed loculated pleural effusion was a large smooth paraspinal mass and likely to be a neurofibroma. This was confirmed at operation. (a and b) Before paracentesis. (c and d) After paracentesis

(*Figure 10.17*). Posterior fossa lesions, such as cerebellar metastases, are very difficult to demonstrate by isotopic methods because of the overlying vascular structures at the base of the cranium.

ARTIFICIAL PNEUMOTHORAX

Isaacs (1925) pointed out that the introduction of 400–600 ml of air into the pleural cavity might give valuable information, especially in obscure cases where one cannot differentiate an interlobar empyema from a lung tumour, or when one desires to know the exact anatomical location of a lesion—that is, whether it is in the lung, the pleura, the mediastinum, the ribs or the chest wall. He thought that a diagnostic pneumothorax was especially indicated when one wished to exclude an interlobar empyema, and stated: 'A bronchial carcinoma leading to atelectasis of an entire lobe of the lung gives a very distinct roentgen ray picture, which is very easily confused with an interlobar empyema, especially if there is, at the same time, a thickening of the pleura. The injection of a few hundred cubic centimetres of air into the pleural cavity helps considerably in making the correct diagnosis in such cases. The complete separation of the lung from the costal pleura speaks for a tiny tumour with secondary atelectasis of the lung, while extensive adhesions (failure of the lung to collapse) speaks more for an interlobar empyema with pleural thickening. Thus it is easily seen that air injected into the pleural cavity gives data as to pleural adhesions and also aids in the differential diagnosis of lung disease.'

Isaacs illustrated his paper with two examples, both of lung tumours. Møller (1950) also gave an example of the use of the technique in excluding neoplasm. The method is now barely mentioned in the literature because, as the lung collapses, a lesion within it tends to become obscured. It does, however, have considerable value in the differentiation of a chest wall mass from an intrapulmonary lesion, and I have used it in occasional cases, employing O_2 or CO_2 rather than air (*Figure 10.18*).

The injection, usually accidental, of air into the pleura during aspiration of a pleural effusion sometimes creates a sufficient pneumothorax to differentiate lung masses from pleural ones (*Figure 10.19*).

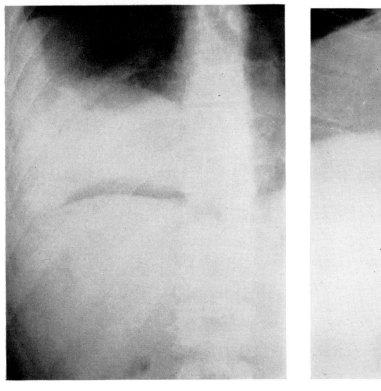
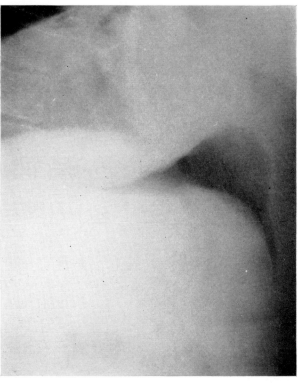

(a)   (b)

Figure 10.20. Pneumoperitoneum (using 1,000 ml CO_2) was used to show that an extensive mass in right side of chest did not extend into the abdomen and that the liver was free from the under-surface of the diaphragm. This was a recurrence of a sarcoma which originated on the upper side of the diaphragm. (a) A.P. view. (b) Lateral view

Occasionally a patient with a lung tumour will develop a spontaneous pneumothorax which may allow a similar differentiation.

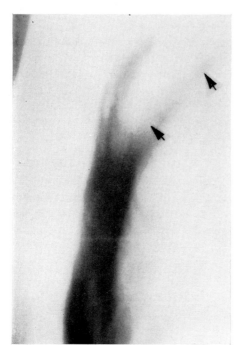

Figure 10.21. Thymus demonstrated by gas mediastinography on lateral tomogram

Figure 10.22. Small pericardial cyst differentiated from the pericardium itself by gas mediastinography. (a) P.A. view. (b) Tomogram in slightly oblique position. A small 'stalk' connects the mass with the pericardium

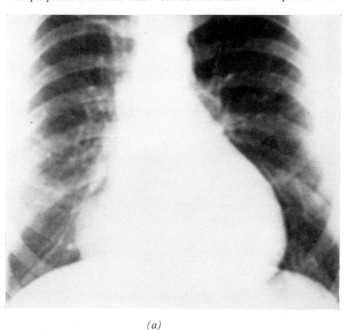

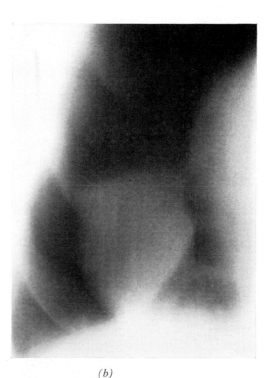

(a)   (b)

ARTIFICIAL PNEUMOPERITONEUM

A gas, usually CO_2 or O_2, introduced into the peritoneal cavity (for a recent paper *see* Lumsden and Truelove, 1957) will usually demonstrate whether the liver is separable from the diaphragm, and may help to indicate whether an intrathoracic tumour which extends down to the diaphragm is operable or not (*Figure 10.20*). Such an examination will also help in assessing whether the tumour arises in or below the diaphragm. In addition, it may show the size of the liver and spleen and demonstrate irregularities of the surface of the liver suggesting metastases or cirrhosis.

MEDIASTINOGRAPHY

As was discussed in Chapter 3, gas mediastinography can be used for the demonstration of thymic masses (Bariety *et al.*, 1965; Pohlenz *et al.*, 1966). It has also been utilized fairly widely to assess the spread of bronchial carcinomas. The first reported use of the method was by Condorelli (1936). Other reports of its use have been by Condorelli, Turchetti and Pidone (1951), Baccaglini (1951), Šimeček and Holub (1961), Hughes, Hanafee and O'Loughlin (1962), Sumerling and Irvine (1966), Ikins *et al.* (1962), and Kreel, Blendis and Piercy (1964). Various ways of introducing the gas have been employed: via the neck (Condorelli and colleagues); trans-sternally (Kreel and co-workers); behind the xiphisternum (Hughes and his associates; Nordenström, 1967b); via a catheter inserted into the wound after scalene node biopsy (Ikins *et al.*, 1962), and pre-sacrally (Baccaglini, 1951).

Most of the above authors claimed that the method gave considerable aid in assessing the involvement of the mediastinal lymph nodes and the extent of mediastinal infiltration, and some claimed that they could differentiate between enlargement of mediastinal lymph nodes due to tumour and that due to other causes. The use of this technique is illustrated in *Figures 10.21* and *10.22*.

Nordenström (1967a, 1969a) has also injected Ultra Fluid Lipiodol into the mediastinum via an anterior percutaneous route from the neck in order to outline enlarged mediastinal lymph nodes, and has obtained biopsies at the same time.

RETROPERITONEAL GAS INSUFFLATION

I have used this method once to demonstrate a large paraspinal mass secondary to bronchial neoplasm

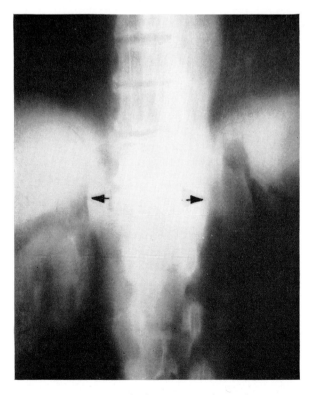

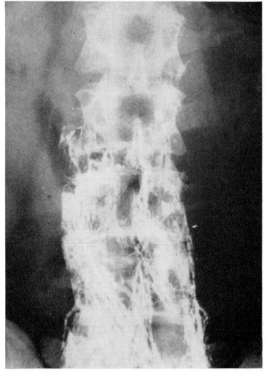

Figure 10.23. Paravertebral extension of spinal metastasis secondary to bronchial carcinoma demonstrated by retroperitoneal gas insufflation (tomogram)

Figure 10.24. Lymphatic block in lumbar region caused by secondary deposits from a bronchial carcinoma. No bone erosion was visible

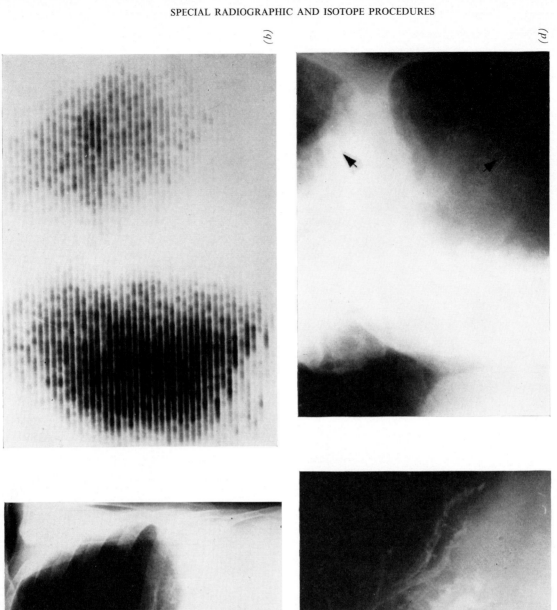

Figure 10.25. Leaking aortic aneurysm at level of diaphragm. This patient presented with repeated syncopal attacks and had a large left-sided pleural effusion which subsequently partly resolved. (a) Plain radiograph showing pleural effusion. (b) Lung scintiscan showing reduced perfusion of left lung secondary to pressure from the effusion. This was carried out to try to confirm or refute the possible diagnosis of pulmonary embolism. (c) Bronchogram showing early bronchiectatic changes in left lower lobe and lingula. (d) Gaseous distension of the stomach, using CO$_2$, shows that the mass at base of left pleural cavity extends below the diaphragm. A little calcification is seen in the wall of the mass. The patient collapsed and died from a further haemorrhage from the aneurysm before any more investigations could be carried out

which was not causing any demonstrable bone erosion on plain radiographs or tomograms (*Figure 10.23*).

GASEOUS DISTENSION OF THE STOMACH

This is occasionally useful in demonstrating retroperitoneal masses which extend down from the thorax into the abdomen (*Figure 10.25*).

Figure 10.26 (below). (a) Small round tumour in right upper lobe with central irregular cavity. (b) There were multiple metastases in the spine mimicking osteoporosis, with vertebral collapse

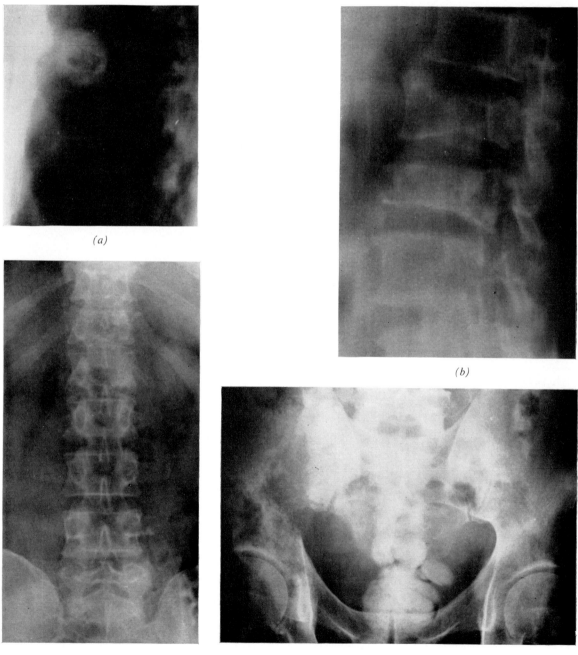

(a)

(b)

Figure 10.27. Absence of left pedicle of L1 vertebra, indicating a secondary deposit

Figure 10.28. Partly osteolytic and partly osteosclerotic secondary deposits in the pelvis from a bronchial carcinoma

SKELETAL SURVEYS AND BONE SCANNING FOR DETECTION OF METASTASES

Skeletal surveys are not carried out on all patients with malignant lung tumours in view of the expense and time involved and the improbability of finding lesions in the absence of symptoms of pain referable to the skeleton. Naturally the ribs, the spine, the clavicles etc. are scrutinized on all chest radiographs, and in some cases unsuspected bone lesions are found. The real problem, as with metastases from other tumours, lies in the demonstration of secondary deposits which have not eroded away sufficient calcium (50–70 per cent in some cases) to render them readily visible on a radiograph. Tomograms may help in

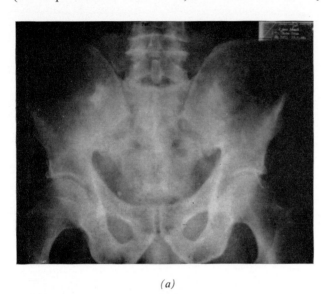

(a)

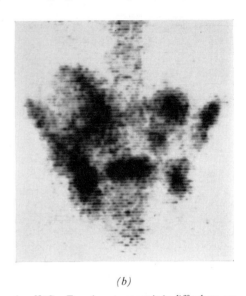

(b)

Figure 10.29. Widespread metastases in the pelvis demonstrated by scintiscanning using ^{87m}Sr. Even in retrospect it is difficult to see the deposits on the radiograph, but note the poor definition of parts of the margins of the right hip and sacro-iliac joints.

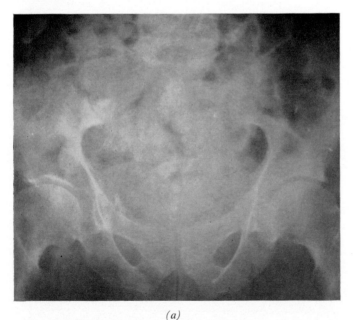

(a)

Figure 10.30. Large metastasis in left acetabular region (also in second lumbar vertebra) demonstrated by scintiscanning using ^{87m}Sr. The deposits were barely visible on the radiographs. Careful scrutiny of the pelvic radiograph shows that the lower part of the left acetabular margin is poorly defined

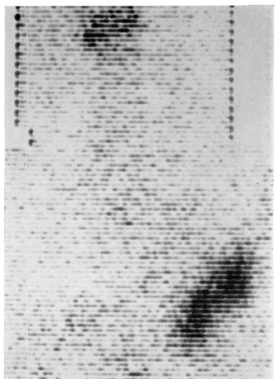

(b)

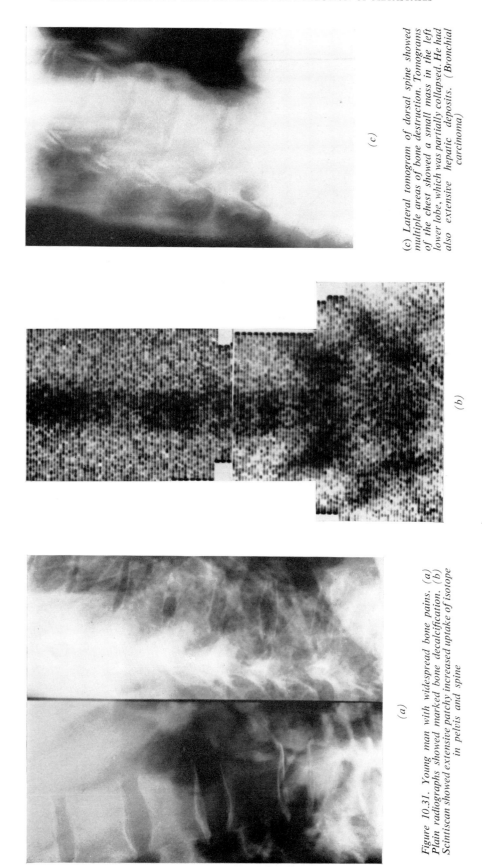

(a)

(b)

(c)

(c) Lateral tomogram of dorsal spine showed multiple areas of bone destruction. Tomograms of the chest showed a small mass in the left lower lobe, which was partially collapsed. He had also extensive hepatic deposits. (Bronchial carcinoma)

Figure 10.31. Young man with widespread bone pains. (a) Plain radiographs showed marked bone decalcification. (b) Scintiscan showed extensive patchy increased uptake of isotope in pelvis and spine

demonstrating that the cortex is incomplete, that bone collapse (for example, of the vertebral column) is present, or that the inner structure of the bone has been destroyed (*Figure 10.26*). The well-known phenomenon of an absent pedicle of a vertebral body is illustrated in *Figure 10.27*. Rarely, secondary deposits from a bronchial neoplasm will cause apparent bone sclerosis (*Figure 10.28*).

Even large areas of bone destruction may, however, be invisible on radiographs, particularly if they lie within the medulla. For this reason, scintiscanning with bone-seeking isotopes has been employed in many centres. The first of these isotopes to be tried was ^{85}Sr, but the long half-life (65 days) of this substance is inconvenient in that one has to scan the patient two to four days after the administration of the isotope, and its excretion into the colon may cause difficulty in interpreting the results. The isotopes now used are ^{87m}Sr and ^{18}F, with half-lives of 2·8 and 1·8 hours respectively. Strontium-87m is derived from a ^{87}Y generator with a half-life of 80 hours and a useful laboratory life of 10 days, whilst ^{18}F is cyclotron-produced and, because of its short half-life, presents transport and management problems. Gallium-67 and ^{113m}In have also occasionally been utilized for bone scanning, but mainly in experimental animals.

I have carried out bone scans on 300 patients with malignant or suspected malignant conditions and in others with benign lesions such as Paget's disease, acute or chronic arthritis or osteoporosis. In 50 cases in which no evidence of bone metastases was reported from the radiographs, scintiscans gave a positive result (*Figure 10.29*). In 30 of these 50 patients, when the radiographs were reassessed in comparison with the scintiscans, many lesions which had initially been undetected on the radiographs could now be seen. The 'hidden areas' appeared to lie especially in the sacrum, or in the pelvis in the fan-shaped part of the ilium or close to the sacro-iliac or hip joints (*Figure 10.30*), and metastases close to these joints were often manifested by a lack of definition of the joint margins. The sacrum in particular is a difficult bone to study by plain radiography, as it is frequently overlaid by bowel shadows which often render large lesions invisible on the routine antero-posterior view.

As with radiography, problems arise with bone scintiscanning. As a scintiscan may be positive in the case of both benign and malignant lesions, it cannot be used to distinguish between them, and such differentiation is better carried out by means of radiography including tomography (*Figure 10.31*). A negative scintiscan may occur in about 5 per cent of patients with disseminated bone lesions (Charkes, Young and Sklaroff, 1968) if there is an absence of any reparative process in the bone at the time of examination. My series contained one patient with a positive radiograph and a negative scintiscan, and two patients had both negative scintiscans and negative radiographs and died within four weeks of these examinations, multiple bony deposits being found at autopsy. Further details of my experience of using scintiscanning to detect bony lesions are given in Wright (1970b, 1971a).

The most recent development is the use of stannous pyrophosphate labelled with ^{99m}Tc, which gives much clearer scintiscans of bones. This complex is cleared rapidly from the blood and shows up much smaller bony deposits than can be visualized with ^{18}F or ^{87m}Sr. For recent work using this agent, *see* Subramanian, McAfee and Bell (1972).

USE OF RADIOACTIVE GALLIUM-67 FOR DETECTION OF TUMOURS

In 1969 Edwards and Hayes, while performing a bone scintiscan, found an unexpected accumulation of ^{67}Ga in a soft tissue tumour in a patient with Hodgkin's disease. (This isotope is produced in a cyclotron and has a half-life of 78 hours.)

For several years many workers have tried to find an isotope which would be selectively concentrated in tumour tissues. An isotope previously tried for this purpose was ^{197}Hg as Neohydrin or mercuric chloride (Sodee, 1964). The report by Edwards and Hayes spurred great activity in the U.S.A., in Japan and in Europe, particularly Holland and Germany, to determine whether it was such an isotope (Higasi *et al.*, 1969; Ando and Hisada, 1970; Edwards and Hayes, 1970a, b; Edwards *et al.*, 1970; Hayes and Edwards, 1972; Higasi *et al.*, 1970; Hisada and Hiraki, 1970; Hör *et al.*, 1970; Winchell *et al.*, 1970). The reports to date have suggested that gallium ions are taken up by rapidly growing tumour cells, though whether by metabolism or by a physical process of diffusion or adhesion remains uncertain (they also adhere to glass surfaces).

Tumours which have been shown to localize the isotope both in the primary growth and in the

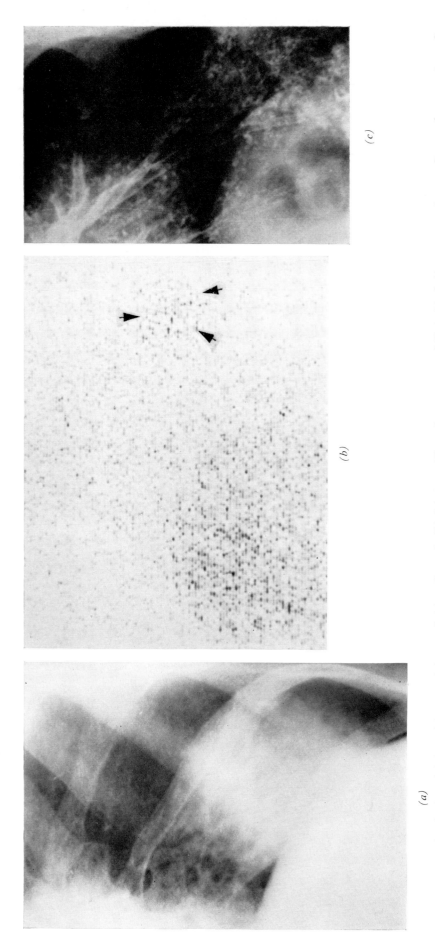

(a)

(b)

(c)

Figure 10.32. Uptake of ^{67}Ga in left lower lobe mass. (a) Part of plain radiograph. (b) Scintiscan. The patient, a woman of 56, had had this asymptomatic mass discovered on a routine radiograph. A tomogram showed that the mass looked like a localized area of consolidation with patent bronchi passing through it. Its edge was not well defined but did not show any 'frayed pattern'. (c) A bronchogram showed the patent bronchi passing through the mass. Some 'bronchiolar filling' had occurred. Due to the consolidation, the view in inspiration appears to show some crowding of the bronchi within the mass, but this area of the lung cannot inflate normally. As discussed in Chapter 9, such an appearance suggests a reticulosis, and a biopsy confirmed the diagnosis of lymphoma. Review of a radiograph taken elsewhere two years previously showed that the lesion was present then though somewhat smaller

metastases include reticuloses, soft tissue and bone sarcomas, lung and thyroid tumours and tumours of the nasal sinuses. Some increased uptake has also been seen in breast, intestinal, oesophageal and abdominal tumours. Poorly differentiated tumours have been reported to concentrate the isotope up to 100 times the concentration seen in blood and muscle, whereas well differentiated or treated tumours display little or no uptake. In addition, some acute or less acute infective processes, such as lung abscess or pneumonia, show an increased uptake of this isotope, and the demonstration of uptake on a single occasion may not by itself be diagnostic of a tumour. In certain cases the apparently large size of a lung tumour on the scintiscan may be largely due to the amount of inflammation present distal to a bronchial block. Another advantage of the isotope seems to be its accumulation by thyroid tumours, which fail to take up ^{131}I or similar substances (*see* Chapter 3). Increased uptake of ^{67}Ga has also been shown in granulomatous processes such as tuberculosis and sarcoidosis.

Experience of the use of the technique in Great Britain has so far been unpromising. Keeling (1970) found that the isotope is often best accumulated by oesophageal tumours or by reticulosis, and Lavender *et al.* (1971) reported that the best example of its accumulation in a chest lesion occurred in relation to a lung abscess with no associated malignancy. My own experience has been limited to a few patients. Two had already diagnosed lung tumours, one of them with a mild associated distal pneumonitis. In one of these two cases there was a faintly positive scintiscan and the excised lobe, when re-scanned the same day, showed a 2:1 uptake of isotope in the tumour compared with the rest of the lung. No uptake was found in a patient with an encysted collection of pleural fluid and a tumour. In another, a patient with a suspected benign lesion (*Figure 10.32*), there was an obvious accumulation of isotope in the mass. This was subsequently shown by lung biopsy to be a primary lung reticulosis. In a young woman with Hodgkin's disease affecting the nodes of the neck, the axillae, the abdomen and the pelvis (as shown by a lymphangiogram) and a mass in the right lung, the neck and axillary nodes and the lung mass were faintly visualized whilst the abdominal and pelvic nodes were not demonstrated.

The greatest practical problem at present with regard to a more general use of ^{67}Ga scanning is the cost of the isotope. As it is cyclotron-produced, each clinical dose is much more expensive than those derived from a generator system (for ^{113m}In the cost is only a few shillings). The present price of the necessary 2–4 mCi for a single examination is of the order of £14 to £28. The technique is also inconvenient in that two to three days have to elapse after the intravenous injection before the scintiscan can be performed. Assessments are at present being carried out of the usefulness of ^{67}Ga scanning in the staging and management of Hodgkin's disease (*see* Kay and McCready, 1972).

Recently, following the demonstration that the antibiotic bleomycin is concentrated in squamous tumours, Merrick *et al.* (1972) have shown that if this antibiotic is labelled with ^{111}In it may be used to show the extent or the metastases of squamous tumours.

II

Value of Radiological Surveys for Detection of Lung Tumours

RESULTS OF MASS SURVEYS

The results have been published of many surveys for the detection of lung tumours, either in the population at large or in selected industries. Whilst I myself have not taken part in any of these surveys, I have followed the various publications with interest and will summarize the principal points made in some of them.

Rigler (1957a), in discussing whether periodic roentgen examination was a drudgery or a challenge, pointed out that most mass surveys, particularly of the chest, have been examinations on a single occasion of a large, usually heterogenous population in which certain disease processes were found and managed to a greater or lesser degree. Furthermore, such surveys have usually been conducted with particular attention to economy and speed, and have often been attended by considerable problems in follow-up. Rigler recognized that much had been achieved in the detection of tuberculosis, but there had been only minor success in cancer of the lung. He advocated periodic x-ray examinations.

Garland (1955) estimated that not more than half the lung cancers present in the examined population had been found by mass surveys. Rigler agreed that such a figure was probably true, but said he did not believe that the error rate was inherent in the method. It merely indicated a misuse of the method. He wrote: 'The personnel is inadequate, rapidity of interpretation is far too great, and there is a lack of interest on the part of the examiners. The examination of 100 or even 200 chest films per hour is not an uncommon procedure*. Such work done hour after hour will invariably lead to a failure to observe the smaller lesions, the very ones that are most likely to be curable.'

Boucot and his colleagues (Boucot, Cooper and Weiss, 1961; Boucot et al., 1964) did a periodic survey in Philadelphia. They took photofluorograms of 6,137 men, aged 45 years and over, every 6 months over periods of 8–10 years. During this time 142 histologically proven lung cancers were found, 66 being seen on the first radiograph after entry into the trial and 76 later. The authors noted that in the cases which presented later, the earliest abnormalities due to lung cancer were variable and often unimpressive (see also page 226).

Bidstrup (1964), presenting the results of routine examinations including full-sized chest radiographs of men working in industries with special hazards associated with lung cancer, reported that in one industry 36 per cent of cases failed to show any evidence of the tumour 1–5 months before the death of the patient. In a further 26 per cent, no evidence was seen 6–10 months before the patient's death. In another industry, Bidstrup found that in 40 per cent of cases death occurred less than 6 months after the diagnosis had been made radiologically.

In order to study whether six-monthly routine examinations could improve the prognosis of bronchial carcinoma, Nash, Morgan and Tomkins (1968) offered such a service by the mass x-ray units in South London to men aged 45 years or over: 67,400 men attended for a first examination, 75 per cent of these returned at least once, and 197,500 repeat examinations were carried out. These revealed 147 patients

---

* I myself think that 100–200 per hour is a very low estimate. Fatigue, however, rapidly comes on, especially when the majority of the radiographs are normal.

with bronchial carcinoma, of whom 27 per cent lived for 4 years or more. Of 83 men undergoing resection, 39 (47 per cent) were alive 4 years later. Men aged 45–54 years, although having as great a proportion of growths resected as the older men, did badly, but the experience with the 84 older men was encouraging. The interval between the penultimate and the ultimate routine films was found to affect survival. Even more striking was the relationship of the interval between examinations to the prognosis after resection. Cancer Registry records revealed that six-monthly routine mass radiography picked up 56 per cent of the bronchial carcinomas which developed in these workers' patients, while 44 per cent of the men became ill and were diagnosed clinically between the routine examinations. The overall four-year survival rate of the whole group was 18 per cent compared with 9 per cent for all patients in the region, the difference being wholly in patients aged 55 years and over. Nash and his colleagues concluded that a mass x-ray unit concentrating on men aged 55 years and over who were smoking 15 cigarettes a day could salvage four-year survivors at a cost of only £300 each, every 1,000 films picking up one potential four-year survivor. Their figures showed a pick-up rate of 0·7 per 1,000 repeat examinations for men smoking 1–4 cigarettes a day, increasing to 2·8 per 1,000 in those who smoked more than 40 cigarettes daily.

More recently Brett (1969), carrying out a controlled study of the relationship between earlier diagnosis and survival in lung cancer in the Mass Radiography Service of the North West Metropolitan Region, found that men whose pulmonary neoplasms had been discovered at six-monthly examinations had considerably increased survival rates. He studied 29,416 men in a test group who were radiographed every six months for three years and compared the results with those in a control group of 25,311 men who had had radiographs only at the beginning and end of the three-year period. Excluding the cases of lung cancer discovered at the first x-ray examination, there were 101 cancer cases in the test series and 76 in the control series, giving an annual incidence of 1·1 and 1·0 per thousand respectively. Of the 101 test series cases, 65 were discovered by six-monthly x-ray examination and 36 by other means between surveys. In the test group as a whole, 43·6 per cent of the patients underwent resection compared with 29 per cent in the control group. Of the 65 patients detected by six-monthly surveys, 65 per cent underwent resection. The five-year survival rate in lung cancer cases discovered by six-monthly examination was 23 per cent compared with 6 per cent in the control series, the average expectation of life after diagnosis being 2·5 years in the test cases and 1·2 years in the controls. Of the patients with resected lung cancers, 32 per cent in the test series and 23 per cent in the control series survived for five years. The five-year survival rates for squamous carcinoma and adenocarcinoma in the test series were 28 and 25 per cent respectively, compared with 15 per cent and nil respectively in the control series. On the basis of these results, Brett concluded that a modest improvement in the prognosis of lung cancer could be achieved through earlier radiological detection*.

Le Roux (1968) found that of 4,000 patients with bronchial carcinoma, 192 (4·8 per cent) presented without symptoms and with an abnormal chest radiograph taken for an unrelated purpose. Such patients were more often suitable for surgical resection of the tumours than those who presented because of symptoms. The proportion of these 192 patients with peripheral tumours (two-thirds) was substantially higher and the proportion with undifferentiated tumours was substantially lower than in the series as a whole. The operative mortality and the rate of non-resectability at exploratory thoracotomy (both 5 per cent) were lower and the long-term survival rate for all resections (4 per cent) was higher than in the rest of the series.

DISCUSSION

The above surveys tend to confirm two points. First, the only measure likely to effect any real decrease in the mortality from lung cancer is the avoidance of smoking. Secondly, examinations relying on low kV large chest radiographs taken in inspiration only may miss lesions hidden behind the ribs, the clavicles or the dome of the diaphragm or situated centrally in the larger air passages, the hilar regions or the mediastinum.

A modest improvement in diagnosis might result from a better interpretation of radiographs and also

---

* Rimington (1971) has shown in 21,579 male mass radiography volunteers that there is a significantly increased incidence of lung cancer in those with chronic bronchitis.

from the use of supplementary films such as lateral, expiration, oblique or lordotic views. However, Boucot and his co-workers discounted the value of these supplementary views in their survey. In our own hospital we always take A.P. as well as P.A. views in patients having miniature radiography. Double reading of radiographs, whether full-sized or miniature films, by more than one observer has been shown to produce a higher pick-up of abnormalities (Smith, 1965).

The present trend towards concentrating the remaining Mass Radiography Service on doctor referrals rather than serving the population at large should result in less fatigue from reading normal films. The phasing out of the service because of the low pick-up rate of disease in the general population is due to economic reasons. The expense of detecting cases of bronchial carcinoma and active tuberculosis by mass radiography techniques is continually increasing. In 1964 Gilbertsen, in the U.S.A., estimated that each examination cost five dollars. Costs in this country have also increased. The present cost of detecting such cases in the general population by mass radiography is of the order of £1,000 to £1,500 per case; for doctor referrals, with their higher pick-up rate, it is much less, being about £300 per case detected (James, 1970, 1971). For simple inflammatory diseases, with their higher incidence, the expense is very much lower still.

The present policy of the Department of Health is to set up static photofluorographic units in all district hospitals which hospital patients, their relatives and the population at large may attend. It is intended that the films should be read by radiologists, and such an arrangement might reduce the fatigue involved in reading large numbers of miniature films. Factories and other commercial enterprises will either have to send their employees to the hospital or have to make their own arrangements for their x-ray examination.

For a discussion of the survival of patients in relation to measurable tumour growth rate, *see* Appendix 5.

12

Summary and Conclusions

I have endeavoured to show the role of diagnostic radiology in the detection, assessment and differential diagnosis of lung and mediastinal tumours and, in particular, of bronchogenic tumours. I have done this with especial reference to plain film appearances, tomograms and bronchograms, and have discussed the development of the latter two techniques and the relevant literature on all three methods of investigation. In addition, I have discussed other radiological and radio-isotope techniques which may be employed.

The following points need re-emphasizing.

PLAIN RADIOGRAPHS

(1) An understanding of the various pathological processes which may occur with a lung tumour is necessary for the proper interpretation of plain radiographs.

(2) Good techniques are required to show areas hidden behind the ribs, in the hilar regions or in the mediastinum.

(3) Suspicious clinical symptoms or signs should always direct further attention to the areas in question.

(4) Bronchial tumours can be grouped into peripheral and central tumours, the earlier manifestations of the two groups being very different.

(5) The presymptomatic detection of the peripheral lesion may enable it to be dealt with at a curable stage.

(6) The use of almost forgotten techniques such as expiration films or fluoroscopy in finding obstructive emphysema is sometimes of value in the detection of central lesions before other signs have developed.

(7) Attention should always be paid to detecting lung collapse before the affected area of the lung becomes abnormally dense. In particular, such signs as rib crowding, slight mediastinal displacement, displacement of fissures or vascular shadows should be carefully sought.

(8) The detailed anatomy of the hilar regions should be more widely known and recognized, and any departure from the normal anatomy should be promptly investigated.

TOMOGRAMS

(9) Tomograms (A.P. and/or lateral) taken with longitudinal movement will define peripheral lung lesions more clearly than plain films and thus allow a more careful study of their morphology.

(10) These tomograms will often show the segmental and sub-segmental bronchi fairly well, but in order to study the larger air passages, the hilar regions and the mediastinum a transverse movement is preferable. Such tomographic movement is most readily achieved by adapting a transverse axial tomo-

graph and taking inclined frontal tomograms in the manner described. These give a very good demonstration of hilar and mediastinal structures not really achievable in any other way.

(11) Inclined frontal tomograms are more easily interpreted than transverse axial tomograms, especially as regards the spread of tumour into the mediastinum.

(12) Inclined frontal tomograms and bronchograms are essentially complementary procedures. The tomograms are more convenient for the patient in that they involve no unpleasant procedure; they also possess the advantage of readily demonstrating soft tissue shadows outside the bronchi.

BRONCHOGRAMS

(13) When required for the detection or assessment of lung tumours, bronchograms should always be carried out by a careful technique employing television fluoroscopy, magnified spot views and large films. Such a careful technique is easy to perform and should cause little inconvenience.

(14) Bronchograms may show filling defects, narrowing or blocks in areas of the bronchial tree. These findings are most valuable in parts of the bronchial tree inaccessible to bronchoscopy.

(15) The limitations of the technique, particularly with regard to the more peripheral tumours, should be understood.

BRONCHOSCOPY

(16) Even in the case of peripheral tumours, bronchoscopy may allow a positive biopsy to be obtained from the central bronchi, either due to their secondary involvement from affected nodes or due to their being affected by spread to the central bronchial walls via the lymphatic system.

OTHER RADIOLOGICAL TECHNIQUES

(17) Angiographic and venographic techniques may assist in assessing the extension of lung tumours into the chest wall or the mediastinum, and hence in deciding the question of operability. They can also be used to show vascular mediastinal tumours or to demonstrate whether a particular mass is an aneurysm.

(18) As extensions of radiological diagnosis, one can pass a small 'flue brush' up and down the bronchi or biopsy a lung lesion under television fluoroscopic control in order to obtain a cytological diagnosis. This may be carried out either percutaneously or transbronchially.

(19) Radiographic techniques involving the injection of a gas may occasionally assist in the locating of tumours or their metastases.

(20) Radio-isotopic procedures are becoming more widely used to detect metastases, particularly those of the brain, liver or bone. They may also help in assessing the decrease in pulmonary vascularity associated with lung tumours.

(21) A specific tumour-seeking isotope would be a great boon in the differential diagnosis of lung and mediastinal masses. Whether this has yet been achieved in the case of ^{67}Ga seems doubtful.

Note.—A recent comparison of treatment policies in cases of inoperable bronchial carcinoma still confined to the chest (Durrant *et al.*, 1971) has suggested that only patients with symptoms should be treated with radiotherapy or anti-tumour chemotherapy and that early treatment in the absence of symptoms does not alter the survival time. This means that the main function of radiology consists in the initial diagnosis of the condition, preferably at an early stage, and the determination of whether or not the tumour is likely to be operable. A visual display of the extent of the disease is also of considerable importance to the radiotherapist when treatment is being planned, as well as in demonstrating any amelioration of the condition.

Postscripts

William Osler (1849–1919, formerly Regius Professor of Medicine at Oxford) observed: 'Syphilis simulates every other disease. It is the only disease necessary to know. One then becomes an expert diagnostician . . .'

If there were at the present time a single chest disease to be studied from a morphological point of view, this would surely be cancer of the lung.

Adler (1912) wrote: 'As at the present the conscientious physician examines every chest for possible tuberculosis, so in the future every chest will have to be examined for possible tumour.' His prediction is unfortunately so true for so many patients that a review of the radiology of lung and mediastinal tumours and other masses seemed to be desirable.

Sir Richard Doll (the present Regius Professor) referred in the Rock Carling Lecture (Doll, 1967) to 'lung cancer—a disease which at present rates can be expected to kill one of every 12 males born in this country'. He found it difficult to see why so much effort should be expended on preventing individuals from having access to marijuana while they were exhorted to smoke tobacco by posters on every public hoarding.

A little progress has been made since then, particularly in regard to the prohibition of smoking in some public buildings and the ban on television advertising of cigarettes. However, until cigarettes are either rendered non-carcinogenic or no longer smoked, radiologists and others examining chest radiographs must always be on the watch for signs of operable and early lung tumours.

Appendices

SUMMARY OF METHODS OF INVESTIGATING LUNG TUMOURS

Clinical methods
  Bronchoscopy
  Thoracotomy
  Node biopsy of neck, mediastinum, etc.

Cytological methods
  Sputum examination
  Bronchial lavage or brushing
  Bronchial biopsy
  Percutaneous biopsy

Radiological methods
  Plain film
    P.A.
    Lateral
    Penetrated or high kV
    With swallowed barium sulphate to show oesophageal displacement
  Bucky film, especially to show rib or other bone erosion
  Tomogram
    A.P. to show
        Lung abnormality
        Bronchial abnormality
        Hilar or mediastinal abnormalities (especially inclined frontal tomogram)
    Lateral
    Transverse axial
  Bronchogram
  Venogram
  Angiogram
  (Biopsy)
  Pneumothorax
  Scintiscan of liver, lung, brain, etc.

Tomogram
  This may define:
    Peripheral mass

TABLE A.3
Site of Lung Mass or Collapse Consolidation in 400 Consecutive Cases

	Number of cases with mass	*Number with collapse or consolidation*
Right lung		3
Right upper lobe	63	32
Right middle lobe	9	4
Right lower lobe	47	13
Right middle and lower lobes in combination		3
Left lung		2
Left upper lobe	56	18
Left lower lobe	49	16
Right hilum	32	
Left hilum	28	
Total	284	91

Note.—Some patients who had both a mass and collapse or consolidation are included in both groups.

When a mass was present, it most commonly showed an irregular border or lobulation. Three patients had very large masses (8 cm or more in diameter) with smooth outer borders. Cavitation was present in 47 masses at the time of diagnosis. In many more cases it developed later in the course of the disease process, either before surgery was undertaken or in patients in whom surgery was impracticable. In 6 patients a second mass was present (? a second primary tumour), and 3 had had lung resections for

TABLE A.4
Stricture or Endobronchial Mass in 400 Consecutive Cases

Site	*Number of cases*
Trachea	1
Right main bronchus	10
Right upper lobe bronchus or its branches	18
Intermediate bronchus	5
Right middle lobe bronchus or its branches	2
Right lower lobe bronchus or its branches	13
Left main bronchus	10
Left upper lobe bronchus or its branches	22
Left lower lobe bronchus or its branches	13
Total	94

TABLE A.5
Other Signs Present in 400 Consecutive Cases

Sign	*Number of cases*	
Hilar or mediastinal node enlargement	87	
Contralateral (left lung to right superior mediastinum)		3
Contralateral (right lung to left superior mediastinum)		1
Superior vena caval obstruction without radiographic evidence of mediastinal enlargement	1	
Mucocoeles or distal bronchiectasis	9	
Satellite masses	4	
Obstructive emphysema	10	
Galaxy or nebula sign	1	
Reduced pulmonary vascularity on plain radiograph	5	
Peribronchial infiltration	3	
Interstitial oedema or lymphangitis	11	
Phrenic nerve involvement	5	
Recurrent laryngeal nerve		3
Pericardial effusion	1	
(Coincident with laryngeal neoplasm)		1
Hypertrophic pulmonary osteo-arthropathy	8	
Involvement of adjacent ribs (including 3 Pancoast tumours)	9	
Pleural effusion or pleural reaction	35	

neoplasm more than five years previously. Six patients had pulmonary metastatic deposits and one had miliary carcinomatosis.

Distal metastases were present as shown in Table A.6.

TABLE A.6

Distal Metastases

Site	Number of cases
Brain	13
Skeleton	10
Liver	15

Tomograms and bronchograms were used as shown in Table A.7.

TABLE A.7

Tomograms and Bronchograms Used

	Number of cases
Conventional antero-posterior tomogram	50
Lateral tomogram	48
Inclined frontal tomogram	80
Transverse axial tomogram	4
Bronchogram	35

Concomitant with the 400 bronchial carcinomas there were four hamartomas, two adenomas and one cylindroma.

(2) Le Roux (1968) in a monograph analysed 4,000 cases of bronchial carcinoma from a clinical point of view. Some of his findings are shown in Table A.8.

TABLE A.8

Findings	Number of cases
Chest wall involved (45 cases resected)	131
Pancoast tumours	37
Cervical nodes positive	579*
Axillary nodes positive	12
Lymphangitis carcinomatosa	24
Left recurrent laryngeal nerve palsy	132
Phrenic palsy	65
Superior vena caval obstruction	183
Oesophageal displacement	138
Pulmono-pulmonary metastases	42
Cerebral secondary deposits	133
Osseous secondary deposits	87†
Hepatic secondary deposits	66†
Cutaneous secondary deposits	38
Hypertrophic pulmonary osteo-arthropathy	49
Complicating tuberculosis	14

* Out of 796 cases, 579 were biopsied (424 on the same side and 77 on the contralateral side, 78 being bilaterally positive).

† As the only signs indicating inoperability.

(3) Bateson (1964) analysed 100 cases of circumscribed bronchogenic carcinoma: 38 patients had no symptoms, and in only 9 could the diagnosis be confirmed by bronchoscopy; 47 of the shadows were under 5 cm in diameter, 36 were between 5 and 7 cm, and 17 had diameters of 7 cm and over.

Bateson's findings were that lung tumours may show ill-defined borders, infiltration, a spreading edge, or a combination of these features. Shadows with well-defined outlines always showed lobulations. The prognosis was better with the well-defined lesions and worse with the very large tumours, which were most commonly squamous cell tumours. Cavitation occurred in all three histological types.

APPENDIX 5

SURVIVAL IN RELATION TO MEASURABLE TUMOUR GROWTH RATE

In 1935 Mottram reported that both benign and malignant warts produced by the application of tar to the skin of mice have very constant growth rates from the time they become of macroscopic size. When size is plotted logarithmically against time, the curve is a straight line. The fact that the length of the invisible growth phase is related to the rate of growth measured during the visible phase and is longer with slower growth rates suggests that invisible growth is also constant.

This concept has been applied to many human tumours, and in particular to bronchial carcinomas (Garland, Coulson and Wollin, 1963; Weiss, Boucot and Cooper, 1966). It is known as the doubling time hypothesis. It assumes that the origin of a tumour is unicellular or nearly so, and that the growth rate is geometric and constant. With these assumptions, the rate of growth can be measured by the time taken by a neoplasm to double its volume. (It should be noted that when a tumour doubles in diameter, its volume is increased eightfold—see also Garland, 1966.)

Such a hypothesis makes no allowance for cellular necrosis or for the shedding of cells into the lumen of a body passage from which they may be excreted (or expectorated in the case of bronchial tumours). Nor does it take into account any depressant effect on the tumour by endogenous or exogenous factors such as host resistance and hormone or other effects, including treatment. Nevertheless it is worth considerable study in relationship to the pre-clinical or invisible lifetime of tumours, since if cancers could be detected when they had a diameter of 1 cm, two-thirds to three-quarters of their lifetime would already have elapsed.

A single malignant cell 10 μ in diameter will produce a nodule 1 mm in diameter in 20 doublings and a nodule 1 cm in diameter in 30 doublings. Ten more doublings will create a mass of approximately 1 kg, and only a few more doublings would produce an insupportable amount of tumour tissue, so that death must supervene after 40 doublings (Collins, Loeffler and Tivey, 1956). These authors also made the following points.

(1) The inadequacy of the five-year cure period in common use may be explained by the fact that slowly growing neoplasms may require many years to reach a discernible size.

(2) The long duration (often years) of invisible growth may explain the failure of 'early' radiographic detection to influence survival, since the diagnosis will not be early in terms of the many doublings which will have occurred by the time the tumour is visible.

(3) Therapeutic measures are undertaken only during the final third or quarter of the cancer's course, and many therapeutic failures are due to metastases which are already present when therapy is instituted. The late appearance of metastases, even after years of survival without evidence of persistent disease at the treated primary site, does not necessarily require the concept of dormant cancer cells. A doubling time of 100 days, a not uncommon occurrence, means that a single cell metastasis would require 8 years to grow into a 1 cm nodule.

(4) The impression of a sudden rapid increase in cancer size is an illusion. When volume increase is plotted arithmetically there appears to be an increasing rapidity of growth, but the rate of change is constant as given by the logarithmic straight line curve.

Weiss, Boucot and Cooper (1966) found in their survey in Philadelphia (see Chapter 11) that out of 76 proven cases of bronchial carcinoma developing during an 8–10 year follow-up period among 6,137 men aged 45 years or over, 12 had had measurable peripheral tumours read as negative 5–7 months before the first radiograph on which the tumour was recognized. There was an inverse correlation between initial size and survival regardless of whether the tumour was resected—that is, the size of the tumour after a 'negative' chest radiograph reflected its rate of growth. This was confirmed in 8 cases by an inverse correlation between initial size and doubling time. The authors concluded that survival may be largely determined by the biological characteristics (such as growth rate) of each tumour, and that even if all other conditions are favourable for resection, such therapy may be effective only in patients whose tumours grow so slowly that there is an opportunity to find them by serial chest radiography while they are still small and have not metastasized. 'A tumour which is large when first seen on semi-annual chest roentgenograms must be growing rapidly, but a tumour which is small may be growing rapidly or slowly.'

Such a concept, however, does not always explain the clinical course of a primary tumour or its metastases. A logarithmic curve plotted back to the origin of the tumour will sometimes suggest that a neoplasm which became clinically apparent in adult life originated in childhood, in foetal life, or even before conception! This is of course absurd, and in many cases the clinical impression is that tumours do have varying growth rates during their clinical course.

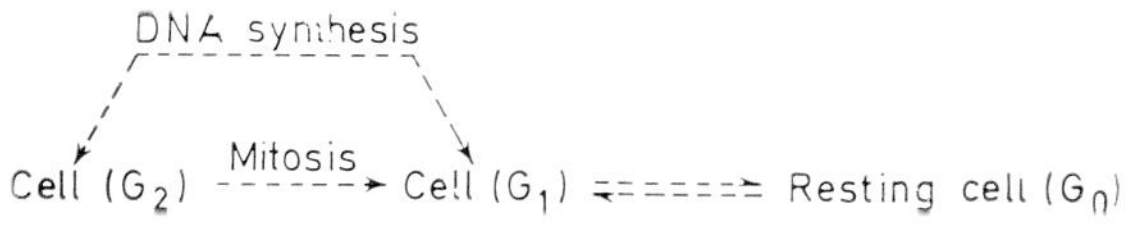

Figure A.1. Diagram of cell cycle of dividing cells, including the concept of resting cells

Lamerton (1972) has pointed out that not all of the cells in a tumour are capable of dividing, and that those which do divide may not do so at the same rate. As in normal intestinal epithelium or bone marrow, there will be 'stem cells' from which are derived the 'intermediate cells' which may rapidly divide, and 'adult cells' which may not undergo division. There are also dormant cells which may not divide without some external stimulus. This theory of a mixed population of cells in a tumour allows a much more rational understanding of the tumour's growth and of its response to treatment, either by radiotherapy or by chemotherapy, than does the hypothesis of a constant rate of division. With treatment there is also an effect produced by the proximity of blood vessels to the cells, in that cells close to the vessels may survive while the more distant ones usually die.

APPENDIX 6

THRESHOLD VISIBILITY OF PULMONARY SHADOWS ON RADIOGRAPHS AND PERCEPTUAL PROBLEMS IN THEIR RECOGNITION

A major problem which arises in viewing radiographs is that sometimes masses or infiltrates are present in the lungs which are invisible or not readily visible on the film. My attention has been particularly directed to the consideration of this problem by the fact that in several patients with advanced and widespread Hodgkin's disease who were radiographed on the day of their deaths or a day or two earlier, the areas of lung disease found at autopsy were not recognized on the radiographs. Some of these lesions measured 2 cm or more in diameter. Certain patients had been radiographed by ward portable apparatus

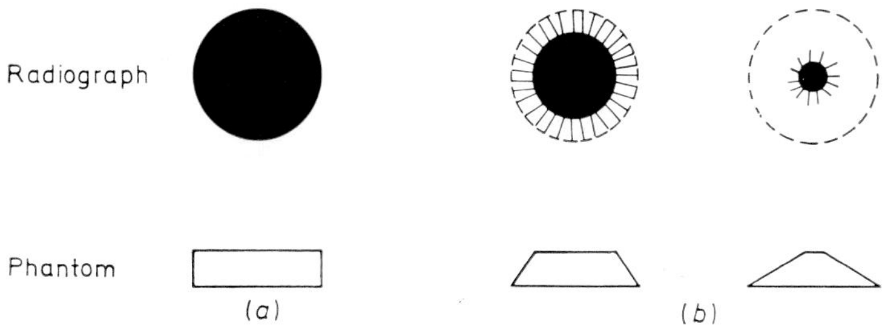

Figure A.2. Appearances of phantoms of lung nodules made from lucite sheets with (a) squared edges and (b) bevelled edges like a mirror

227

with some movement blurring, but others had had good quality departmental radiographs taken. Areas of consolidation due to infective processes are sometimes similarly invisible, whereas rounded secondary deposits are usually visible if they are larger than 1 cm in diameter.

Even small shadows such as linear shadows (e.g. septal lines) with a repetitive pattern may be readily visible, as in miliary tuberculosis or the fine iron deposits seen in some patients with haemosiderosis, while much larger lesions up to the size of a collapsed lobe (for example, the right middle lobe) may be invisible on a single view if a flat border of the collapsed lung is not tangential to the radiographic beam.

Newell and Garneau (1951) radiographed lucite objects of diverse shapes and sizes as well as various seeds such as turnip and millet. They found that the visibility of a sharp shadow was unaffected by its size if over 0·5 cm, all simple shapes (circle, square, triangle, etc.) being equally visible. Fuzziness of the outline of an object lessened its visibility, and unsharpness made faint shadows less visible. If square or rounded lucite sheets had their edges bevelled, then as the bevelled edges became thinner the sheets became less visible on the radiographs and almost disappeared, although the central thickness of the blocks remained the same. Newell and Garneau considered that tiny shadows became visible because of their repetitive pattern and/or because of a summation of the shadows. They pointed out that when objects were radiographed through the chest, the contrast required for threshold visibility was about ten times that required for radiography in air. It made little difference to the visibility of faint shadows whether the chest film was heavily or lightly exposed within reasonable limits. They also observed that the 'hardness' of the x-ray beam used for chest radiography had little effect on the visibility of faint pulmonary shadows, but that what difference there was favoured higher voltage and heavy filtration.

Tuddenham (1957, 1963) similarly studied the problems of perception in chest radiographic diagnosis. He held the view that the perception of a lesion depends on the rate of change of illumination produced by that lesion on a radiograph when it is read, expressed as a function of distance across the viewer's retina. The 'visual stimulus' of such a shadow depends upon the retinal illumination gradient that corresponds to its border, the gradient in turn being determined by the radiographic contrast across the shadow's border and by the width of the latter, or the unsharpness of the shadow expressed in terms of the visual angle it subtends at the observer's eye.

Under-exposure of radiographs is much more of a problem than over-exposure. Moderate over-exposure can be a benefit in that the density of the lung fields will then be above unity and mediastinal and otherwise hidden shadows may be revealed. A chest radiograph is not a work of art; it is merely a means of recording and recognizing information. Under-exposed films in which insufficient of the silver has been affected to record useful information frequently fail to show abnormalities which would otherwise have been recorded. With moderately over-exposed films, on the other hand, all that is required is a bright illuminator to bring out the information.

Further study of the perception of shadows possessing poor contrast explains why minification may be of assistance in the initial detection of disease in the lungs or bronchi. It also helps to explain the usefulness of photofluorograms not only in reducing cost but in simplifying the problem of visual search, in that the whole of the shadow can be appreciated in a single fixation. The reduced size of the image of an abnormality may also increase its apparent density. On enlargement the shadows, having little contrast difference, become less clearly distinguishable. However, magnification is of considerable value in distinguishing between shadows in which the contrast difference is greater, such as those seen in studies employing positive contrast agents or on tomograms, where the contrast difference between soft tissues and gas is increased. On chest radiographs the contrast difference between abnormal shadows and the multiplicity of anatomical background structures is often poor, and much will depend on the viewer's method of scrutiny and his knowledge of normal anatomy if disease abnormalities are to be appreciated. The reading of all chest radiographs by two observers will facilitate the visual perception of a higher proportion of abnormalities.

To demonstrate that the sharpness of an object and the presence of a well-defined edge tangential to the x-ray beam is of paramount importance in rendering the object visible on a chest radiograph, I radiographed a loaf of bread (which has an air-filled cellular structure) into which three glycerine suppositories had been inserted and water containing a thickening agent had been injected (*Figure A.3*). It was clearly apparent that the water, which had partially diffused into the bread and had an unsharp edge, had become almost invisible. From this model it would seem reasonable to suppose that certain lung lesions with unsharp edges—such as Hodgkin's infiltration, some consolidations produced by infections, and tumours surrounded by infection—may not be easily seen. Rounded lesions such as most secondary or primary tumours above 1 cm in diameter, lying peripherally in the lung substance, should be readily visible.

The consideration of this problem is of great practical importance. Recently Rigler (1969) observed 'It is common to see the statement that nodular lesions of the lung less than 1 cm in size are extremely difficult to detect and that those under 5 mm are practically never found'. He radiographed patients with known primary tumours at monthly intervals to see how early he could detect a pulmonary metastasis, and on retrospectively reviewing the radiographs he found that he was able to discern 1–2 mm lesions as beading along vessels. The low density of a tumour makes its detection difficult if it is small, and even a 2 cm mass may be missed because of superimposed rib shadows. High kV and a very fine focal spot may permit better demonstration of small asymptomatic tumours.

Improved techniques for chest radiography certainly seem to avoid the gross errors caused by failure to observe fairly large lesions. In the retrospective study of radiographs of patients with carcinoma of the bronchus carried out by Tala (1967), 168 out of 632 cases had shown radiographic evidence of the disease 6 months to (in one case) 9 years before the condition was recognized. The average period during which the lesion was present but unrecognized was 2·4 years.

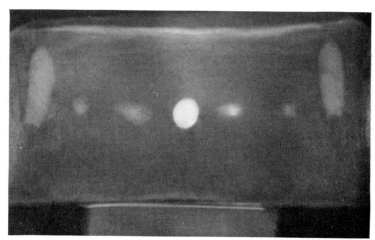

Figure A.3. A square-shaped loaf of bread was used as a lung phantom and 'lesions' were placed within it. It was radiographed by a similar technique to that used for patients (see Figure 3.2). The outermost and the central lesion are glycerin suppositories ('water density jellied structures' approximately 1 cm in diameter); the central one is 'end-on', while the outer ones are shown in their long axes. Between these have been injected lesions consisting of 1 ml (those adjacent to the middle suppository) or 0·5 ml water with carboxy-methyl-cellulose (KY Jelly) as a thickening agent. These latter are much less visible than the suppositories because they have a less definite edge

APPENDIX 7

BRONCHOGRAPHIC TECHNIQUE AND INSTRUMENTS

Technique of bronchography by crico-thyroid route (*see also Figure 8.4 and pages 161–165*)

After preliminary local anaesthesia of the skin and trachea—for the latter I use 1–4 ml of 4 per cent topical prilocaine hydrochloride 40 mg/ml (Citanest), which is much less toxic than cocaine—the larynx is steadied with the left hand and the needle is inserted through the crico-thyroid membrane into the trachea. Aspiration of air from the trachea establishes that the needle is lying within it.

The patient is asked to breathe shallowly during the injection of the medium and not to cough. He leans towards the side being examined and posteriorly while 4–5 ml of contrast medium are injected, and then takes 2–3 maximum inspirations. This procedure is repeated with the patient leaning sideways and anteriorly. He then has 2 ml injected while lying on his side. He is next rotated backwards 30–40 degrees and takes two large breaths to fill the apical bronchus of the lower lobe. After this, 8 ml are injected and allowed to run down into the main and upper lobe bronchi. The needle and syringe are removed. The patient is tilted head downward in an oblique prone position (the side being examined is lowermost); he takes two or three deep breaths before being turned supine, when the deep respirations are repeated. A total of 20 ml of contrast medium is usually employed, but for some patients with large bronchi, more is needed. When much collapse is present or a limited examination is required, 10 ml may suffice. Details of a similar technique are given by Saxton and Strickland (1964).

Instruments which have been used for bronchography

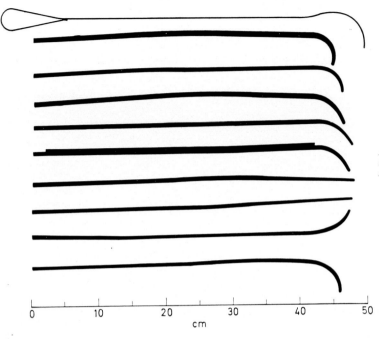

Figure A.4. Métras sounds for endobronchial injection. Note.—Similar catheters have been used by Tsuboi (1970) in performing transbronchial biopsies of peripheral lung lesions

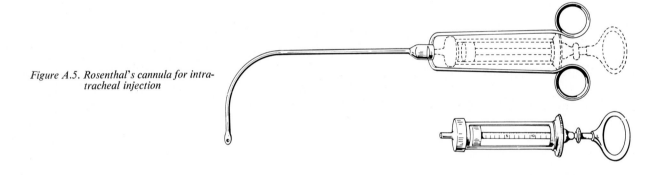

Figure A.5. Rosenthal's cannula for intra-tracheal injection

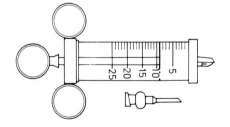

Figure A.6. Syringe and needle used for crico-thyroid injection

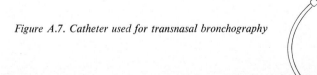

Figure A.7. Catheter used for transnasal bronchography

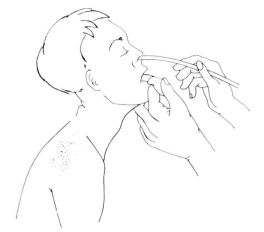

Figure A.8. Position of patient during intubation of the larynx. The tongue is pulled well forward

APPENDIX 8

RADIATION DOSAGE FROM CHEST RADIOGRAPHY AND TOMOGRAPHY

The measurements at the Churchill Hospital are shown in Tables A.9–A.11.

TABLE A.9
Radiography

Chest radiography

kV	mAs	Filtration	Focus–film distance (ft)	P.A. or lateral	Skin exposure with back scatter (mr)
150	8 10–12 15	1·2 mm brass added	11	P.A. P.A. Lateral	5* 7–9† 12†
110	7	2 mm aluminium (inherent tube)	11		20
100	4·5	2 mm aluminium (inherent tube)	6		32

Note.—Three-phase 10,000 rev. tubes. With 200 kV, 11 ft f.fd. and 2 mm aluminium filter the skin exposure is 3–5 mr.

Mass radiography using Odelca camera (single phase)

| 80 | 36 | 2 mm aluminium added | 6 | P.A. | 250* |
| 90 | 36 | 2 mm aluminium added | 6 | P.A. | 280† |

* Average female.
† Average male.
Note.—Before the 2 mm aluminium were added, the incident skin dose with the Odelca camera varied between 380 and 560 mr.

TABLE A.10
Rotational Tomography

Using Radiotome (single phase)

kV	mA	Time (sec)	Tomographic technique	Skin exposure with back scatter (mr)
90	75	1	Inclined frontal	300
100	75	1	Inclined frontal	350
90	50	4	Transverse axial	800

TABLE A.11
Linear Tomography

Using Siemens Planigraph (single phase)

kV	mA	Time (sec)	Region	Skin exposure with back scatter (mr)
70	75	1	Apex of lung	150
80	75	1	Apex of lung	210
90	75	1	Apex of lung	280
100	75	1	Hilum or mediastinum	330

Note.—56 in (1·4 m) focus–table top distance.

Using Siemens Multiplanigraph (three-phase)

kV	mA	Time (sec)	Region	Skin exposure with back scatter (mr)
70	80	0·4		210
80	80	1		520
90	80	1		650
100	80	1		800

Note.—43 in (1 m) focus–table top distance.

APPENDIX 9

METHODS OF PRODUCING ^{113m}In COMPLEXES FOR SCANNING PROCEDURES

The generator containing the parent isotope, ^{113}Sn (half-life 118 days), has a useful life of 9 months. Each time it is used it is eluted with 5 ml N/20 HCl at pH 1·4. The eluate is collected in a glass bottle and the procedures shown in Table A.12 are carried out in order to produce the required substances for scintiscanning (^{113m}In has a half-life of 1·7 hours and a γ energy emission of 380 keV).

TABLE A.12
Production of ^{113m}In Isotope Complexes for Scintiscanning (*see also* Wagner, 1968)

	For lung	For liver	For brain	For blood pool
How used	Particles 50–100 μ	Particles under 1 μ	Chelate	Binding to transferrin
Eluate volume	3 ml	3 ml	3 ml	4 ml
Add	0·6 ml FeCl$_3$ in 0·1 N HCl	1 ml gelatin 5 per cent; 5 ml phosphate buffer* to achieve pH of 7·9	0·2 ml FeCl$_3$ in 0·1 N HCl + 2·0 ml DTPA (1·6 mg/ml)	0·5 ml gelatin 20 per cent
Add 0·5 N NaOH to adjust pH to	12	—	5·0–5·5	—
Heat	Boiling water 5–10 minutes and shake	—	—	—
Add	1 ml gelatin 20 per cent	—	—	—
Autoclave for 20 minutes at 15 p.s.i.				

* 8·8 g Na$_2$HPO$_4$ + 0·6 g KH$_2$PO$_4$ in 1 litre H$_2$O.

232

APPENDIX 10
MEDICAL BULLETINS ON KING GEORGE VI

SEPT. 29, 1951 THE KING'S HEALTH BRITISH MEDICAL JOURNAL 793

THE KING'S HEALTH

OPERATION FOR LUNG RESECTION

Below we print the bulletins which have been issued since the King's illness in May. The first was made public on Friday, June 1, and read:

The King has been confined to his room for the past week with an attack of influenza.

There is now a small area of catarrhal inflammation in the lung, but the constitutional disturbance is slight.

DANIEL DAVIES. GEOFFREY MARSHALL.
HORACE EVANS. JOHN WEIR.

On Monday, June 4, the next bulletin stated:

The catarrhal inflammation in the King's lung has not entirely disappeared, though his Majesty's general condition has improved.

A period of complete rest will be essential to his Majesty's recovery, and on the advice of his doctors he has reluctantly decided to cancel all his public engagements for at least four weeks.

DANIEL DAVIES. GEOFFREY MARSHALL.
HORACE EVANS. JOHN WEIR.

A further bulletin issued on Wednesday, June 6, read:

The King's progress both in the local and general condition continues to be satisfactory.

DANIEL DAVIES. GEOFFREY MARSHALL.
HORACE EVANS. JOHN WEIR.

A bulletin issued on Tuesday, June 12, stated:

The King continues to make good progress. The temperature has been normal for the past week, and the inflammation in the lung has subsided.

In view of the attacks of catarrhal infection his Majesty has suffered this year we have advised that a prolonged convalescence is essential.

DANIEL DAVIES. GEOFFREY MARSHALL.
HORACE EVANS. JOHN WEIR.

The next bulletin was issued on Tuesday, September 18.

During the King's recent illness a series of examinations have been carried out, including radiology and bronchoscopy. These investigations now show structural changes to have developed in the lung. His Majesty has been advised to stay in London for further treatment.

G. MATHER CORDINER. GEOFFREY MARSHALL.
DANIEL DAVIES. C. PRICE THOMAS.
THOMAS DUNHILL. JOHN WEIR.
PETER KERLEY. ROBERT A. YOUNG.

A bulletin on Friday, September 21, stated:

The condition of the King's lung gives cause for concern.

In view of the structural changes referred to in the last bulletin we have advised his Majesty to undergo an operation in the near future. This advice the King has accepted.

DANIEL DAVIES. C. PRICE THOMAS.
GEOFFREY MARSHALL HORACE EVANS.
ROBERT A. YOUNG. JOHN WEIR.
THOMAS DUNHILL.

At 4.30 p.m. on Sunday, September 23, a bulletin was issued which stated:

The King underwent an operation for lung resection this morning. Whilst anxiety must remain for some days, his Majesty's immediate post-operative condition is satisfactory.

DANIEL DAVIES. C. PRICE THOMAS.
GEOFFREY MARSHALL. R. MACHRAY.
ROBERT A. YOUNG. HORACE EVANS.
THOMAS DUNHILL. JOHN WEIR.

Later on the same day, at 9.15 p.m., a further bulletin stated:

The King's condition continues to be as satisfactory as can be expected.

DANIEL DAVIES. JOHN WEIR.
GEOFFREY MARSHALL. C. PRICE THOMAS.
HORACE EVANS.

A bulletin issued on Monday, September 24, stated:

The King has had a restful night. His Majesty's condition this morning continues to be as satisfactory as can be expected.

DANIEL DAVIES. JOHN WEIR.
HORACE EVANS. C. PRICE THOMAS.
GEOFFREY MARSHALL.

A second bulletin, issued on the same day at 7 p.m., stated:

The King has gained strength during the day.

DANIEL DAVIES. C. PRICE THOMAS.
HORACE EVANS. JOHN WEIR.
GEOFFREY MARSHALL.

The latest bulletin before going to press, issued at 11 a.m. on Tuesday, September 25, stated:

After another restful night the King continues to gain strength.

DANIEL DAVIES. C. PRICE THOMAS.
HORACE EVANS. JOHN WEIR.
GEOFFREY MARSHALL.

Numb. 39457 755

The London Gazette

EXTRAORDINARY

Published by Authority

Registered as a Newspaper

WEDNESDAY, 6 FEBRUARY, 1952

Whitehall, February 6, 1952

The King, who retired last night in his usual health, passed peacefully away in his sleep at Sandringham early this morning.

(*a*) (*b*)

Figure A.9. (a) Reports on the King's health (reproduced by courtesy of the Editor of British Medical Journal*). (b) Report of the King's death (Crown copyright, reproduced with the permission of the Controller of Her Majesty's Stationery Office)*

References

Abbey Smith, R. (1966). 'Development and treatment of fresh lung carcinoma after successful lobectomy.' *Thorax* **21**, 1–20.

Abeles, H. and Chaves, A. D. (1952). 'The significance of calcification in pulmonary coin lesions.' *Radiology* **58**, 199–203.

— and Ehrlich, D. (1951). 'Single, circumscribed, intrathoracic densities.' *New England Journal of Medicine* **244**, 85–88.

Ackery, D. M. (1971). 'The gamma camera and chest diseases.' Lecture quoted in *Proceedings of the Royal Society of Medicine*, 1972, **65**, 705.

Adami, J. G. and Nicholls, A. G. (1909). *The Principles of Pathology*. Philadelphia: Lea & Febiger.

Adler, I. (1912). *Primary Malignant Growths of the Lungs and Bronchi*. New York: Longmans Green.

Aeby, C. (1880). *Der Bronchialbaum der Säugethiere und des Menschen* (The Bronchial Tree of Mammals and Men). Leipzig: Engelmart.

Albrecht, E. (1904). 'Ueber Hamartome' (About hamartomas). *Verhandlungen der deutschen pathologischen Gellschaft* **7**, 153–157.

Alè, G. and Macchi, L. (1963). 'Studio morfologico e topografico degli aneurismi dell'aorta toracica mediante la tomografia assiale transversa.' *Annali di radiologia diagnostica* **36**, 303–328.

Alexander, C. (1966). 'Diaphragm movements and the diagnosis of diaphragmatic paralysis.' *Clinical Radiology* **17**, 79–83.

Amisano, P. (1946). 'La stratigrafia toracica a strato-transverso.' *La radiologia medica* **32**, 418.

— Piazza, A. and Oliva, L. (1950). 'La technique de la stratigraphie axiale transversale.' *Journal de radiologie et de l'électrologie* **31**, 459–460.

Amundsen, P. (1953). 'Planigraphy in Müller and Valsalva experiments.' *Acta radiologica* **40**, 387–394.

— and Sörensen, E. (1956). 'Angiocardiography in intrathoracic tumours with particular reference to the question of operability.' *Acta radiologica* **45**, 185–198.

Anaker, H. (1955). *Lungenkrebs und Bronchographie* (Lung Cancer and Bronchography). Stuttgart: Thieme.

Ando, A. and Hisada, K. (1970). 'Affinity of gallium-67 for malignant tumour.' *Radioisotopes, Japan* **19**, 239–246.

Andrews, J. R. (1936). 'Planigraphy.' *American Journal of Roentgenology* **36**, 575–587.

Ansell, G. (1968). 'A national survey of radiological complications: Interim report.' *Clinical Radiology* **19**, 175–191.

Ardran, G. M. and Crooks, H. E. (1964). 'The reduction of scatter fog in chest radiography.' *British Journal of Radiology* **37**, 477–479.

— and Emrys-Roberts, E. (1965). 'Tomography of the larynx.' *Clinical Radiology* **16**, 369–376.

Assman, H. (1914). *Erfahnungen über die Röntgenuntersuchung der Lungen* (Experiences regarding x-ray investigations of the lungs). Jena: Fischer.

Azzopardi, J. G., Freeman, E. and Poole, G. (1970). 'Endocrine and metabolic disorders in bronchial carcinoma.' *British Medical Journal* **4**, 528–529.

Baccaglini, M. (1951). 'Pneumo-médiastin par voie rétropéritoneale.' *Journal de radiologie et de l'électrologie* **32**, 753–756.

Baetjer, A. M. (1950). 'Pulmonary carcinoma in chromate workers.' *Archives of Industrial Hygiene* **2**, 487–516.

Balestra, G. and Oliva, L. (1953). 'De la conduite de la couche fixe et de l'effacement des images parasites du thorax selon les différentes techniques stratigraphiques.' *Journal de radiologie et de l'électrologie* **34**, 813–815.

— Passeri and Macarini (1950). 'La stratigraphie axiale transversale dans la pathologie de l'appareil pulmonaire.' *Journal de radiologie et de l'électrologie* **31**, 462–463.

Ball, K. (1970). 'Cigarette smoking and the responsibility of the physician.' *British Journal of Hospital Medicine* **4**, 865–866.

Bamberger, E. (1890). 'Ueber Knochenveränderungen bei chronischen Lungen und Herzkrankheiten' (Concerning bone changes in chronic lung and heart diseases). *Zeitschrift für klinische Medezin* **18**, 193–217.

Barden, R. P. (1967). 'Para-endocrine syndromes associated with carcinoma of the lung.' *American Journal of Roentgenology* **100**, 626–630.

Bariety, M., Coury, C., Monod, O., Gimbert, J-L. and Wargon, H. (1965). 'Twelve years' experience with gas mediastinography (770 cases).' *Diseases of the Chest* **48**, 449–454.

Barjon, F. (1921). 'Étude clinique et radiologique du cancer médiastino-pleuro-pulmonaire.' *Journal de radiologie et de l'électrologie* **5**, 241–248.

Barnard, W. G. (1952). 'Embryoma of lung.' *Thorax* **7**, 299–301.

Baron, M. G. and Whitehouse, W. M. (1961). 'Primary lymphosarcoma of the lung.' *American Journal of Roentgenology* **85**, 294–308.

Bartelink, D. L. (1932). 'Roentgen section.' *Nederlandsch Tijdschrift voor Geneeskunde* **76**, 23.

Bartholinus, T. (1653). *Vasa Lymphatica*. London: Pulleyn.

Bartley, O. (1960). 'The isometric relaxation phase of the left ventricle.' *Acta radiologica*, Supplement **198**.

Bartram, C. and Strickland, B. (1971). 'Pulmonary varices.' *British Journal of Radiology* **44**, 927–935.

Bates, M. (1970). 'Pericardial aspiration.' *British Journal of Hospital Medicine* **4**, 323–326.

Bateson, E. M. (1964). 'The solitary circumscribed bronchogenic carcinoma.' *British Journal of Radiology* **37**, 598–607.

Becker, F. G. (1826). *De glandulis thoracis lymphaticis atque thymo*. These, Berlin.

Belcher, J. R. and Anderson, R. (1965). 'Surgical treatment of carcinoma of the bronchus.' *British Medical Journal* **1**, 948–954.

Berkman, Y. M. (1969). 'The many facets of alveolar cell carcinoma of the lung.' *Radiology* **92**, 793–798.

Beyreuther, H. (1924). 'Multiplicität von Carcinomen bei einem Fall von sog. "Schneeberger" Lungenkrebs mit Tuberkulose' (Multiple carcinomas in one case of so-called 'Schneeberg' lung cancer with tuberculosis). *Virchows Archiv für Pathologische Anatomie und Physiologie und für klinische Medizin* **250**, 230–243.

Bidstrup, P. L. (1964). 'The use of radiology in the early detection of lung cancer as an industrial disease.' *British Journal of Radiology* **37**, 337–344.

Bignall, J. R., Martin, M. and Smithers, D. W. (1967). 'Survival in 6,086 cases of bronchial carcinoma.' *Lancet* **2**, 1067–1070.

Binns, T. B. (1954). 'Bronchography with Dionosil.' *Lancet* **1**, 163.

Bjork, L. and Lodin, H. (1955). 'The reaction of the rabbit lung on bronchography with viscous contrast media.' *Acta Societatis medicorum upsaliensis* **60**, 61–67.

Black, J. M. and Poole, G. (1955). 'A study of tuberculous round foci.' *American Review of Tuberculosis and Pulmonary Diseases* **73**, 805–817.

Blackman, S. (1960). 'Rotational tomography of the face.' *British Journal of Radiology* **33**, 408–418.

Bleyer, J. M. and Marks, J. H. (1957). 'Tuberculomas and hamartomas of the lung.' *Radiology* **77**, 1013–1022.

Bluth, I. (1966). 'Laminagraphic studies of the vascular patterns in cancer of the lung with special reference to the "circumscribed" variety.' *American Journal of Roentgenology* **98**, 397–403.

Bocage, A. E. M. (1922). French Patent No. 536464.

Boijsen, E. and Reuter, S. R. (1966). 'Subclavian and internal mammary angiography in the evaluation of anterior mediastinal masses.' *American Journal of Roentgenology* **98**, 447–450.

— and Zsigmond, M. (1965). 'Selective angiography of bronchial and intercostal arteries.' *Acta radiologica* (diagnosis) **3**, 513–528.

Bonne, C. (1939). 'Morphological resemblance of pulmonary adenomatosis (Jaagsiekte) in sheep and certain cases of cancer of the lung in man.' *American Journal of Cancer* **35**, 491–501.

Bonte, G., Brenot, M. et Trinéz, G. (1955). *La tomographie axiale transversale*. Paris: Doin.

Botenga, A. S. J. (1970). *Selective Bronchial and Intercostal Arteriography*. Leiden, Netherlands: Stenfert Kroese.

Boucot, K. R., Cooper, D. A. and Weiss, W. (1961). 'The Philadelphia pulmonary neoplasm research project: An interim report.' *Annals of Internal Medicine* **54**, 363–386.

— — — and Carnadan, W. J. (1964). 'Appearance of first roentgenographic abnormalities due to lung cancer.' *Journal of the American Medical Association* **190**, 1103–1106.

Boyd, J. T., Doll, R., Faulds, J. S. and Leiper, J. (1970). 'Cancer of the lung in iron ore (haematite) miners.' *British Journal of Industrial Medicine* **27**, 97–105.

Boyd, W. (1950). *The Pathology of Internal Diseases*, 5th edn, p. 234. London: Kimpton.

Bozzetti, G. (1935). 'La realizzazione practica della stratigrafia.' *Radiologia medica* **22**, 257–267.

Bret, P. and Chollat, L. (1964). Personal communication to F.P.G. in Greenwell and Wright (1965).

Brett, G. Z. (1969). 'Earlier diagnosis and survival in lung cancer.' *British Medical Journal* **4**, 260–263.

Bridge, J. C. and Henry, S. A. (1928). 'Industrial cancers.' In *Report of International Conference on Cancer*, London.

British Medical Journal (1951). Bulletins: 'The King's health.' **2**, 279.

— (1952). 'King George the Sixth, "Our most illustrious doctor".' **1**, 386–388.

— (1961). Leading article: 'Early detection of lung cancer.' **2**, 818–819.

— (1969). 'Points from Parliament' (reply by Secretary of State for Social Services) **2**, 258.

— (1971). 'Questions in the Commons' (reply by Secretary of State for Social Services) **4**, 501.

Britt, C. I., Christoforidis, A. J. and Andrews, N. C. (1960). 'Bilateral simultaneous squamous cell carcinoma of the lung.' *Journal of Thoracic and Cardiovascular Surgery* **40**, 102–106.

Brock, R. C. (1946). *The Anatomy of the Bronchial Tree*. London: Oxford University Press. (2nd edn 1954.)

Browder, J. and De Veer, J. A. (1935). 'The varied pathologic basis for the symptomatology produced by tumours in the region of the pulmonary apex and upper mediastinum.' *American Journal of Cancer* **24**, 507–521.

Burcharth, F. and Axelsson, C. (1972). 'Bronchial adenomas.' *Thorax* **27**, 442–449.

Burger, G. C. E. (1949). 'Perceptibility of details in roentgen examination of the lung.' *Acta radiologica* **31**, 193–222.

Buzzi, G. (1950). 'La stratigraphie axiale transversale dans la pathologie du mediastin.' *Journal de radiologie et de l'électrologie* **31**, 146–153.

Carman, R. D. (1921). 'Primary cancer of the lung from a roentgenologic viewpoint.' *Medical Clinics of North America* **5**, 307–354.

Carr, J. C. (1973). 'The Mallory–Weiss syndrome.' *Clinical Radiology* **24**, 107–112.

Chandler, F. G. (1932). 'Bronchiectasis and lung abscess.' *British Journal of Radiology* **5**, 721–722.

Charkes, N. D., Young, I. and Sklaroff, D. M. (1968). 'The pathologic basis of the strontium bone scan.' *Journal of the American Medical Association* **206**, 2482–2488.

Chaudhuri, M. R. (1971). 'Independent bilateral primary bronchial carcinomas.' *Thorax* **26**, 476–480.

Christiansen, K. H. and Smith, D. E. (1962). 'Bronchogenic carcinoma: a sixteen year study.' *Journal of Thoracic and Cardiovascular Surgery* **43**, 267–275.

Christie, A. C. (1937). 'The diagnosis and treatment of primary cancer of the lung.' *British Journal of Radiology* **10**, 141–158.

Cimmino, C. V. (1961). 'Further notes on the esophageal–pleural stripe.' *Radiology* **77**, 974–977.

Clagett, O. T., McDonald, J. R. and Schmidt, H. W. (1952). 'Localised fibrous mesothelioma of the pleura.' *Journal of Thoracic Surgery* **24**, 213–230.

Clerf, L. H. and Crawford, B. L. (1936). 'Benign glandular tumours of the bronchus.' *Transactions of the College of Physicians of Philadelphia*, 4th series, **4**, 6–8.

Cliffton, E. E., Das Gupta, T. and Pool, J. L. (1964). 'Bilateral pulmonary resection for primary or metastatic lung cancer.' *Cancer* **17**, 86–94.

Collins, J. D., Furmanski, S., Steckel, R. J. and Snow, H. D. (1972). 'Minimum calcification demonstrable in pulmonary nodules.' *Radiology* **105**, 49–50.

Collins, V. P., Loeffler, R. K. and Tivey, H. (1956). 'Observations on growth rates of human tumors.' *American Journal of Roentgenology* **76**, 988–1000.

Condorelli, L. (1936). 'Il pneumomediastino artificiale; ricerche anatomiche preliminari.' *Minerva Medica* **1**, 81–86.

— Turchetti, A. and Pidone, G. (1951). 'Il pneumomediastino posteriore.' *Annali di radiologia diagnostica* **23**, 33–54.

Cordier, G., Papamiltiades, M. and Cedard, C. (1958). 'Les lymphatiques des bronches et des segments pulmonaires.' *Bronches* **8**, 8–52.

Cordingley, J. L. (1972). 'Pores of Kohn.' *Thorax* **27**, 433–441.

Cordova, J. F., Tesluk, H. and Knudtson, K. P. (1962). 'Asbestos and carcinoma of the lung.' *Cancer* **15**, 1181–1187.

Cotton, R. E. (1959). 'The bronchial spread of lung cancer.' *British Journal of Diseases of the Chest* **53**, 142–150.

Councilman, W. T. (1900). 'The lobule of the lung and its relation to lymphatics.' *Journal of the Boston Society of Medical Sciences* **4**, 165–168.

Court, P., Binet, J., Lemoine, G. and Mathey, J. (1964). 'Syndrome de Pierre Marie–Bamberger et cancer du poumon.' *Journal français de médecine et chirurgie thoracique* **18**, 69–85.

Craig, J. W. (1937). 'Hypertrophic pulmonary osteoarthropathy as the first symptom of pulmonary neoplasm.' *British Medical Journal* **1**, 750–752.

Cranz, H. J. and Pribram, H. F. W. (1965). 'The pulmonary vessels in the diagnosis of lobar collapse.' *American Journal of Roentgenology* **94**, 665–673.

Craven, J. D. (1965). 'A new method of bronchography.' *British Journal of Radiology* **38**, 395–397.

Cruikshank, W. (1786). *The Anatomy of the Absorbing Vessels of the Human Body.* London: G. Nicol.

Cudkowicz, L. and Armstrong, J. B. (1953). 'The blood supply of malignant pulmonary neoplasms.' *Thorax* **8**, 152–156.

Dahlgren, S. E. and Overfors, C-O. (1969). 'Primary malignant lymphosarcoma of the lung.' *Acta radiologica* (diagnosis) **8**, 401–408.

Darke, C. S. and Lewtas, N. A. (1968). 'Selective bronchial arteriography in the demonstration of abnormal systemic circulation in the lung.' *Clinical Radiology* **19**, 357–367.

Davidson, M. (1932). 'Intrathoracic new growths.' *British Journal of Radiology* **5**, 725–726.

Davies, D. (1970). 'Aspergilloma and residual tuberculous cavities—the results of a resurvey.' *Tubercle* **51**, 227–245.

Deasy, J. B. (1970). 'Mass radiography.' *British Medical Journal* **3**, 48.

de Maestri, A. (1950). 'La stratigraphie transversale du thorax en pédiatrie.' *Journal de radiologie et de l'électrologie* **31**, 464–466.

de Vulpian and Réjou (1960). 'Notes sur la technique tomographique.' *Journal de radiologie et de l'électrologie* **41**, 483–487.

di Chiro, G. (1964). 'Axial transverse encephalography.' *American Journal of Roentgenology* **92**, 441–447.

— (1965). 'Axial transverse encephalography with the Radiotome.' *Medica mundi* **10**, 92.

di Guglielmo, L. (1971). 'Radiocontrast agents for bronchography.' In *International Encyclopedia of Pharmacology and Therapeutics*, Section 76, Chapter 10, pp. 395–411. Oxford: Pergamon.

di Rienzo, S. (1949). *Radiologic Exploration of the Bronchus.* Springfield, Ill.: Thomas.

Dijkstra, C. (1958). *Bronchography.* Oxford: Blackwell.

Doll, R. (1953). 'Mortality from lung cancer among non-smokers.' *British Journal of Cancer* **7**, 303–312.

— (1954). 'The mortality of doctors in relation to their smoking habits. Preliminary report.' *British Medical Journal* **1**, 1451–1455.

— (1955). 'Mortality from lung cancer in asbestos workers.' *British Journal of Industrial Medicine* **12**, 81–86.

— (1956). 'Lung cancer and other causes of death in relation to smoking. A second report on the mortality of British doctors.' *British Medical Journal* **2**, 1071–1081.

— (1964). 'Mortality in relation to smoking. Ten years' observations of British doctors.' *British Medical Journal* **1**, 1399–1410 and 1460–1467.

236

Doll, R. (1967). *Prevention of Cancer: Pointers from Epidemiology*. Rock Carling Fellowship Lecture. London: Nuffield Provincial Hospitals Trust.

— and Hill, A. B. (1952). 'A study of the aetiology of carcinoma of the lung.' *British Medical Journal* 2, 1271–1286.

— — and Kreyberg, L. (1957). 'The significance of cell type in relation to the aetiology of lung cancer.' *British Journal of Cancer* 11, 43–48.

Don, C. (1952). 'A new medium for bronchography.' *British Journal of Radiology* 25, 573–578.

Doppman, J. L., Hammond, W. G., Melson, G. L., Evans, R. G. and Ketcham, A. S. (1969). 'Staining of parathyroid adenomas by selective angiography.' *Radiology* 92, 527–530.

Dotter, C. T., Steinberg, I. and Holman, C. W. (1950). 'Lung cancer operability: Angiocardiographic study of 53 consecutive proved cases of lung cancer.' *American Journal of Roentgenology* 64, 222–238.

Doub, H. P. (1950–51). 'Mediastinal cysts of embryologic origin.' *Journal of the Faculty of Radiologists* 2, 302–310.

Doyle, L. (1970). Letter. *British Medical Journal* 4, 686.

Drevvatne, T. and Frimann-Dahl, J. (1961). 'Peripheral bronchial carcinomas: A radiological and pathological study.' *British Journal of Radiology* 34, 180–186.

Dudley, N. E. (1971). 'Methylene blue for rapid identification of the parathyroids.' *British Medical Journal* 3, 680–681.

Durrant, K. R., Berry, R. J., Ellis, F., Ridehalgh, F. R., Black, J. M. and Hamilton, W. S. (1971). 'Comparison of treatment policies in inoperable bronchial carcinoma.' *Lancet* 1, 715–719.

Düx, A., Felix, E., Bücheler, E., Sobbe, A. and Paquet, K. J. (1969). 'Angiographic diagnostic methods in bronchial carcinoma: Arteriography, azygography, cavography, pulmonary angiography before and after unilateral pulmonary exclusion.' *Fortschritte auf dem Gebiete der Röntgenstrahlen* 111, 731–749.

Dziadiw, R., Kinkhabwala, M. and Rabinowitz, J. G. (1972). 'Pulmonary gumma.' *Radiology* 103, 59–60.

Edholm, P. (1960). 'The tomogram, its formation and content.' *Acta radiologica*, Supplement 193.

Edwards, C. L. and Hayes, R. L. (1969). 'Tumor scanning with ^{67}Ga citrate.' *Journal of Nuclear Medicine* 10, 103–105.

— — (1970a). 'Scanning malignant neoplasms with gallium-67.' *Journal of the American Medical Association* 212, 1182–1190.

— — (1970b). 'Scanning tumors of soft tissue and bone with ^{67}Ga citrate.' *Journal of Nuclear Medicine* 11, 332.

— — Nelson, B. M. and Tehranian, N. (1970). 'Clinical investigation of ^{67}Ga for tumor scanning.' *Journal of Nuclear Medicine* 11, 316.

Edwards, M. H. and Ahmad, A. (1972). 'Epicardial cyst—a case report.' *Thorax* 27, 503–506.

Ellis, F. (1947). 'Needle biopsy in the diagnosis of tumour.' *British Journal of Surgery* 34, 240–261.

— Feldman, A. and Oliver, R. (1964). 'Compensation for tissue inhomogeneity in cobalt 60 therapy.' *British Journal of Radiology* 37, 795–798.

Elson, L. (1972). Report in London *Evening News*, 17 November 1972, p. 3.

Engel, S. (1926). 'Die Topographie der bronchialen Lymphknoten und ihre präparatorische Darstellung' (The topographical anatomy of the bronchial lymph nodes and their dissection). *Beitrage zur Klinik der Tuberkulose* 64, 468–481.

Fariñas, L., Zaldivar, R. G., Llambes, J. and Fariñas, L. M. (1955). 'Evaluation of the different radiologic methods in the diagnosis of carcinoma of the lung.' *Acta radiologica interamericana* 5, 54–64 (abstract in *Radiology*, 1957, 68, 889).

Fariñas, P. L. (1933). 'Serien-Bronchographien zur Frühdiagnose des Bronchialkarzinoms' (Serial bronchography in the early diagnosis of bronchial carcinoma). *Fortschritte auf dem Gebiete der Röntgenstrahlen* 48, 330–338.

— (1934). 'Serial bronchography in the early diagnosis of bronchial carcinoma.' *American Journal of Roentgenology* 32, 757–762.

Farr, R. F., Scott, A. C. H., Ollerenshaw, R. and Everard, G. J. H. (1964). *Transverse Axial Tomography*. Oxford: Blackwell.

Fayos, J. V. and Lampre, I. (1971). 'Cardiac apical mass in Hodgkin's disease.' *Radiology* 99, 15–18.

Feldman, F., Kanter, I. E., Fleming, R. J. and Seaman, W. B. (1971). 'Simultaneous arterial and venous angiography in the evaluation of anterior mediastinal tumors.' *Radiology* 93, 1281–1289.

Felson, B. (1960). *Fundamentals of Chest Roentgenology*, pp. 31–49 and 85–91. Philadelphia: Saunders.

— and Felson, H. (1950). 'Localization of intrathoracic lesions by means of the P.A. roentgenogram: the silhouette sign.' *Radiology* 55, 363–373.

Fennessy, J. J. (1966). 'Bronchial brushing in diagnosis of peripheral lung lesions.' *American Journal of Roentgenology* 98, 474–481.

— (1967). 'Transbronchial biopsy of peripheral lung lesions.' *Radiology* 88, 878–882.

Fetterman, L. E. (1969). 'Brief note on bronchography.' *Radiology* 93, 770.

Feyrter, F. (1959). 'Über das Bronchus Carcinoid' (About the bronchial carcinoid). *Virchows Archiv für pathologische Anatomie und Physiologie* 332, 25–43.

Flavell, G. (1954). 'The problem of the "small round lesion".' *Tubercle* 35, 54–62.

Fleischner, F. G. and Reiner, L. (1964). 'Linear x-ray shadows in acquired pulmonary haemosiderosis and congestion.' *New England Journal of Medicine* 250, 900–904.

— and Sachsse, E. (1963). 'Retrotracheal lymphadenopathy in bronchial carcinoma, revealed by barium-filled oesophagus.' *American Journal of Roentgenology* 90, 792–798.

Flynn, M. W. and Felson, B. (1970). 'The roentgen manifestations of thoracic actinomycosis.' *American Journal of Roentgenology* 110, 707–716.

Hör, G., Glaubitt, D., Grebe, S. F., Hampe, J., Haubold, U., Kaul, A., Koeppe, P., Koppenhagen, J., Langhammer, H. and van der Schoot, J. B. (1970). *Gallium 67 for Tumour Scanning.* Lecture to Gesellschaft für Nuklear-Medizin, Hanover.

Howells, J. B. (1964). 'Alveolar cell carcinoma of the lung.' *Clinical Radiology* **15**, 112–122.

Hueper, W. C. (1957). In *Cancer*, Vol. 1, Part 1, pp. 412, 438 and 456. Ed. by R. W. Raven. London: Butterworths.

Hughes, D. L., Hanafee, W. and O'Loughlin, B. J. (1962). 'Diagnostic pneumomediastinum.' *American Journal of Roentgenology* **78**, 12–18.

Hughes, R. K. and Blades, B. (1961). 'Multiple primary bronchogenic carcinoma.' *Journal of Thoracic and Cardiovascular Surgery* **41**, 421–429.

Huguenin, R. (1928). *Le cancer primitif du poumon.* Paris: Masson.

— and Delarue, J. (1933). 'Importance diagnostique de la bronchoscopie radiologique dans les cancers primitifs du poumon.' *Paris médicale* **1**, 167–172.

Huizinga, E. and Smelt, G. J. (1950). *Bronchography.* Assen, Netherlands: Van Gorcum.

Ingram, F. L. (1950). 'Gummatous stenosis of the bronchus.' *British Journal of Radiology* **23**, 116–118.

Ikins, P. M., Berne, A. S., Strachley, C. J. and Bugden, W. F. (1962). 'Carbon dioxide pneumomediastinography as aid in evaluation of resectability of bronchogenic carcinoma.' *Journal of Thoracic and Cardiovascular Surgery* **44**, 793–800.

Isaacs, H. J. (1925). 'Diagnostic pneumothorax.' *American Journal of Roentgenology* **13**, 250–253.

Jackson, C. (1918). 'The bronchial tree: Its study by insufflation of opaque substances in the living.' *American Journal of Roentgenology* **5**, 454–455.

James, R. T. (1970). *Annual Report of the Director of the Oxford Regional Mass Radiography Service.*

— (1971). Personal communication.

Janover, M. L., Dreyfuss, J. R. and Skinner, D. B. (1966). 'Azygography and lung cancer.' *New England Journal of Medicine* **275**, 803–808.

Kassay, D. (1960). *Clinical Applications of Bronchology.* New York: McGraw-Hill.

Kaufmann, E. (1911). *Lehrbuch der spiellen pathologischen Anatomie.* Berlin: Reimer.

Kay, D. N. and McCready, V. R. (1972). 'Clinical isotope scanning using ^{67}Ga citrate in the management of Hodgkin's disease.' *British Journal of Radiology* **45**, 437–443.

Keal, E. E. (1960). 'Asbestosis and abdominal neoplasms.' *Lancet* **2**, 1211.

Keeling, P. (1970). Lecture to British Nuclear Medicine Society.

Kemp, F. H., Morely, H. M. C. and Emrys-Roberts, E. (1948). 'A sail-like triangular projection from the mediastinum: A radiographic appearance of the thymus gland.' *British Journal of Radiology* **21**, 618–624.

Kerley, P. (1925). 'Neoplasms of lungs and bronchi.' *British Journal of Radiology* (old series) **30**, 333–349.

— (1933). 'Radiology in heart disease.' *British Medical Journal* **2**, 594–597.

— (1951). *In Textbook of X-ray Diagnosis by British Authors*, Vol. 2. 2nd edn (*see also* 3rd edn, 1962). Ed. by S. C. Shanks and P. Kerley. London: Lewis.

— (1954). 'The nature of round intrapulmonary tumours.' *Acta radiologica*, Supplement **116**, 256–262.

Kieffer, J. (1929). U.S. Patent No. 1954321.

— (1938). 'The laminagraph and its variations.' *American Journal of Roentgenology* **39**, 497–513.

Kirklin, B. R. and Paterson, R. (1928). 'The roentgenologic manifestations of carcinoma of the lung. 1: Parenchymal type. 2: Bronchial type.' *American Journal of Roentgenology* **19**, 20–27, 126–133.

Kjellberg, S. R. (1960). Personal communication.

Klemperer, P. and Rabin, C. B. (1931). 'Primary neoplasms of the pleura.' *Archives of Pathology* **11**, 385–412.

Knoblich, R. (1960). 'Extramedullary hematopoiesis presenting as intrathoracic tumors. Report of a case in a patient with thalassemia minor.' *Cancer* **13**, 462–468.

Knox, R. (1909). 'Two cases of thoracic disease presenting similar appearances on radiographic examination.' *Archives of the Roentgen Ray* **14**, 236–238.

— (1917). *Radiography and Radio-therapeutics. Part I: Radiography.* London: Black.

Koerner, H. J. and Sun, D. I.-C. (1966). 'Mediastinal lipomatosis secondary to steroid therapy.' *American Journal of Roentgenology* **98**, 461–464.

Köhler, R. (1969). 'Pulmonary sequestration.' *Acta radiologica* (diagnosis) **8**, 337–351.

Korol, E. and Scott, H. A. (1934). 'Use of chest roentgenograms taken with breath held in expiration.' *American Journal of Roentgenology* **31**, 266–270.

Korsten, J., Grossman, H., Winchester, P. H. and Canale, V. C. (1970). 'Extramedullary hematopoiesis in patients with thalassemia anaemia.' *Radiology* **95**, 257–263.

Kováts, F. and Zsebök, Z. (1959). *Roentgenanatomische Grundlagen der Lungenuntersuchung* (Basic X-ray Anatomy of Lung Investigation). Budapest: Akademia Kiadó.

Kramer, R. (1930). 'Adenoma of bronchus.' *Annals of Otorhinolaryngology* **39**, 689–695.

— and Som, M. L. (1936). 'Bronchochoscopic study of carcinoma of the lung: Analysis of three hundred cases of bronchial carcinoma with one hundred post mortem examinations.' *Archives of Otolaryngology* **23**, 526–543.

Kreel, L. (1967). 'Selective thymic venography—a new method for visualization of the thymus.' *British Medical Journal* **1**, 406–407.

— Blendis, L. M. and Piercy, J. C. (1964). 'Pneumomediastinography by trans-sternal method.' *Clinical Radiology* **15**, 219–223.

Kreyberg, L. (1962). 'Histological lung cancer types. A morphological and biological correlation.' *Acta pathologica microbiologica scandinavica*, Supplement 157.

Kreyberg, L. (1969). *Aetiology of Lung Cancer: A Morphological, Epidemiological and Experimental Analysis.* Oslo: Universitetsforlaget.

Küss, G. (1898). *De l'hérédité parasitaire de la tuberculose humaine.* Paris: Asselin & Houzeau.

Lamerton, L. F. (1972). 'Cell proliferation and the differential response of normal and malignant tissues.' Thompson Memorial Lecture. *British Journal of Radiology* **45**, 161–170.

Lange-Cordes, E. (1956–57). 'Über die intramuköse Ausbreitung der Bronchialcarcinome' (About the intramucosal spread of bronchial carcinomas). *Thoraxchirurgie* **4**, 327–331.

Langston, H. T. and Sherrick, J. C. (1962). 'Bilateral simultaneous bronchogenic carcinoma. Report of a case of surgical excision.' *Journal of Thoracic and Cardiovascular Surgery* **43**, 742–751.

Larkin, J. C. and Phillips, S. (1955). 'Carcinoma complicating cyst of the lung.' *Diseases of the Chest* **27**, 453–457.

Laubenberger, T. (1965). 'The diagnosis of tumours of the thorax with inclined tomography.' *American Journal of Roentgenology* **94**, 681–688.

Lavender, J. P. and Doppman, J. (1962). 'The hilum in pulmonary venous hypertension.' *British Journal of Radiology* **35**, 303–313.

— — Shawdon, H. and Steiner, R. E. (1962). 'Pulmonary veins in left ventricular failure and mitral stenosis.' *British Journal of Radiology* **35**, 293–302.

— Lowe, J., Barker, J. R., Burn, J. I. and Chaudri, M. A. (1971). 'Gallium 67 citrate scanning in neoplastic and inflammatory lesions.' *British Journal of Radiology* **44**, 361–366.

Lawther, P. J. (1971). 'Asbestosis and allied diseases.' *Proceedings of the Royal Society of Medicine* **64**, 833–834.

Leaf, C. H. (1898). *The Surgical Anatomy of the Lymphatic Glands.* London: Constable.

Leafstedt, S. W., Sweetman, W. R., Chester, C. L. and Thorpe, J. D. (1968). 'Multiple primary neoplasms of the lung.' *Journal of Thoracic and Cardiovascular Surgery* **55**, 626–633.

Le Gal, Y., and Bauer, W. C. (1961). 'Second primary bronchogenic carcinoma. A complication of successful lung cancer surgery.' *Journal of Thoracic and Cardiovascular Surgery* **41**, 114–124.

Leigh, T. F. (1963). 'Mass lesions of the mediastinum.' *Radiologic Clinics of North America* **1**, 377–394.

— and Weens, H. S. (1959). *The Mediastinum.* Springfield, Ill.: Thomas.

Lemine, P., Trepanier, A. and Hebert, G. (1970). 'Bronchocele and blocked bronchiectasis.' *American Journal of Roentgenology* **110**, 687–693.

Lemon, W. E. and Good, C. A. (1950). 'Hamartoma of lung: Improbability of preoperative diagnosis.' *Radiology* **55**, 692–699.

Lenk, R. (1954). 'Morphologic and functional symptomatology of primary cancer of the lung as seen in routine roentgenograms.' *Acta radiologica*, Supplement **116**, 247–255.

Le Roux, B. T. (1962). 'Pleural tumours.' *Thorax* **17**, 111–119.

— (1968). *Bronchial Carcinoma.* Edinburgh: Livingstone.

— (1971). 'Opacities of the middle and upper lobes in combination.' *Thorax* **26**, 55–61.

— and Duncan, J. G. (1964). 'Bronchography with Hytrast.' *Thorax* **19**, 37–43.

— Rogers, M. A. and Gotsman, M. S. (1971). 'Aneurysms of the thoracic aorta.' *Thorax* **26**, 638–651.

Lian, C., Huguenin, R., and Brawermann, M. (1933). 'Valeur de l'éxploration lipiodolée dans le diagnostic différentiel entre anéurisme de l'aorte et cancer du poumon.' *Bulletin de l'Association française par l'étude du cancer* **22**, 692–700.

Liebow, A. A. (1955). 'Pathology of carcinoma of the lung as related to the roentgen shadow.' *American Journal of Roentgenology* **74**, 383–401.

Light, J. P. and Oster, W. F. (1964). 'The study of the clinical and pathological reaction to the bronchographic agent Hytrast.' *American Journal of Roentgenology* **92**, 615–662.

Lindgren, E. (1946). 'Roentgen diagnosis of arterio-venous aneurysm of the lungs.' *Acta radiologica* **27**, 585–600.

Lissner, J. (1962). *Flachen- und Elektrokymographie.* Stuttgart: Thieme.

Locke, G. B. (1953–54). 'Carcinoma of the middle lobe bronchus.' *Journal of the Faculty of Radiologists* **5**, 1–18.

Lodge, T. (1950). 'Primary bronchogenic carcinoma: A review of 130 cases.' *Journal of the Faculty of Radiologists* **2**, 118–123.

— (1960). 'The changing pattern of chest disease.' In *Modern Trends in Diagnostic Radiology—3*, pp. 26–38. Ed. by J. W. McLaren. London: Butterworths.

Lodin, H. (1953). 'The value of tomography in examination of the intrapulmonary bronchi.' *Acta radiologica*, Supplement **101**.

— (1957). 'Mediastinal herniation and displacement studied by transversal tomography.' *Acta radiologica* **48**, 337–349.

— (1961). 'Transversal tomography of the descending aorta.' *Acta radiologica* **56**, 251–256.

— (1962). 'Transversal tomography in the examination of thoracic deformities (funnel chest and kyphoscoliosis).' *Acta radiologica* **57**, 49–56.

Lubert, M. and Krause, G. R. (1951). 'Patterns of lobar collapse as observed radiographically.' *Radiology* **56**, 166–182.

— — (1956). 'Total unilateral pulmonary collapse: a study of the roentgen appearance in the lateral view.' *Radiology* **67**, 175–185.

— — (1958). 'Gross anatomico-spatial changes occurring in lobar collapse: A demonstration by means of three-dimensional plastic models.' *American Journal of Roentgenology* **79**, 258–268.

— — (1963). 'Further observations on lobar collapse.' *Radiologic Clinics of North America* **1**, 331–346.

Ludin, H. and Künzli, H. F. (1969). 'Resolution of angiography in detecting liver metastases.' *British Journal of Radiology* **42**, 145–151.

Lumsden, K. and Truelove, S. C. (1957). 'Diagnostic pneumoperitoneum.' *British Journal of Radiology* **30**, 516–523.

241

Lynah, H. L. and Stewart, W. H. (1921). 'Roentgenographic studies of bronchiectasis and lung abscess after direct injection of bismuth mixture through the bronchoscope.' *American Journal of Roentgenology* **8**, 49–61.

Lyons, H. A. and Vertova, F. (1958). 'Angiocardiography: An aid for the early diagnosis of bronchogenic carcinoma.' *American Journal of Medical Science* **236**, 147–155.

McBurney, R. P., Claggett, O. T. and McDonald, J. R. (1952). 'Obstructive pneumonitis secondary to bronchial adenoma.' *Journal of Thoracic Surgery* **24**, 411–419.

McCort, J. J. and Robbins, L. L. (1951). 'Roentgen diagnosis of intrathoracic lymph node metastases in carcinoma of the lung.' *Radiology* **57**, 339–360.

McDonald, C. J., Castellino, R. A. and Blank, N. (1970). 'The aortic "nipple". The left superior intercostal vein.' *Radiology* **96**, 533–536.

McKinlay, A. K. and Wright, F. W. (1967). 'Inclined frontal (rotational) tomography of the sternum.' *Clinical Radiology* **18**, 460–462.

Macleod, W. M., Murray, I. G., Davidson, J. and Gibbs, D. D. (1972). 'Histoplasmosis: A review and account of three patients diagnosed in Great Britain.' *Thorax* **27**, 6–17.

Manges, W. F. (1922). 'Roentgen ray diagnosis of non-opaque foreign bodies in the air passages.' *American Journal of Roentgenology* **9**, 288–304.

— (1926). 'Non-opaque foreign bodies in the air passages: X-ray diagnosis and localisation.' *British Journal of Radiology* **31**, 119–149.

Mapp, M. M., Krouse, T. B., Fox, E. F. and Voci, G. (1969). 'Chemodectoma of the anterior mediastinum.' *Radiology* **92**, 547–548.

Marchal, M. and Marchal, M. T. (1963). *Encycl. Med. Chir.* **32**, 326A. (Cited by Sutherland, Leask and Samuel, 1968.)

Marie, P. (1890). 'De l'osteo-arthropathie hypertrophiante pneumique.' *Revue médicale* **10**, 1–36.

Markovits, P. and Desprez-Curely, J. P. (1962). 'Inclined frontal tomography in the examination of the mediastinum.' *Radiology* **78**, 371–380.

Marlois, R. (1956). *Exploration tomographique de l'arbre trachéo-bronchique à l'aide d'un balayage horizontal.* Thèse, Paris.

Martin, P. L. and Broussin, J. (1958). 'Tomographie de médiastin selon la technique de Frain.' *Journal de radiologie et de l'électrologie* **39**, 656–658.

— and Broussin, J. (1961). 'Nouvelles observations de cancers broncho-pulmonaires étudies par tomographies, selon la technique de Frain.' *Journal de radiologie et de l'électrologie* **42**, 69–70.

Mascagni, P. (1787). *Vasorum lymphaticorum corporis humani historia et ichnographia.* Senis.

Mason, W. E. and Templeton, A. W. (1966). 'Bronchographic signs useful in diagnosis of lung cancer.' *Diseases of the Chest* **49**, 284–288.

Mattina, M., Curicale, G. and Cricchio, A. (1964). 'La tomografia transversale nello studio del mediastino.' *Radiologica pratica* **14**, 93.

Maxwell, D. R., Reid, Lynne, and Simon, G. (1961). 'Properties of a new contrast medium for bronchography: n-propyl 2,4,6,tri-iodi-3-diacetamidobenzoate (propyl docetrizoate).' *British Journal of Radiology* **34**, 744–747.

Mayall, G. F. (1965). 'Inclined frontal tomography using the Polytome.' *Clinical Radiology* **16**, 390–391.

Maynard, C. D., Miller, R. P., Heaphy, L. J. and Whitty, J. E. (1969). 'Pulmonary scanning in bronchogenic carcinoma.' *Radiology* **92**, 903–907.

Meighan, J. W. (1972). 'Pulmonary cryptococcosis mimicking carcinoma of the lung.' *Radiology* **103**, 61–62.

Merrick, M. V., Gunasekera, S. W., Lavender, J. P., Nunn, A. D., Thakur, M. L. and Williams, E. D. (1972). 'A comparison of several chelates with gallium[67] in inflammatory and neoplastic lesions, with a note on indium[111] labelled bleomycin.' *Proceedings of the Symposium on Medical Radioisotope Scintigraphy*, Monte Carlo. Vienna: International Atomic Energy Agency.

Métras, H. (1947). 'Une sonde pour le cathétérisme des bronches du lobe supérieur.' *Presse médicale* **55**, 198.

— (1948). *L'arbre bronchique.* Paris: Vigot Frères.

Middlemass, I. B. D. (1953). 'Deformity of the oesophagus in bronchogenic carcinoma.' *Journal of the Faculty of Radiologists* **5**, 121–125.

Milani, E. (1954). 'Les tumeurs primitives du poumon.' *Acta radiologica*, Supplement **116**, 340–346.

Miller, W. S. (1937). *The Lung.* Springfield, Ill.: Thomas. (2nd edn 1947.)

Møller, P. F. (1950). 'The value of roentgen diagnosis of bronchogenic cancer.' *Journal of the Faculty of Radiologists* **2**, 102–117.

Molnar, W. and Riebel, F. A. (1963). 'Bronchography: An aid to the diagnosis of peripheral pulmonary carcinoma.' *Radiologic Clinics of North America* **1**, 303–314.

Morel, J. M. (1965). 'Tomography device.' *National Institutes of Health* (*N.I.H.*) *Record*, Bethesda, Maryland, March 23, pp. 3–4.

Morlock, H. V. (1934). 'Obstructive emphysema due to bronchial carcinoma.' *Post-Graduate Medical Journal* **10**, 408–409.

Mottram, J. C. (1935). 'On origin of tar tumours in mice, whether from single cells or many cells.' *Journal of Pathology and Bacteriology* **40**, 127–139.

Müller, H. (1882). *Zur Entstehungsgeschichte der Bronchialerweiterungen* (The pathogenesis of bronchiectasis). Ermslieben: Busch.

Munro, A. H. G. and Crompton, G. K. (1972). 'Inappropriate antidiuretic hormone secretion in oat-cell carcinoma of bronchus. Aggravation of hyponatraemia by intravenous cyclophosphamide.' *Thorax* **27**, 640–642.

Myddleton, G. (1964). 'Deaths from smoking.' *British Medical Journal* **2**, 58.

Naclerio, E. A. and Langer, L. (1948). 'Adenoma of the bronchus: Review of fifteen cases.' *American Journal of Surgery* **75**, 532–547.

Nadel, J. A., Walfe, W. G. and Graf, P. D. (1968). 'Powdered tantalum as a medium for bronchography in canine and human lungs.' *Investigative Radiology* **3**, 229–238.

Nash, F. A., Morgan, J. M. and Tomkins, J. G. (1968). 'South London lung cancer study.' *British Medical Journal* **2**, 715–721.

Nelson, S. W., Christoforidis, A. J. and Pratt, P. C. (1964). 'Further experience with barium sulphate as a bronchographic contrast medium.' *American Journal of Roentgenology* **92**, 594–614.

Newell, R. R. and Garneau, R. (1951). 'The threshold visibility of pulmonary shadows.' *Radiology* **56**, 409–415.

Newton, T. H. and Preyer, L. (1965). 'Selective bronchial arteriography.' *Radiology* **84**, 1043–1051.

Nissenbaum, J. (1964). 'Bronchography in diagnosis of bronchogenic carcinoma.' *Diseases of the Chest* **46**, 331–338.

Nohl, H. C. (1962). *The Spread of Carcinoma of the Bronchus.* London: Lloyd-Luke.

Nohl-Oser, H. C. (1972). 'An investigation of the anatomy of the lymphatic drainage of the lungs as shown by the lymphatic spread of bronchial carcinoma.' *Annals of the Royal College of Surgeons of England* **51**, 157–176.

Noonan, C. D., Margulis, A. R. and Wright, R. (1965). 'Bronchial arterial patterns in pulmonary metastases.' *Radiology* **84**, 1033–1042.

Nordenström, B. (1965a). 'A new technique for transthoracic biopsy of lung changes.' *British Journal of Radiology* **38**, 550–553.

— (1965b). 'Therapeutic roentgenology: A preliminary report on the selective application of cryostatics and the transthoracic needle coagulation of bronchial carcinomas.' *Acta radiologica* **3**, 115–128.

— (1967a). 'Transjugular approach to the mediastinum for mediastinal needle biopsy: A preliminary report.' *Investigative Radiology* **2**, 134–140.

— (1967b). 'Paraxiphoid approach to the mediastinum for mediastinography and mediastinal needle biopsy.' *Investigative Radiology* **2**, 141–146.

— (1967c). 'Selective catheterization and angiography of bronchial and mediastinal arteries in man.' *Acta radiologica* **6**, 13–25.

— (1969a). 'New trends and techniques of roentgen diagnosis of bronchial carcinoma.' In *Frontiers of Pulmonary Radiology*, pp. 380–404. Ed. by M. Simon, E. J. Potchen and M. Le May. New York: Grune & Stratton.

— (1969b). 'Bronchial arteriography.' *Les bronches* **19**, 368–391.

— (1971). 'Electric potentials in pulmonary lesions.' *Acta radiologica* (diagnosis) **11**, 1–16.

— and Carlens, E. (1964). 'Bronchial biopsy in connection with bronchoscopy. *Acta radiologica* (diagnosis) **3**, 37–40.

— and Novek, J. (1960). 'The atelectatic complex of the left lung.' *Acta radiologica* **53**, 177–183.

Oeser, H., Ernst, H. and Gerstenberg, E. (1969). 'Das "paradoxe Hiluszeichen" beim zentralen Bronchuskarzinom' (The paradoxial 'hilus sign' of central bronchial carcinomas). *Fortschritte auf dem Gebiete der Röntgenstrahlen* **110**, 205–208.

O'Keefe, M. E., Good, C. A. and McDonald, J. R. (1957). 'Calcification in solitary nodules of the lung.' *American Journal of Roentgenology* **77**, 1023–1033.

Oliva, L. (1950). 'Lo studio stratigrafico assiale transverso dell'aorta toracica patologica.' *Radiologia* **6**, 649–665.

Olympus Optical Co. Ltd. (1970). Advertisement. *British Journal of Hospital Medicine* **4**, 2.

Onuigbo, W. I. B. (1962). 'Contralateral cervical node metastases in lung cancer.' *Thorax* **17**, 201–204.

Ormond, R. S., Jaconette, J. R. and Templeton, A. W. (1963). 'The pleural esophageal reflection: An aid in the evaluation of esophageal disease.' *Radiology* **80**, 738–742.

Osler, W. (1849–1919). *Aphorisms from his Bedside Teachings and Writings*, No. 301. Ed. by W. D. Bean. New York: Henry Schuman. (Published 1950).

Ott, A. and Titscher, R. (1969). 'Das primare Dopelkarzinom der Lunge' (Double primary carcinoma of the lung). *Fortschritte auf dem Gebiete der Röntgenstrahlen* **110**, 793–799.

Overholt, R. H., Bougas, J. A. and Woods, F. M. (1955). 'Surgical treatment of lung cancer found on x-ray survey.' *New England Journal of Medicine* **252**, 432–442.

Paatero, Y. V. (1954). 'Pantomography in theory and use.' *Acta radiologica* **41**, 321–335.

Palmer, P. E. S., Barnard, P. J., Cushman, R. P. A. and Crawshaw, G. R. (1967) 'Bronchography with Hytrast.' *Clinical Radiology* **18**, 94–100.

Pancoast, H. K. (1932). 'Superior pulmonary sulcus tumors (Tumors characterized by pain, Horner's syndrome, destruction of bone and atrophy of hand muscles).' *Journal of the American Medical Association* **99**, 1391–1396.

Parrot, J. M. (1876). In *Compte rendu des séances de la Société de biologie* **28**, 308.

Paterson, R. (1928). 'Roentgen-ray treatment of primary carcinoma of the lung.' *British Journal of Radiology* **1**, 90–96.

Paulson, D. L. (1957). 'Importance of pulmonary nodule.' *Minnesota Medicine* **39**, 127–136.

Payne, W. S., Clagett, O. T. and Harrison, E. G. (1962). 'Surgical management of bilateral malignant lesions of the lung.' *Journal of Thoracic and Cardiovascular Surgery* **43**, 279–290.

Peabody, J. W., Katz, S. and Davis, E. W. (1957). 'Bronchial carcinoma arising in a lung cyst.' *American Journal of Roentgenology* **77**, 1048–1050.

— Rupnik, E. J. and Hanner, J. W. (1957). 'Bronchial carcinoma masquerading as a thin walled cyst.' *American Journal of Roentgenology* **77**, 1051–1054.

Peterson, B. E., Pirogov, A. I. and Smulevich, V. B. (1963). 'Simultaneous bilateral lobectomy in a case of bilateral primary cancer of the lungs.' *Journal of Thoracic and Cardiovascular Surgery* **45**, 705–712.

Pfahler, G. E. (1919). 'Malignant disease of the lungs: Its early recognition and progressive development, as studied by roentgen rays.' *American Journal of Roentgenology* **6**, 575–580.

Pfister, R. C., Oh, K. S. and Ferrucci, J. T. (1970). 'Retrosternal density: A radiologic evaluation of the retrosternal–paramediastinal space.' *Radiology* **96**, 317–324.

Pohl, E. (1927). Imperial German Patent No. 544200.

Pohlenz, O., Feindt, H. R., Hauch, H. F. and Nitschke, M. (1966). 'Zur differential Diagnose des prominenten Pulmonalisbogens mit Hilfe des Pneumomediastinum' (About differential diagnosis of the prominent pulmonary conus by the help of pneumomediastinography). *Fortschritte auf dem Gebiete der Röntgenstrahlen* **104**, 468–494.

Pollard, A., Grainger, R. G., Fleming, O. and Meachim, G. (1962). 'An unusual case of metastasising bronchial "adenoma" associated with the carcinoid syndrome.' *Lancet* **2**, 1084–1086.

Pompili, G. and Alè, G. (1961). 'Morfologia degli strumi tiroidei cervicotoracici ed endotoracici in stratigrafia assiale transversa.' *Annali di radiologia diagnostica* **34**, 191–211.

Poppe, J. K. (1948). 'Bronchography in early diagnosis of bronchiectasis and bronchogenic carcinoma.' *Northwest Medicine* **47**, 735–737.

Portes, F. and Chausse, M. (1922) French Patent No. 541941.

Price, J. E. and Rigler, L. G. (1970). 'Widening of the mediastinum resulting from fat accumulation.' *Radiology* **96**, 497–500.

Rabin, C. B. and Neuhof, H. (1934). 'Topographic classification of primary cancer of lung: Its application to operative indication and treatment.' *Journal of Thoracic Surgery* **4**, 147–164.

— Selikoff, I. J. and Kramer, R. (1952). 'Paracarinal biopsy in evaluation of operability of carcinoma of the lung.' *A.M.A. Archives of Surgery* **65**, 822–836.

Ramchand, S. and Baskerville, L. (1969). 'Multiple hamartomas of the lung.' *American Review of Respiratory Diseases* **99**, 932–935.

Randall, W. S. and Blades, B. (1946). 'Primary bronchogenic leiomyosarcoma.' *Archives of Pathology* **42**, 543–548.

Ransome, J. (1964). 'Effect of injecting Dionosil into the soft tissues of the neck.' *Journal of Laryngology and Otology* **78**, 220–223.

Raphael, M. J. (1963). 'Mediastinal haematoma.' *British Journal of Radiology* **36**, 921–924.

— (1970). 'Pulmonary angiography.' *British Journal of Hospital Medicine* **3**, 377–390.

Raven, R. W. (Ed.) (1960). *Cancer Progress*. Industrial Aspects, p. 81. London: Butterworths.

Rayl, D. F. and Spjut, H. J. (1963). 'Bronchographic crystalline inclusion pneumonia due to Hytrast.' *Radiology* **80**, 588–604.

Rees, D. O. and Ruttley, M. S. T. (1970). 'The bronchocele in bronchial neoplasm.' *Clinical Radiology* **21**, 62–67.

Reich, S. B. and Abouav, J. (1965). 'Interalveolar air drift.' *Radiology* **85**, 80–87.

Reisner, D. (1928). 'Intrabronchial polypoid adenoma.' *Archives of Surgery* **16**, 1201–1213.

Rigler, L. G. (1955). 'The roentgen signs of carcinoma of the lung.' *American Journal of Roentgenology* **74**, 415–428.

— (1957a). 'Periodic roentgen examination—drudgery or challenge?' *Journal of the American Medical Association* **163**, 530–534.

— (1957b). 'A roentgen study of the evolution of carcinoma of the lung.' *Journal of Thoracic Surgery* **34**, 283–297.

— (1965). Personal communication.

— (1966). 'The earliest roentgenographic signs of carcinoma of the lung.' *Journal of the American Medical Association* **195**, 655–657.

— (1969). Panel discussion: 'The future of pulmonary radiology.' In *Frontiers of Pulmonary Radiology*, p. 405. Ed. by S. Simon, E. J. Potchen and M. Le May. New York: Grune & Stratton.

— and Kelby, G. M. (1947). 'Emphysema. Early roentgen sign of bronchogenic carcinoma.' *Radiology* **49**, 578–586.

Rimington, J. (1971). 'Smoking, chronic bronchitis and lung cancer.' *British Medical Journal* **2**, 373–375.

Rinker, C. T., Garrotte, L. J., Lee, K. R. and Templeton, A. W. (1968). 'Bronchography: Diagnostic signs and accuracy in pulmonary carcinoma.' *American Journal of Roentgenology* **104**, 802–807.

— Templeton, A. W., MacKenzie, J., Ridings, G. R., Almond, C. H. and Kiphart, R. (1967). 'Combined superior vena cavography and azygography in patients with suspected lung carcinoma.' *Radiology* **88**, 441–446.

Robbins, L. L. (1954). 'The roentgenographic appearance of benign lesions of the bronchus and lung.' *Acta radiologica*, Supplement **116**, 263–275.

— and Hale, C. H. (1945a). 'The roentgen appearance of lobar and segmental collapse of the lung: A preliminary report.' *Radiology* **44**, 107–114.

— — (1945b). 'Techniques of examination.' *Radiology* **44**, 471–476.

— — (1945c). 'The normal chest as it pertains to collapse.' *Radiology* **44**, 543–547.

— — (1945d). 'Collapse of an entire lung or major part thereof.' *Radiology* **45**, 23–26.

— — (1945e). 'Collapse of the lower lobes.' *Radiology* **45**, 120–127.

— — (1945f). 'Collapse of the right middle lobe.' *Radiology* **45**, 260–266.

— — (1945g). 'Collapse of the upper lobes.' *Radiology* **45**, 347–355.

Robinson, C. L. N. and Jackson, C. A. (1958). 'Multiple primary cancer of the lung.' *Journal of Thoracic Surgery* **36**, 166–173.

Rosenthal, G. (1928). 'La cure de la dilatation des bronches et la rôle des injections intratrachéales et de la trachéo-fistulisation emploi des boues antiseptiques.' *Paris médecine* **1**, 134–137.

Rossi, P., Shahinfor, A. H. and Ruzcika, F. F. (1965). 'Transtracheal selective bronchography.' *Radiology* **85**, 829–833.

— Tracht, D. G. and Ruzicka, F. F. (1971). 'Thyroid angiography—techniques, anatomy and indications.' *British Journal of Radiology* **44**, 911–926.

Rostoski, O., Saupe, E. and Schmorl, G. (1926). 'Die Bergkrankheit der Erzbergleute in Schneeberg in Sachsen ("Schnee-berger Lungenkrebs")' (Mountain sickness of miners of Schneeberg in Saxony (lung cancer in Schneeberg)). *Zeitschrift für Krebsforchung* **23**, 360–384.

Rouvière, H. (1932). *Anatomie des lymphatiques de l'homme.* Paris: Masson.

Royal College of Physicians (1962). *Report on Smoking.* London: Pitman.

— (1971). *Smoking and Health Now.* London: Pitman.

Rubin, P. (1966). 'Bronchogenic carcinoma.' *Journal of the American Medical Association* **195**, 643–653.

Rudler, J. C., Frain, C., Roujeau, J. and Bardessoule, P. (1955). 'L'intérêt de la tomographie frontale-oblique dans l'appréciation de l'extension des cancer bronchiques.' *Poumon et cor* **11**, 477–486.

Rybadova, N. I. and Kutznetsov, S. A. (1968). 'Concerning the method of tomographic examination of the bronchial tree.' *Vestnik rentgenolii i radiologii* **43**, 36–43 (abstract in *Radiology* **91**, 1249).

Salzer, G. (1951). 'Vorschlag einer Einteilung des Bronchus-Karzinoms nach pathologisch-anatomisch-klinischen Gesichtepunkten' (A proposed classification of bronchial tumours by their pathological, anatomical and clinical appearances). *Wiener medizinische Wochenschrift* **101**, 102–103.

Samuel, E. (1969). 'Radiology of serosal malignancy.' *Clinical Radiology* **20**, 113–123.

Samuels, B. I., Dowdy, A. H. and Lecky, J. W. (1972). 'Parathyroid thermography.' *Radiology* **104**, 575–578.

Sanders, D. E., Delarue, N. C. and Lau, G. (1962). 'Angiocardiography as a means of determining resectability of primary lung cancer.' *American Journal of Roentgenology* **87**, 884–891.

— — and Silverberg, S. A. (1970). 'Combined angiography and mediastinoscopy in bronchogenic carcinoma.' *Radiology* **97**, 331–339.

Sargent, E. N. and Turner, F. (1970). 'Needle holder and guide for pulmonary aspiration biopsy.' *Radiology* **96**, 346.

— Barnes, R. A. and Schwinn, C. P. (1970). 'Multiple pulmonary fibroleiomyomatous hamartomas.' *American Journal of Roentgenology* **110**, 694–700.

Saxton, H. M. and Strickland, B. (1964). *Practical Procedures in Diagnostic Radiology.* London: H. K. Lewis. (2nd edn 1972).

Schaudig, E. and Kirst, J. (1960). 'Das Transversalschichtbild des Mediastinum beim Bronchialkarzinom' (Transverse axial tomography of the mediastinum in bronchial carcinoma). *Radiologia diagnostica* **1**, 404–413.

Scheff, S. and Laforet, E. G. (1966). 'The internal thoracic muscle and the lateral chest roentgenogram.' *Radiology* **86**, 27–30.

Schinz, H. R., Baensch, W. E., Friedl, F. and Uehlinger, E. (1953). *Roentgen Diagnostics,* Vol. 3. 1st American edn, translated by J. T. Case. London: Heinemann.

Schmorl, G. (1928). In *Report of the International Conference on Cancer,* London, p. 272.

Schoenbaum, S. and Viamonte, M. (1971). 'Subepithelial endobronchial metastases.' *Radiology* **101**, 63–69.

Secker Walker, R. H. and Goodwin, J. (1971). 'Quantitative aspects of lung scanning.' *Proceedings of the Royal Society of Medicine* **64**, 344–347.

— and Provan, J. L. (1969). 'Scintillation scanning of lungs in pre-operative assessment of carcinoma of bronchus.' *British Medical Journal* **3**, 327–330.

— — Jackson, J. A. and Goodwin, J. (1971). 'Lung scanning in carcinoma of the bronchus.' *Thorax* **26**, 23–32.

Seldinger, S. I. (1954). 'Localisation of parathyroid adenomata by arteriography.' *Acta radiologica* **42**, 353–366.

Sheehan, V. A. and Schonfeld, M. D. (1963). 'Mucoid impaction simulating tumor.' *Radiology* **80**, 811–812.

Sherman, I. S. and Malone, B. H. (1950). 'Roentgen study of muscle tumors primary in lung.' *Radiology* **54**, 507–515.

Sherman, R. S. and Phillips, S. J. (1968). 'Radiologic diagnosis of pulmonary neoplasms.' In *Lung Cancer: A Study of Five Thousand Memorial Hospital Cases,* pp. 151–197. Ed. by W. L. Watson. St. Louis: Mosby.

Shields, T. W., Drake, C. T. and Sherrick, J. C. (1964). 'Bilateral primary bronchogenic carcinoma.' *Journal of Thoracic and Cardiovascular Surgery* **48**, 401–417.

Shimkin, P. M., Doppman, J. L., Powell, D., Marx, S. J. and Ketcham, A. S. (1972). 'Demonstration of parathyroid adenomas by retrograde thyroid venography.' *Radiology* **103**, 63–67.

Shopfner, C. E., Jansen, C. and O'Kell, R. T. (1968). 'Roentgen significance of the transverse thoracis muscle.' *American Journal of Roentgenology* **103**, 140–148.

Sicard, J. A. and Forestier, J. E. (1922). 'L'huile iodée en clinique. Applications therapeutiques et diagnostiques.' *Bulletin et mémoires de la Société d'hôpitaux de Paris* **36**, 463.

— — (1932). *The Use of Lipiodol in Diagnosis and Treatment.* London: Oxford University Press.

Šimeček, C. and Holub, E. (1961). 'Pneumomediastinography in carcinoma of lung.' *Thorax* **16**, 65–67.

Simon, G. (1950). 'The x-ray appearance of acquired atelectasis of the upper lobes.' *Journal of the Faculty of Radiologists* **1**, 223–230.

— (1956). *Principles of Chest X-ray Diagnosis.* London: Butterworths. (2nd edn 1962; 3rd edn 1971.)

Sinclair, D. J. and Gravelle, I. H. (1967). 'Abdominal presentation of bronchogenic carcinoma.' *British Journal of Radiology* **40**, 441–445.

Smith, M. J. (1965). 'Errors in diagnostic radiology.' *American Journal of Roentgenology* **84**, 689–703.

Snider, G. L. and Placik, B. (1967). 'The relationship between pulmonary tuberculosis and bronchogenic carcinoma.' *American Review of Respiratory Diseases* **99**, 229–236.

Sodee, D. B. (1964). 'Selective neoplasm localisation with mercury-197 neohydrin.' In *Medical Radioisotope Scanning,* Vol. 2, pp. 147–157. Vienna: I.A.E.A.

Spencer, H. (1968). *Pathology of the Lung,* 2nd edn. Oxford: Pergamon.

Stein, J. and Poppel, M. H. (1955). 'Hamartoma of lung.' *American Journal of Surgery* **89**, 439–446.

Steinberg, I. (1966). 'SVC syndrome due to tuberculosis.' *American Journal of Roentgenology* **98**, 440–446.

— and Finby, N. (1959). 'Great vessel involvement in lung cancer: Angiographic report on 250 consecutive proved cases.' *American Journal of Roentgenology* **81**, 807–818.

Steiner, P. E. and Francis, B. F. (1934). 'Primary apical lung carcinoma.' *American Journal of Cancer* **22**, 776–785.

Steiner, R. E. (1958). 'Radiological appearances of pulmonary vessels in pulmonary hypertension.' *British Journal of Radiology* **31**, 188–200.

Steinert, R. (1928). 'Untersuchungen des Lymphsystems der Lunge, zugleich ein Beitrag zur Frage der Topographie der bronchialen Lymphknoten' (Examination of the lymph systems of the lungs with a discussion of the anatomy of the bronchial lymph nodes). *Beitrage zur Klinik der Tuberculose* **68**, 497–510.

Stern, H. S., Goodwin, D. A., Wagner, H. N. and Kramer, H. H. (1966). 'In¹¹³ᵐ—a short-lived isotope for lung scanning.' *Nucleonics* **11**, 57–59.

Stern, W. Z., Richardson, J. O. and Wolfe, R. (1970). 'Multiple calcified aneurysms in coarctation of the aorta.' *Radiology* **96**, 331–334.

Stevenson, J. J. (1950). 'Horizontal body section radiography.' *British Journal of Radiology* **23**, 319–324.

Stocks, P. (1947). 'Regional and local differences in cancer death rates.' In *Studies on Medical and Population Subjects.* London: H.M.S.O.

Storey, C. F., Grant, R. A. and Rothman, B. F. (1953). 'Coin lesions of the lung.' *Surgery, Gynecology and Obstetrics* **97**, 95–104.

Stout, A. P. and Murray, M. R. (1942). 'Localized pleural mesothelioma.' *Archives of Surgery* **43**, 951–964.

Stradling, P. (1968). *Diagnostic Bronchoscopy: An Introduction.* Edinburgh: Livingstone.

Stuts, E. and Vieten, H. (1955). *Die Bronchographie.* Stuttgart: Thieme.

Subramanian, G., McAfee, J. G. and Bell, E. G. (1972). '⁹⁹ᵐTc-labelled pyrophosphate as a skeletal imaging agent.' *Radiology* **102**, 701–704.

Sukiennikow, W. (1903). 'Topographische Anatomie der bronchialen und trachealen Lymphdrüsen' (Topographic anatomy of bronchial and tracheal lymph nodes). *Berliner Klinische Wochenschrift* **15**, 316–318, 347–349 and 369–372,

Sumerling, M. D. and Irvine, W. J. (1966). 'Pneumediastinography.' *American Journal of Roentgenology* **98**, 451–460.

Surmont, J., Markovits, P. and Desprez-Curely, J. P. (1961). 'Tomographies frontales inclinées (T.F.I.) dans les affections tumorales du médiastin.' *Gazette médicale de France* **68**, 1885–1904.

— — — (1962). 'Étude tomographique frontale inclinée de l'arbre tracheo-bronchique dans les affections bronchomédiastinales. Resultats portant sur 498 observations.' *Journal de radiologie et de l'électrologie* **48**, 80–81.

Sutherland, G. R., Leask, E. and Samuel, E. (1968). 'Pulmonary vascular and venilatory changes in bronchial carcinoma studied by fluorodensitometry.' *Clinical Radiology* **19**, 269–277.

Taetes, C. D. (1970). 'Steroid induced mediastinal lipomatosis.' *Radiology* **96**, 501–502.

Takahashi, S. (1969). *An Atlas of Axial Transverse Tomography and its Clinical Application.* Berlin: Springer.

— and Matsuda, T. (1960). 'Axial transverse laminagraphy applied to rotational therapy.' *Radiology* **74**, 61–64.

Tala, E. (1967). 'Carcinoma of the lung: A retrospective study with special reference to pre-diagnosis period and roentgenographic signs.' *Acta radiologica*, Supplement **268**.

Talner, L. B., Gmelich, J. T., Liebow, A. A. and Greenspan, R. H. (1970). 'The syndrome of bronchial mucocoele and hyperinflation of the lung.' *American Journal of Roentgenology* **110**, 675–686.

Terry, L. (1964). *Smoking and Health.* Report of the Advisory Committee to the Surgeon General of the Public Health Service. Publication 1103, U.S. Department of Health, Education and Welfare.

Therkelsen, F. and Sorensen, H. R. (1953). 'Diagnosis, determination of operability and differential diagnosis in bronchogenic carcinoma.' *Acta chirurgica scandinavica* **106**, 1–23.

Thomas, C. Price (1954). 'Benign tumours of the lung.' *Lancet* **1**, 1–7.

Thomas, G. and Stecken, A. (1961). 'Transversaltomographie normaler und pathologischer Befunde der Lungengefäße und der Aorta' (Transverse tomography of normal and pathological findings of the pulmonary vessels and the aorta). *Radiologia diagnostica* **2**, 375–382.

— — (1962). 'Transversaltomographie normaler und pathologischer Befunde der Lungengefäße und der Aorta. Erweiterung der Diagnostik pathologischer Aorten Befunde durch das Schichtverfahren unter besonderer Berücksichtigung der Transversaltomographie' (Transverse tomography of normal and pathological findings of the pulmonary vessels and the aorta. Better diagnosis of pathological findings of the aorta by tomography, especially transverse axial tomography). *Radiologia diagnostica* **3**, 447–461.

Trapnell, D. H. (1963). 'The peripheral lymphatics of the lung.' *British Journal of Radiology* **36**, 660–670.

— (1964a). 'Recognition and incidence of intrapulmonary lymph nodes.' *Thorax* **19**, 44–50.

— (1964b). 'Radiological appearances of lymphangitis carcinomatosa of the lung.' *Thorax* **19**, 251–262.

— (1964c). 'Septal lines in pneumoconiosis.' *British Journal of Radiology* **37**, 805–810.

— (1964d). 'Septal lines in sarcoidosis.' *British Journal of Radiology* **37**, 811–813.

— (1967). *Principles of X-ray Diagnosis.* London: Butterworths.

— (1970). 'The blood vessels and lymphatics of the lung.' In *Modern Trends in Diagnostic Radiology—4.* London: Butterworths.

— (1972). Personal communication.

Tsuboi, E. (1970). *Atlas of Transbronchial Biopsy.* Stuttgart: Thieme.

Tuddenham, W. J. (1957). 'The visual physiology of roentgen diagnosis. Basic concepts.' *American Journal of Roentgenology* **78**, 116–123.

Tuddenham, W. J. (1963). 'Problems of perception in chest roentgenology: Facts and fallacies.' *Radiologic Clinics of North America* 1, 277–289.

Turner-Warwick, M. (1963). 'Precapillary systemic–pulmonary anastomosis.' *Thorax* 18, 225–237.

Tuttle, W. McK. and Womack, N. A. (1934). 'Bronchogenic carcinoma: A classification in relation to treatment and prognosis.' *Journal of Thoracic Surgery* 4, 125–146.

Twining, E. W. (1937). 'Tomography by means of a single attachment to the Potter–Bucky couch.' *British Journal of Radiology* 10, 332–347.

Vallebona, A. (1930). 'Una modalità di tecnica per la dissociazione radiografica delle ombre applicata alto studio del cranio.' *La radiologia medica* 17, 1090–1097.

— (1947a). 'Vecci e nuovi methodi stratigrafici.' *La radiologia medica* 33, 601.

— (1947b). 'Nouvelle méthode roentgenstratigraphique.' *Radiologia clinica* 16, 279.

— (1948). 'Inuovi orizzonti della stratigrafia nei vari campi della medicina: l'esplorazione stratigrafica tridimensionale.' *Informatore medico* 2, 3–159.

— (1949). 'Stratigraphie 1930. Stratigraphie 1947.' *Journal de radiologie et de l'électrologie* 30, 308–309.

— (1950a). 'Axial transverse laminagraphy.' *Radiology* 55, 271–273.

— (1950b). 'La stratigraphie axiale transversale au point de vue pratique.' *Journal de radiologie et de l'électrologie* 31, 460–462.

— (1953). *Tratto di stratigrafia*. Milan: Francesco Vallardi.

Van Allen, C. M., Lindskog, C. F. and Richter, H. G. (1930). 'Gaseous interchange between adjacent lung lobules.' *Yale Journal of Biology and Medicine* 2, 297–300.

— — — (1931). 'Collateral respiration. Transfer of air collaterally between pulmonary lobules.' *Journal of Clinical Investigation* 10, 559–590.

Viamonte, M. (1964). 'Selective bronchial arteriography in man.' *Radiology* 83, 830–839.

— (1965). 'Angiographic evaluation of lung neoplasms.' *Radiologic Clinics of North America* 3, 529–542.

Vickers, A. A. (1949). 'Bronchography: The methods by which it may be performed.' *British Journal of Radiology* 22, 137–151 and 224–233.

Voigt, O. (1964). 'Eine einfache Technik zur Anfertigung von Tracheobronchotomogrammen mit normalen Schichtgenäten' (A simple technique for performing tracheobronchial tomograms with common tomographic apparatus). *Röntgen Blätter* 17, 33–42.

Vix, V. A. and Klatte, E. C. (1970). 'The lateral chest radiograph in the diagnosis of hilar and mediastinal masses.' *Radiology* 96, 307–316.

Wagner, H. N. (1968). *Principles of Nuclear Medicine*. Philadelphia and London: Saunders.

Wagner, J. C., Sleggs, C. A. and Marchland, P. (1960). 'Diffuse pleural mesothelioma and asbestos exposure in the North West Cape Province.' *British Journal of Industrial Medicine* 17, 260–271.

— Gilson, J. C., Berry, G. and Timbrell, V. (1971). Epidemiology of asbestos cancers.' *British Medical Bulletin* 27, 71–76,

Walker, D. and Wilson, I. V. (1967). 'Pulmonary infarction simulating bronchial carcinoma.' *Clinical Radiology* 18, 218–224.

Walter, J. B. and Pryce, D. M. (1955). 'The site of origin of lung cancer and its relation to histological type.' *Thorax* 10, 117–126.

Warren, S. and Gates, O. (1932). 'Multiple primary malignant tumours. A survey of the literature and a statistical study.' *American Journal of Cancer* 16, 1358–1414.

Waters, C. A., Baynes-Jones, L. S. and Rowntree, L. G. (1917). 'Roentgenography of the lungs (Roentgenographic studies in living animals after intra-tracheal injection of iodoform emulsion).' *Archives of Internal Medicine* 19, 538–549.

Watson, A. J., Cameron, E. A. and Percy, J. S. (1964). 'Multiple primary bronchial carcinoma. Report of two cases and a review.' *British Journal of Diseases of the Chest* 58, 181–197.

Watson, W. (1936). British Patent No. 480,459.

— (1937). British Patent No. 508,381.

— (1939). 'Differential radiography.' *Radiography* 5, 81–88.

— (1940). 'Differential radiography.' *Radiography* 6, 161–172.

— (1943). 'Body section radiography in practice.' *Radiography* 9, 33–38.

— (1953). 'Simultaneous multisection radiography.' In *Modern Trends in Diagostic Radiology—2*. Ed. by J. W. McLaren. London: Butterworths.

— (1958). 'Gridless radiography at high voltage with air-gap technique.' *X-ray Focus* 2, 12–13.

— (1962). 'Axial transverse tomography.' *Radiography* 28, 179–189.

Watson, W. L. (1968). *See* Sherman and Phillips (1968), pp. 524–525.

Weiss, W., Boucot, K. R. and Cooper, D. A. (1966). 'The survival of men with measurable proved lung cancer in relation to growth rate.' *American Journal of Roentgenology* 98, 404–415.

Wenckebach, K. F. (1913). 'The radiology of the chest.' *Archives of the Roentgen Ray* 18, 169–182.

Wessler, H. and Jaches, L. (1923). *Clinical Roentgenology of Diseases of the Chest*. Troy, U.S.A.: Southworth Co.

West, J. and Van Schoonhoven, P. (1957). 'Carcinoma of the lung developing in a congenital cyst.' *Surgery* 42, 1071–1076.

Westermark, N. (1938). 'On bronchostenosis: A roentgenographic study.' *Acta radiologica* 19, 285–335.

— (1944). 'On the influence of the intra-alveolar pressure on the normal and pathological structure of the lungs.' *Acta radiologica* 25, 874–882.

Westra, D. (1966). *Zonography: The Narrow-angle Tomography*. Amsterdam: Excerpta Medica Foundation.

Williams, E. O. and Azzopardi, J. G. (1960). 'Tumours of the lung and the carcinoid syndrome.' *Thorax* **15**, 30–36.

Williams, R. B. and Daniel, R. A. (1950). 'Leiomyoma of the lung.' *Journal of Thoracic Surgery* **19**, 806–810.

Willis, R. A. (1948). *Pathology of Tumours*, 1st edn. London: Butterworths. (2nd edn 1953.)

Willis, T. (1679). *Pharmaceutice rationalis*. London: Dring, Harper & Leigh.

Willner, O. (1956). 'On the thickness of the layer in rectilinear tomography.' *Acta radiologica* **46**, 511–517.

Willson, J. K. U. (1961). 'Cricothyroid bronchography with a polyethylene catheter.' *Radiology* **81**, 305–311.

Wilt, K. E., Andrews, N. C., Meckstroth, C. V., Molnar, W. and Klassen, K. P. (1959). 'The role of bronchography in the diagnosis of bronchogenic carcinoma.' *Diseases of the Chest* **35**, 517–523.

Winchell, H. S., Sanchez, P. D., Watanabe, C. K., Hollander, L., Anger, H. O. and McRae, J. (1970). 'Visualization of tumours in humans using ^{67}Ga-citrate and the Anger whole-body scanner, scintillation camera and tomographic scanner.' *Journal of Nuclear Medicine* **11**, 459–466.

Wolfel, D. A., Linberg, E. J. and Light, J. P. (1966). 'The abnormal azygogram.' *American Journal of Roentgenology* **97**, 933–938.

Wood, D. A. and Miller, M. (1938). 'The rôle of the dual pulmonary circulation in various pathologic conditions of the lungs.' *Journal of Thoracic Surgery* **7**, 649–670.

— and Pierson, P. H. (1945). 'Pulmonary alveolar adenomatosis in man. Is this the same disease as Jaagsiekte in sheep?' *American Review of Tuberculosis and Respiratory Diseases* **51**, 205–224.

Woodburn Morison, J. M. (1923). 'Elevation of the diaphragm. Unilateral phrenic paralysis. A radiological study with special reference to the differential diagnosis.' *Archives of Radiology and Electrotherapy* **28**, 72–83.

Woodruff, J. H., Ottman, R. E. and Isaac, F. (1958). 'Bronchiolar cell carcinoma.' *Radiology* **70**, 335–348.

Wormer, D. C. (1969). 'Cavitary bronchiolar carcinoma.' *American Review of Respiratory Diseases* **99**, 773–776.

Wright, F. W. (1965). 'Bronchography with Hytrast.' *British Journal of Radiology* **38**, 791–795.

— (1970a). 'Accidental injection of Dionosil into the neck during bronchography.' *Clinical Radiology* **21**, 384–389.

— (1970b). 'Some observations on bone scanning, mainly using Sr^{87m}.' In *Proceedings of the Symposium Ossium*, 1968, pp. 35–39. Edinburgh: Livingstone. (*See also* papers by other authors on the detection of bone lesions and metastases in the same symposium.)

— (1970c). 'Placental localisation by isotope scanning with In^{113m}. Results in 200 patients.' *British Medical Journal* **2**, 636–639.

— (1971a). 'A comparison of conventional skeletal radiography with isotope bone scans using Sr^{87m}.' *British Journal of Radiology* **44**, 898.

— (1971b). 'Bronchial mucocoele and endobronchial tumours.' *British Medical Journal* **4**, 112.

— (1972). 'The diagnosis of free and loculated pericardial effusions during haemodialysis treatment by diagnostic radiology, isotope scintiscanning and ultrasound.' *British Journal of Clinical Practice* **26**, 143–149.

— (1973a). 'Experience with a gamma camera compared with a double headed scanner.' *British Journal of Radiology* **46**, 77.

— (1973b). 'Spontaneous pneumothorax and pulmonary malignant disease (report of five cases, three with metastatic disease and two with primary lung tumours), a syndrome which may be associated with cavitating lung masses.' In the press.

— and Ardran, G. M. (1971). 'Clinical uses and hazards of radiocontrast agents.' In *International Encyclopedia of Pharmacology and Therapeutics*, Section 76, pp. 551–685. Oxford: Pergamon.

— and Bishop, M. C. (1973). 'Pulmonary and renal tumours in the same patient, metastases or double primary neoplasm. Methods of spread of these tumours.' In the press.

— MacLarnon, J. C. and Morrison, P. J. M. (1972). 'Rotational tomography of hilar and vascular abnormalities.' *Clinical Radiology* **23**, 26–36.

— Ledingham, J. G. G., Dunnill, M. S. and Grieve, N. W. T. (1973). 'Polycystic kidneys, renal hamartomas, their variants and complications.' *Clinical Radiology* (in the press).

Xanthakis, D., Efthimiadis, M., Papadakis, G., Primikinios, N., Chassapakis, G., Roussaki, A., Veranis, N., Akravikis, A. and Aligizakis, C. J. (1972). 'Hydatid disease of the chest.' *Thorax* **27**, 517–528.

Yeh, S. H., de la Hay, J. E. and Kriss, J. P. (1968). 'Tc^{99m} labelled toluidine blue O for liver scintillography.' *International Journal of Applied Radiation and Isotopes* **19**, 885–887.

Young, D. A. and Simon, G. (1972). 'Certain movements measured on inspiration–expiration chest radiography correlated with pulmonary function studies.' *Clinical Radiology* **23**, 37–41.

— Yune, H. Y. and Klatte, E. C. (1970). 'Thymic venography.' *Radiology* **96**, 521–526.

Zavala, D. C., Bedell, G. N. and Rossi, N. P. (1972). 'Trephine lung biopsy with a high speed air drill.' *Journal of Thoracic and Cardiovascular Surgery* **64**, 220–228.

Zellos, S. (1962). 'Bronchial adenoma.' *Thorax* **17**, 61–68.

Zheutlin, N., Lasser, E. C. and Rigler, L. G. (1954). 'Bronchographic abnormalities in alveolar cell carcinoma of lung. New diagnostic sign.' *Diseases of the Chest* **25**, 542–549.

Ziedses des Plantes, B. G. (1931). 'Een bijzondere methods voor het maken van Röntgenphotos van schedel en wervelkolm' (A special method for taking x-ray pictures of the skull and spine). *Nederlandsch Tijdschrift voor Geneeskunde* **75**, 5218–4222.

Zuckerman, S. C. and Jacobson, G. (1962). 'Transtracheal bronchography. Complications of injection outside the trachea.' *American Journal of Roentgenology* **87**, 840–843.

Index